MOTIVATIONAL INTERVIEWING

APPLICATIONS OF MOTIVATIONAL INTERVIEWING
Stephen Rollnick and William R. Miller, Series Editors
www.guilford.com/d/pp/AMI_series

Since the publication of Miller and Rollnick's classic *Motivational Interviewing*, now in its third edition, MI has been widely adopted as a tool for facilitating change. This highly practical series includes general MI resources as well as books on specific clinical contexts, problems, and populations. Each volume presents powerful MI strategies that are grounded in research and illustrated with concrete "how-to-do-it" examples.

Motivational Interviewing in the Treatment of Psychological Problems
Hal Arkowitz, Henny A. Westra, William R. Miller,
and Stephen Rollnick, Editors

Motivational Interviewing in Health Care:
Helping Patients Change Behavior
Stephen Rollnick, William R. Miller,
and Christopher C. Butler

Building Motivational Interviewing Skills:
A Practitioner Workbook
David B. Rosengren

Motivational Interviewing with Adolescents and Young Adults
Sylvie Naar-King and Mariann Suarez

Motivational Interviewing in Social Work Practice
Melinda Hohman

Motivational Interviewing in the Treatment of Anxiety
Henny A. Westra

Motivational Interviewing: Helping People Change, Third Edition
William R. Miller and Stephen Rollnick

Motivational Interviewing in Groups
Christopher C. Wagner and Karen S. Ingersoll,
with Contributors

MOTIVATIONAL INTERVIEWING

Helping People Change

THIRD EDITION

William R. Miller
Stephen Rollnick

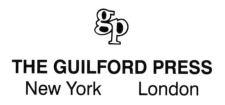

THE GUILFORD PRESS
New York   London

© 2013 The Guilford Press
A Division of Guilford Publications, Inc.
72 Spring Street, New York, NY 10012
www.guilford.com

Printed in the United States of America

This book is printed on acid-free paper.

Last digit is print number: 9 8 7 6 5 4 3 2 1

The authors have checked with sources believed to be reliable in their efforts to provide
information that is complete and generally in accord with the standards of practice
that are accepted at the time of publication. However, in view of the possibility of
human error or changes in behavioral, mental health, or medical sciences, neither the
authors, nor the editor and publisher, nor any other party who has been involved in the
preparation or publication of this work warrants that the information contained herein
is in every respect accurate or complete, and they are not responsible for any errors
or omissions or the results obtained from the use of such information. Readers are
encouraged to confirm the information contained in this book with other sources.

Library of Congress Cataloging-in-Publication Data

Miller, William R. (William Richard)
  Motivational interviewing : helping people change / by William R. Miller and Stephen
Rollnick.—3rd ed.
    p. cm.—(Applications of motivational interviewing)
  Includes bibliographical references and index.
  ISBN 978-1-60918-227-4 (hard cover : alk. paper)
  1. Compulsive behavior—Treatment. 2. Substance abuse—
Treatment. 3. Substance abuse—Patients—Counseling of. 4. Compulsive
behavior—Patients—Counseling of. 5. Motivation (Psychology) 6. Interviewing in
psychiatry. I. Rollnick, Stephen, 1952– II. Title.
  RC533.M56 2013
  616.85′84—dc23
                                                          2012024802

About the Authors

William R. Miller, PhD, is Emeritus Distinguished Professor of Psychology and Psychiatry at the University of New Mexico. He introduced motivational interviewing in a 1983 article in the journal *Behavioral Psychotherapy* and in the first edition of *Motivational Interviewing*, written with Stephen Rollnick, in 1991. Dr. Miller's research has focused particularly on the treatment and prevention of addictions, with broader implications for the psychology of change. He is a recipient of the international Jellinek Memorial Award, two career achievement awards from the American Psychological Association, and an Innovators in Combating Substance Abuse Award from the Robert Wood Johnson Foundation, among many other honors. The Institute for Scientific Information lists Dr. Miller as one of the world's most cited scientists.

Stephen Rollnick, PhD, is Professor of Health Care Communication in the School of Medicine, at Cardiff University, Cardiff, Wales, United Kingdom. He worked as a clinical psychologist in mental health and in primary health care for many years, and then turned to how motivational interviewing could be used to improve challenging consultations in health and social care. Dr. Rollnick's research and guidelines for good practice have been widely published, and his work on implementation continues, with a focus on children with HIV/AIDS in Africa and on pregnant teens in deprived communities. Drs. Rollnick and Miller are corecipients of the Engel Award from the American Academy on Communication in Healthcare.

Preface to the Third Edition

This edition appears 30 years after motivational interviewing (MI) first emerged. The concept of MI grew out of conversations in Norway in 1982, which led to the 1983 journal article in which MI was originally described. The first edition of this book, which focused primarily on addictions, was published in 1991. The second edition, published in 2002, was quite a different book, addressed to preparing people for change across a broad range of problem areas. Another decade later, this third edition is as different from the second as the second was from the first. More than 25,000 articles citing MI and 200 randomized clinical trials of MI have appeared in print, most of them published since the second edition. Research has provided important new knowledge on MI processes and outcomes, the psycholinguistics of change, and how practitioners learn MI.

With all these developments, it became clear that it was time to write a new edition. How we conceptualize and teach MI has evolved substantially. Like the second edition, this edition is about facilitating change across a wide range of topics and settings. It offers our most complete explication of MI to date, beyond its more specific applications in particular settings that are addressed elsewhere (Arkowitz, Westra, Miller, & Rollnick, 2008; Hohman, 2012; Naar-King & Suarez, 2011; Rollnick, Miller, & Butler, 2008; Westra, 2012).

Quite a lot is different in this edition, and more than 90% of the writing is new. Instead of proposing phases and principles of MI, in this edition we describe four broad processes that this approach comprises—engaging, focusing, evoking, and planning—and have organized this book around them. We hope this four-process model helps to clarify how MI unfolds in actual practice. We explore how the processes of MI may be used throughout the course of change, and not only in behavior change. Important new knowledge on the underlying processes and training of MI has been incorporated. We have explicated sustain talk as the opposite of change talk and differentiated it from signs of discord in the counseling relationship, abandoning our earlier reliance on the concept of resistance. We also address two special counseling situations that differ somewhat from mainstream MI, but nevertheless make use of its conceptual framework and methods: counseling with neutrality (Chapter 17) and developing discrepancy with people who are not (yet) ambivalent (Chapter 18). There are new case examples, a glossary of MI terms, and an updated bibliography. Additional resources are available at *www.guilford.com/p/miller2*. We have intentionally given priority to the practical core and application of MI, placing our discussion of the history, theory, evidence base, and fidelity assessment at the end of the book.

While we know much more than we did a decade ago about the methodology of MI, what has not changed (and must not) is the underlying spirit of MI, the mind-set and heart-set with which it is practiced. Like a musical theme and variations, there is a consistent motif running through these three editions, even though the particular descriptions of MI evolve over time. We continue to emphasize that MI involves a collaborative partnership with clients, a respectful evoking of their own motivation and wisdom, and a radical acceptance recognizing that ultimately whether change happens is each person's own choice, an autonomy that cannot be taken away no matter how much one might wish to at times. To this we have added an emphasis on *compassion* as a fourth element of the fundamentally humane spirit with which we wish MI to be practiced. Erich Fromm has described a selfless unconditional form of loving that seeks the other's well-being and growth. In medical ethics it is called beneficence, in Buddhism *metta*, in Judaism *hesed* (a characteristic of a mensch), in Islam *rahmah*, and in first-century Christianity *agape* (Lewis, 1960; Miller, 2000; Richardson, 2012). Whatever the name, it involves relating to those we serve in what Buber (1971) described as an *I–Thou* valuing manner and never as objects to be manipulated (*I–It*). Some of the interpersonal influence processes described in MI occur (often without awareness) in everyday discourse, and some are intentionally applied in contexts such as sales, marketing, and politics, where compassion may not be at the heart (although it is possible). In spirit, MI overlaps with millennia-old wisdom on compassion that crosses time and cultures and on how people negotiate with each other about change. Perhaps this is why clinicians who encounter MI sometimes have a feeling of *recognizing* it, as if it were something they had known all along. In a way, it is. What we have sought to do with MI is to make it specifiable, learnable, observable, and useful.

ABOUT LANGUAGE

MI is now applied in quite a wide variety of settings. Depending on the context, the recipients of MI might be referred to as clients, patients, students, supervisees, consumers, offenders, or residents. Similarly, the providers of MI might be counselors, educators, therapists, coaches, practitioners, clinicians, or nurses. In this text we have sometimes used a specific contextual term, but most of our discussion of MI is generic and could apply across many settings. As a writing convention, we have usually used the terms *counselor*, *clinician*, or *practitioner* to refer to generic providers and *client*, or simply *person*, as general terms for those served by MI. For consistency in the many examples of clinical dialogue provided throughout this book, we have marked them as exchanges between an interviewer and a client, regardless of the setting.

The term *motivational interviewing* occurs more than a thousand times throughout this book, and we have chosen to use the simple abbreviation "MI" rather than spell the term out each time, although we recognize that this abbreviation has other specific meanings as well. A variety of other terms that occur in everyday language have particular meanings within the context of MI. Most readers will readily understand these meanings from our initial explanation and subsequently from context and can consult the glossary of MI terms in Appendix A when in doubt.

ACKNOWLEDGMENTS

We are indebted to the remarkable community of colleagues known as MINT—the Motivational Interviewing Network of Trainers—for stimulating discussions that have informed us over the years as we developed the second and third editions of *Motivational Interviewing*. Jeff Allison has been a flowing fountain of inspiration and creative thinking about MI, contributing metaphors, conceptual clarity, and so many good ideas about how to convey MI to others. The psycholinguist Paul Amrhein has contributed key insights regarding the language processes underlying MI, substantially influencing how we now understand change talk. Professor Theresa Moyers has been at the forefront of MI process and training research, advancing our understanding of how MI works by applying the scientific method while also clearly recognizing its limitations.

This is the ninth book that we have personally authored or edited with The Guilford Press, in addition to serving as series editors for other Guilford books on MI. Having worked with many other publishers, we continue to be impressed with and grateful for the outstanding level of care, quality editing, and attention to detail that has been our consistent experience with

Guilford. It has been a great pleasure over the years to work with editors like Jim Nageotte and Kitty Moore—not necessarily when in the midst of yet another rewrite, but always in the quality of the final product. As before, the copy editor for this book, Jennifer DePrima, was greatly helpful in getting the language just right. Finally, we are grateful again to Theresa Moyers for her careful review of the manuscript, offering suggestions to improve its flow and clarity.

Contents

A more comprehensive bibliography of MI, two annotated case examples, reflection questions for each chapter, the personal values card sort, and a glossary of MI terms are available at *www.guilford.com/p/miller2*.

PART I

WHAT IS
MOTIVATIONAL INTERVIEWING?

Our discussion begins at the broadest level by defining, delimiting, and describing the clinical method of motivational interviewing (MI). Within the context of these chapters we offer not one but three definitions of increasing complexity. In Chapter 1 we provide a layman's definition to address the question "What is it for?" Chapter 2 describes the underlying spirit or mindset of MI, which we regard to be essential to good practice. Here we offer a pragmatic practitioner's definition of MI that is pertinent to the question "Why would I want to learn this and how would I use it?" Then in Chapter 3 we give an overview of the clinical method itself, describing a new framework for understanding MI and offering a technical therapeutic definition that addresses how it works.

CHAPTER 1

Conversations about Change

Things do not change: We change.
—HENRY DAVID THOREAU

A fool takes no pleasure in understanding,
but only in expressing personal opinion.
—PROVERBS 18:2

They happen naturally every day: conversations about change. We ask things of each other and are keenly attuned to the aspects of natural language that signal reluctance, willingness, and commitment. In fact, a primary function of language, besides conveying information, is to motivate, to influence each other's behavior. It can be as simple as asking someone to pass the salt or as complex as negotiating an international treaty.

There are also particular conversations about change that occur as consultations with a professional, where one person seeks to help another to make changes. Counselors, social workers, clergy, psychologists, coaches, probation officers, and teachers all regularly engage in such conversations. A large proportion of health care is concerned with managing chronic conditions for which people's own behavior and lifestyle determine their future health, quality of life, and longevity. Thus physicians, dentists, nurses, dietitians, and health educators are also regularly engaged in conversations about behavior and lifestyle change (Rollnick, Miller, & Butler, 2008).

Other professional conversations focus on change that is not so directly about behavior, unless "behavior" is defined in so broad a manner as to encompass all of human experience. Forgiveness, for example, is a significant psychological issue with broad health implications (Worthington, 2003, 2005). The focus of forgiveness may be someone who has died, and its impact more on internal mental and emotional health than on overt behavior. Self-concept, decisions, chosen attitudes, grief, and acceptance are all common clinical issues that can influence behavior, but are themselves more matters of internal resolution. In this edition we explicitly include such change as a worthy potential focus of MI (Wagner & Ingersoll, 2009).

MI involves attention to natural language about change, with implications for how to have more effective conversations about it, particularly in contexts where one person is acting as a helping professional for another. Our experience is that many such conversations occur in a rather dysfunctional way, albeit with the best of intentions. MI is designed to find a constructive way through the challenges that often arise when a helper ventures into someone else's motivation for change. In particular, MI is about arranging conversations so that people talk themselves into change, based on their own values and interests. Attitudes are not only reflected in but are actively shaped by speech.

A CONTINUUM OF STYLES

It is possible to think about helping conversations as lying along a continuum (see Box 1.1). At one end is a *directing* style, in which the helper is providing information, instruction, and advice. A director is someone who tells people what to do and how to proceed. The implicit communication in directing is "I know what you should do, and here's how to do it." A directing style has complementary roles for the recipient of direction, such as obeying, adhering, and complying. Common examples of directing are a physician explaining how to take a medication properly, or a probation officer explaining the contingencies and consequences imposed by the court.

At the opposite end of this continuum is a *following* style. Good listeners take an interest in what the other person has to say, seek to understand, and respectfully refrain (at least temporarily) from inserting their own material. The implicit communication of a helper in a following style is "I trust your own wisdom, will stay with you, and will let you work this out in your own way." Some complementary roles to a following style are taking the lead, going ahead, and exploring. There are times in most practices when following is appropriate—simply to listen as a human companion,

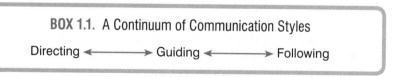

BOX 1.1. A Continuum of Communication Styles

Directing ⟷ Guiding ⟷ Following

for example, with a dying patient for whom everything necessary has been done, or a client who enters a session with strong emotion.

In the middle is a *guiding* style. Imagine going to another country and hiring a guide to help you. It is not the guide's job to order you when to arrive, where to go, and what to see or do. Neither does a good guide simply follow you around wherever you happen to wander. A skillful guide is a good listener and also offers expertise where needed. MI lives in this middle ground between directing and following, incorporating aspects of each. Helping a child to learn a new task involves guiding—not doing too much or too little to help. Box 1.2 provides some verbs associated with each of these three styles of communication, all of which occur naturally in everyday life.

THE RIGHTING REFLEX

We appreciate and admire those who choose to be helpers. Henri Nouwen (2005) observed that "anyone who willingly enters into the pain of a stranger is truly a remarkable person," and we agree (p. 16). A life of

---

BOX 1.2. Some Verbs Associated with Each Communication Style

Directing style	Guiding style	Following style
Administer	Accompany	Allow
Authorize	Arouse	Attend
Command	Assist	Be responsive
Conduct	Awaken	Be with
Decide	Collaborate	Comprehend
Determine	Elicit	Go along with
Govern	Encourage	Grasp
Lead	Enlighten	Have faith in
Manage	Inspire	Listen
Order	Kindle	Observe
Prescribe	Lay before	Permit
Preside	Look after	Shadow
Rule	Motivate	Stay with
Steer	Offer	Stick to
Run	Point	Take in
Take charge	Show	Take interest in
Take command	Support	Understand
Tell	Take along	Value

service to others is a profound gift. A variety of selfless motives can draw people into helping professions: a desire to give back, to prevent and alleviate suffering, to manifest the love of God, or to make a positive difference in the lives of others and in the world.

Ironically, these very same motives can lead to the overuse of a directing style in an ineffective or even counterproductive way when the task is helping people to change. Helpers want to help, to set things right, to get people on the road to health and wellness. Seeing people head down a wrong path stimulates a natural desire to get out in front of them and say, "Stop! Go back! Don't you see? There is a better way over there!," and it is done with the best of intentions, with one's heart in the right place. We call this the "righting reflex"—the desire to fix what seems wrong with people and to set them promptly on a better course, relying in particular on directing. What could possibly be wrong with that?

AMBIVALENCE

Consider next that most people who need to make a change are ambivalent about doing so. They see both reasons to change and reasons not to. They want to change and they don't want to, all at the same time. It is a normal human experience. In fact, it is an ordinary part of the change process, a step along the way (DiClemente, 2003; Engle & Arkowitz, 2005). If you're ambivalent, you're one step closer to changing.

There are also some people who need to make a change (at least in the opinion of others), but themselves see little or no reason to do so. Perhaps they like things just the way they are, or maybe they've tried to change in the past and given up. For them, *developing* ambivalence about change would be a step forward! (We address this in Chapter 18.)

But far and away the most common place to get stuck on the road to change is ambivalence. Most people who smoke, drink too much, or exercise too little are well aware of the downside of their behavior. Most people who have had a heart attack know full well that they ought to quit smoking, exercise regularly, and eat more healthily. Most people with diabetes can recite the dreadful consequences that can ensue from poorly controlled blood glucose. On the positive side, most people can also describe the merits of saving money, being physically active, recycling, eating lots of fruits and vegetables, and being kind to others. Yet other motives conflict with doing the right thing, even when you know what it is. Ambivalence is simultaneously wanting and not wanting something, or wanting both of two incompatible things. It has been human nature since the dawn of time.

> The most common place to get stuck on the road to change is ambivalence.

It is therefore normal when a person is ambivalent to hear two kinds of talk mixed together. One type is *change talk*—the person's own statements that favor change. In our first edition (Miller & Rollnick, 1991) we called these "self-motivational statements." The opposite type is *sustain talk*—the person's own arguments for *not* changing, for sustaining the status quo. If you simply listen to a person who is ambivalent, both change talk and sustain talk occur naturally, often within the same sentence: "I need to do something about my weight [change talk] but I've tried about everything and it never lasts [sustain talk]. I mean, I know I need to lose weight for my health [change talk] but I just love to eat [sustain talk]." "Yes, but . . . " is the cadence of ambivalence.

There is something peculiarly sticky about ambivalence, even though it can also be an uncomfortable place to be. People can remain stuck there for a long time, vacillating between two choices, two paths, or two relationships. Take a step in one direction and the other starts looking better. The closer you get to one alternative, the more its disadvantages become apparent while nostalgia for the other beckons. A common pattern is to think of a reason for changing, then think of a reason not to change, then stop thinking about it. The path out of ambivalence is to choose a direction and follow it, to keep moving in the chosen direction.

Now consider what happens when an ambivalent individual meets a helper with the righting reflex. Arguments both for and against change already reside within the ambivalent person. The helper's natural reflex is to take up the "good" side of the argument, explaining why change is important and advising how to do it. Talking with an alcohol-dependent person, a helper might say, "You have a serious drinking problem and you need to quit." The fantasized reply is "Oh, I see. I just didn't realize how serious it is. OK, that's what I'm going to do!"; the more likely response, however, is "No I don't." Similarly, the helper's natural righting reflex when counseling a pregnant drinker is to educate her about the dangers of alcohol to the unborn child.

> Arguments both for and against change already reside within the ambivalent person.

Chances are, however, that the person has already heard the "good" arguments, not only from others but also from a voice within. Ambivalence is a bit like having a committee inside your mind, with members who disagree on the proper course of action. A helper who follows the righting reflex and argues for change is siding with one voice on the person's internal committee.

So what happens next? There is a rather predictable response when a person who feels two ways about something hears one side of the picture being emphasized: "Yes, but . . . " or maybe just "But . . . " without the "Yes." (This also happens in committees where there is disagreement.) Argue for one side and the ambivalent person is likely to take up

BOX 1.3. Personal Reflection: On the Origins of Motivational Interviewing

It is no coincidence that MI emerged in the context of addiction treatment. I was puzzled that the writings and opinions of practitioners in this field were so disparaging of people with substance use disorders, characterizing them as being pathological liars with formidable immature personality defenses, in denial and out of touch with reality. This had not been my experience in working with such people, and there was precious little scientific evidence that as a group they had abnormal personality or defensive structures any different from normal people. So if these people walked through the doors of addiction clinics just as diverse as a general population, how could it happen that clinicians came to see them as so inexorably alike and difficult? When similarity in behavior is not accounted for by preexisting characteristics, a natural place to look for an explanation is in the context, the environment. Could the apparent homogeneity of abnormal behavior be due to how people were being treated?

One did not need to look far in the 1980s. Addiction treatment in the United States was often highly authoritarian, confrontational, even demeaning, relying on a heavily directing style of counseling. In my own first experience in treating people with alcohol problems I had the good fortune of working on a unit where this was not the case, and because I knew very little about alcoholism I relied heavily on listening to clients on the ward, learning from them and trying to understand their dilemma. I found them usually to be open, interesting, thoughtful people well aware of the chaos ensuing from their drinking. That's why, when I began reading clinical descriptions, I thought, "That doesn't sound at all like the same people I've been seeing!"

It soon became apparent that client openness versus defensiveness, change talk versus sustain talk, is very much a product of the therapeutic relationship. "Resistance" and motivation occur in an interpersonal context. This is now well demonstrated by research, and it is easy to observe in ordinary practice. By the way in which one counsels it is possible to increase and decrease client motivation (or reticence) like the volume control on a radio. "Denial" in addiction treatment is often not so much a client problem as a counselor skill issue. Counsel in a way that evokes defensiveness and counter-argument and people are less likely to change. It also confirms the clinician's belief that these people are difficult, resistant, and intractable. It is a self-fulfilling prophecy.

I set out, then, to discover how to counsel in a way that evokes people's own motivation for change rather than putting them on the defensive. A simple principle that emerged from our earliest discussions was to have the client, not the counselor, voice the reasons for change. As it turned out, overreliance on a directing style was not the exclusive property of addiction treatment, and MI began to find applications in other fields such as health care, corrections, and social work.

—WRM

(cont.)

BOX 1.3. *(cont.)*

Before I read that first article about MI I had an experience that sowed the seed for my later interest in it. I was working as a nurses' aide in a treatment center for people with drinking problems. The center had a forceful philosophy, quite intimidating at the time for a 23-year-old. The message was that we needed to help the clients to face their denial about the severity of their problem because otherwise they would continue to lie to themselves and others about their destructive habit. It didn't take long to ascertain in case discussions and in the coffee room who were the particularly "resistant" clients. One of them was assigned to a group that I ran for young people. One evening, after saying virtually nothing in the group meeting, he went out and shot his wife and then himself in front of their two young children.

Some years later I read this paper (Miller, 1983) suggesting that "denial" could be viewed as the expression of a dysfunctional relationship and damaged rapport and could be transformed in a positive direction by using a more collaborative style with clients. I realized with some shock that the personal and professional inclination to blame, judge, and label others for being "resistant" and "not motivated" was not confined to the addiction field. It popped up in just about every care setting I came across. MI provided a different way of approaching these conversations about change.

—SR

---

and defend the opposite. This sometimes gets labeled as "denial" or "resistance" or "being oppositional," but there is nothing pathological about such responses. It is the normal nature of ambivalence and debate.

This debate process might seem therapeutic—a kind of psychodramatic acting out of the person's ambivalence with the helper simply representing the pro-change side—were it not for another principle of human nature, which is that most people tend to believe themselves and trust their own opinions more than those of others. Causing someone to verbalize one side of an issue tends to move the person's balance of opinion in that direction. In other words, people learn about their own attitudes and beliefs in the same way that others learn them: by hearing themselves talk (Bem, 1967, 1972). From this perspective, if you as a helper are arguing for change and your client is arguing against it, you've got it exactly backward. Ideally, the client should be voicing the reasons for change. Any successful salesperson knows this. People are quite sensitive to how they are spoken to about an ambivalent topic, in part because

> If you are arguing for change and your client is arguing against it, you've got it exactly backward.

they have already been having these same discussions about change within themselves. The righting reflex and associated directing style tends to set up an oppositional pattern of conversation. How constructive is this, and what's the likely outcome?

THE DYNAMICS OF CHANGE CONVERSATIONS

The righting reflex involves the belief that you must *convince* or *persuade* the person to do the right thing. You just need to ask the right questions, find the proper arguments, give the critical information, provoke the decisive emotions, or pursue the correct logic to make the person see and change. This assumption was rife in the addiction treatment field during much of the latter half of the 20th century: that people with such problems were incapable of perceiving reality themselves and their pathological defenses had to be broken down before they could change. This perspective calls forth a massive righting reflex from the helper: confront the person with reality, provide the solution, and when you meet resistance turn up the volume (White & Miller, 2007). Clients tend to respond in the predictable way, thus leading to the erroneous conclusion that all people with addictions are characterologically immature, fiercely defended, and "in denial" (Carr, 2011). This phenomenon is not unique to addiction treatment. Echoes of this pattern, and the associated judgments and labels about poor motivation, can be found in many settings across health and social care and criminal justice.

Try this thought experiment, or better still, have a friend try it with you. Choose something that you have been thinking about changing, should change, perhaps want or need to change, but haven't done so yet. In other words, think of a change about which you are ambivalent. We all have them. Now have (or imagine) a "helper" who tells you how much you need to make this change, gives you a list of reasons for doing so, emphasizes the importance of changing, tells you how to do it, assures you that you can do it, and exhorts you to get on with it. How would you be likely to respond? We have used this exercise all over the world, and people's responses are remarkably consistent. A few find it helpful, perhaps one in 20 (just enough to keep helpers doing it), but most often the "helped" person feels some if not all of the following:

Angry (agitated, annoyed, irritated, not heard, not understood)
Defensive (discounting, judged, justifying, oppositional, unwilling to change)
Uncomfortable (ashamed, overwhelmed, eager to leave)
Powerless (passive, one-down, discouraged, disengaged)

In fact, sometimes in this interaction the person being "helped" concludes that he or she actually *doesn't* want to make the change! That was not usually the helper's intention, of course. It's just how people normally respond to the righting reflex, to being told what to do and why and how they should do it. People tend to feel bad in response to the righting reflex, and causing people to feel bad doesn't help them to change.

Now try it again, but this time your friend will act differently. Again, you are to talk about something you want to change, should change, need to change, have been thinking about changing, but haven't changed yet. This time your friend gives you no advice at all, but instead asks you a series of questions and listens respectfully to what you say. We developed these five questions in 2006 to give beginners a feeling for the process of MI:

1. "Why would you want to make this change?"
2. "How might you go about it in order to succeed?"
3. "What are the three best reasons for you to do it?"
4. "How important is it for you to make this change, and why?"

Your friend listens patiently, and then gives you back a short summary of what *you* have said: why you want to change, why it's important, what the best reasons are, and how you could do it in order to succeed. Then your friend asks one more question, and again simply listens as you reply:

5. "So what do you think you'll do?"

That's it. We haven't explained yet what's going on in this conversation about change or given you any theory or guidelines. The questions themselves are not the method, but they do provide a sense of the person-centered spirit and style of MI. We have also used this exercise all over the world, and again people tend to respond to their listener (regardless of the helper's prior education or experience) in similar ways. They usually say that they felt:

> Engaged (interested, cooperative, liking the counselor, ready to keep talking)
> Empowered (able to change, hopeful, optimistic)
> Open (accepted, comfortable, safe, respected)
> Understood (connected, heard, listened to)

In both cases the subject of the conversation is the same—a possible change characterized by ambivalence—but the outcomes tend to be quite different. So which would you rather spend your time working with: (1) angry, defensive, uncomfortable, and passive people who don't like you; or (2) people who feel engaged, empowered, open, and understood and rather like their time with you? They are *the same people*. The difference is in the dynamics of the conversation.

A BEGINNING DEFINITION

So what exactly is MI? It's certainly not a simple five-step sequence of questions for promoting change. Skillful MI involves a lot more than asking questions, and it requires high-quality listening. In our first edition (Miller & Rollnick, 1991) we provided no definition at all. Since then we have offered various approximations (Miller & Rollnick, 2002, 2009; Rollnick & Miller, 1995). The problem in part is the complexity of MI. For this third edition we offer three different *levels* of definition, one in each of the first three chapters. The first of these is a layperson's definition that focuses on its purpose:

> *Motivational interviewing is a collaborative conversation style for strengthening a person's own motivation and commitment to change.*

MI is, first and foremost, a conversation about change. If we had called it anything else it probably would have been "motivational conversation." It can be brief or prolonged, and it may occur in many different contexts, with individuals or groups, but it is always a collaborative conversation, never a lecture or monologue. It is more a matter of guiding than directing. Also, as the name implies, its primary purpose is to strengthen motivation for change—the person's *own* motivation. Being motivated is incomplete without commitment, and in this edition we devote more attention to how MI connects with planning and implementing change (Part V). In Chapter 3 we offer an overview of the method of MI, but first we turn to the underlying spirit that guides good practice.

KEY POINTS

✓ *Motivational interviewing is a collaborative conversation style for strengthening a person's own motivation and commitment to change.*

✓ The overall style of MI is one of *guiding*, which lies between and incorporates elements of *directing* and *following* styles.

✓ Ambivalence is a normal part of preparing for change and a place where a person can remain stuck for some time.

✓ When a helper uses a directing style and argues for change with a person who is ambivalent, it naturally brings out the person's opposite arguments.

✓ People are more likely to be persuaded by what they hear themselves say.

CHAPTER 2

The Spirit
of Motivational Interviewing

> If you treat an individual as he is, he will stay as he is, but
> if you treat him as if he were what he ought to be and could
> be, he will become what he ought to be and could be.
> —JOHANN WOLFGANG VON GOETHE

> Compassion is the wish to see others free from suffering.
> —THE DALAI LAMA

When we began teaching MI in the 1980s we tended to focus on technique, on *how* to do it. Over time we found, however, that something important was missing. As we watched trainees practicing MI, it was as though we had taught them the words but not the music. What had we failed to convey? This is when we began writing about the underlying *spirit* of MI, its mind-set and heart-set (Rollnick & Miller, 1995).

What we mean by this is the underlying perspective with which one practices MI. Without this underlying spirit, MI becomes a cynical trick, a way of trying to manipulate people into doing what they don't want to do: the expert magician skillfully steers the hapless client into the right choice. In short, it becomes just another version of the righting reflex, a battle of wits in which the goal is to outsmart your adversary. Our first edition reflected a bit of this language and perspective.[1]

---

[1] A recent book (Pantalon, 2011) reflects a mirror opposite of the spirit of MI, promising on the cover that open questions like those described in Chapter 1 represent a way to "get anyone to do anything" in less than 7 minutes. The same notion of MI as a simple trick is implicit in the invitations that we receive periodically to teach a staff MI over pizza during the lunch hour. We accept some responsibility for this misunderstanding from our early presentations of MI.

So what is this underlying spirit, the set of heart and mind with which one enters into the practice of MI? That is the primary focus of this chapter. We begin with four key interrelated elements of the spirit of MI: partnership, acceptance, compassion, and evocation. For each of these there is an experiential as well as a behavioral component. One can, for example, experience acceptance or compassion for others, but without behavioral expression it does them no good.

We hasten to add that these are not prerequisites for the practice of MI. If one first had to become profoundly accepting and compassionate before being able to practice MI, the wait could be lifelong. It is our experience that the practice of MI itself teaches these four habits of the heart.

PARTNERSHIP

The first of four vital aspects of the spirit of MI is that it involves *partnership*. It is not something done by an expert to a passive recipient, a teacher to a pupil, a master to a disciple. In fact it is not done "to" or "on" someone at all. MI is done "for" and "with" a person. It is an active collaboration between experts. People are the undisputed experts on themselves. No one has been with them longer, or knows them better than they do themselves. In MI, the helper is a companion who typically does less than half of the talking. The method of MI involves exploration more than exhortation, interest and support rather than persuasion or argument. The interviewer seeks to create a positive interpersonal atmosphere that is conducive to change but not coercive.

> MI is done "for" and "with" a person.

We have found that it is helpful sometimes to use metaphors and similes when explaining what MI is like, and we will do so throughout this book. A good one here is that MI is like dancing rather than wrestling.[2] One moves with rather than against the person. It is not a process of overpowering and pinning an adversary. A good MI conversation looks as smooth as a ballroom waltz. Someone is still leading in the dance, and skillful guiding is definitely part of the art of MI, without tripping or stepping on toes. Without partnership there is no dance.

Why is this important? One simple reason is that when the goal is for another person to change, the counselor can't do it alone. The client has vital expertise that is complementary to your own. Activation of that expertise is a key condition for change to occur (Hibbard, Mahoney, Stock, & Tusler, 2007; Hibbard, Stockard, Mahoney, & Tusler, 2004). MI is not a way of tricking people into changing; it is a way of activating their own motivation and resources for change. A pitfall to avoid here is the expert

---

[2]This metaphor was originally suggested by Jeff Allison.

trap, communicating that, based on your professional expertise, you have the answer to the person's dilemma. Avoiding this trap includes letting go of the assumption that you are *supposed to* have and provide all the right answers. In truth, you don't necessarily have them when the topic is personal change. The expert trap is fertile ground for the righting reflex to spring up. Many professionals during postgraduate training were taught and expected to come up with the right answer and to provide it promptly. Willing suspension of this reflex to dispense expertise is a key element in the collaborative spirit of MI.

> MI is not a way of tricking people into changing; it is a way of activating their own motivation and resources for change.

The partnership nature of MI implies being attuned to and monitoring your own aspirations as well as your client's. The interpersonal process of MI is a meeting of aspirations that, as in any partnership, may differ. Without awareness of one's own opinion and investment, one has only half the picture. We regard honesty about these aspirations to be essential in MI. Sometimes the provider's agenda can be presumed from the context. When a person walks through the door of a "smoking cessation clinic" or an "alcohol/drug treatment program," the intended topic of conversation and direction of change are no mystery. Those who staff a suicide prevention hotline seek to prevent suicide, and probation officers are about preventing illegal behavior. In many settings, the client sets the agenda for change, presenting specific problems and concerns. It does happen, however, that a provider's priorities for change differ from the client's, a scenario that we consider in more detail in Chapter 10. Our emphasis here is on awareness and honesty regarding one's own values and agenda in conversations about change.

This partnership aspect of MI spirit bespeaks a profound respect for the other. In a way, the MI practitioner is a privileged witness to change, and the conversation is a bit like sitting together on a sofa while the person pages through a life photo album. You ask questions sometimes, but mostly you listen because the story is the person's own. Your purpose is to understand the life before you, to see the world through this person's eyes rather than superimposing your own vision.

ACCEPTANCE

Related to this spirit of partnership is an attitude of profound *acceptance* of what the client brings. To accept a person in this sense does not mean that you necessarily approve of the person's actions or acquiesce to the status quo. The interviewer's personal approval (or disapproval) is irrelevant here.

What we mean by acceptance has deep roots in the work of Carl Rogers and contains at least four aspects (see Box 2.1).

Absolute Worth

First, acceptance involves prizing the inherent worth and potential of every human being. Rogers (1980b) referred to this attitude as nonpossessive caring or unconditional positive regard, "an acceptance of this other individual as a separate person, a respect for the other as having worth in his or her own right. It is a basic trust—a belief that this other person is somehow fundamentally trustworthy" (p. 271). It was one of his necessary and sufficient therapeutic conditions for change to occur. Fromm (1956, p. 23) described this as a respect that is "the ability to see a person as he is, to be aware of his unique individuality. Respect means the concern that the other person should grow and unfold as he is. Respect thus implies the absence of exploitation."

The opposite of this attitude is one of judgment, placing conditions on worth: "I will decide who deserves respect and who does not." There is a fascinating paradox here. We concur with Rogers that when people experience themselves as unacceptable they are immobilized. Their ability to

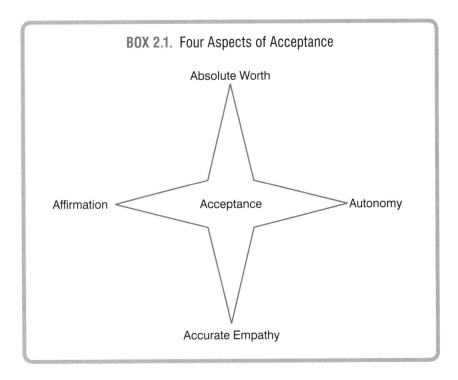

BOX 2.1. Four Aspects of Acceptance

Absolute Worth

Affirmation   Acceptance   Autonomy

Accurate Empathy

change is diminished or blocked. When, on the other hand, people experience being accepted as they are, they are freed to change.

Rogers (1959) took this *Menschenbild*, this view of human nature, a step further, positing that, when given critical therapeutic conditions, people will naturally change in a positive direction. This tendency toward "self-actualization" (Maslow, 1943, 1970) is as natural as a plant's growth upward toward the light when given adequate soil, water, and sunshine. It is as if each person has a natural mature end-state or purpose (*telos*, in Greek) toward which he or she will grow given optimal conditions. The *telos* of an acorn is an oak tree. Are people also inherently self-actualizing, naturally inclined to grow toward a positive *telos*? We cannot know for sure, but we *can* choose our own *Menschenbild*,[3] the way in which we decide to view people and human nature—a view that tends to become a self-fulfilling prophecy (Leake & King, 1977; Miller, 1985a).

Accurate Empathy

A second key aspect of acceptance (and another of Rogers's critical conditions for change) is accurate empathy, an active interest in and effort to understand the other's internal perspective, to see the world through her or his eyes. We don't mean sympathy, a feeling of pity for or camaraderie with the person. Neither do we mean identification: "I've been there and I know what you're experiencing. Let me tell you my story." Those may or may not be present, but empathy is an ability to understand another's frame of reference and the conviction that it is worthwhile to do so. Rogers and his students described well the therapeutic skill of accurate empathy (Rogers, 1965; Truax & Carkhuff, 1967). It is "to sense the client's inner world of private personal meanings as if it were your own, but without ever losing the 'as if' quality" (Rogers, 1989, pp. 92–93). The opposite of empathy is the imposition of one's own perspective, perhaps with the assumption that the other's views are irrelevant or misguided.

Autonomy Support

Third, acceptance involves honoring and respecting each person's autonomy, their irrevocable right and capacity of self-direction (Deci & Ryan, 1985; Markland, Ryan, Tobin, & Rollnick, 2005). Viktor Frankl (2006) observed:

> We who lived in concentration camps remember the men who walked through the huts comforting others, giving away their last piece of bread.

---

[3]Thanks to Joachim Koerkel for suggesting this helpful term and concept.

They may have been few in number, but they offer sufficient proof that everything can be taken from a man but one thing: the last of the human freedoms—to choose one's attitude in any given set of circumstances, to choose one's own way. (pp. 65–66)

Rogers (1962) sought in his client-centered approach to offer people "complete freedom to be and to choose" (p. 93). His confidence in doing so was related, no doubt, to his view of human nature as essentially "positive, forward moving, constructive, realistic, trustworthy" (p. 91). He believed that, when given the essential therapeutic conditions, people will naturally grow in a positive direction. His perspective was in part a contrast to the Freudian view that people are fundamentally self-serving pleasure seekers mostly unconscious of the dark drives that shape their lives.

The opposite of autonomy support is the attempt to *make* people do things, to coerce and control. A probation officer who says "You can't leave the county" is not literally telling the truth, nor is a counselor who tells an alcohol-dependent person "You can't drink." What they mean is that certain behavior is likely to have negative consequences, but the choice always remains with the individual. There is also a paradox here. Telling someone that "You can't," and more generally trying to constrain someone's choices typically evokes psychological reactance (Dillard & Shen, 2005; Karno & Longabaugh, 2005a, 2005b), the desire to reassert one's freedom. On the other hand, directly acknowledging a person's freedom of choice typically diminishes defensiveness and can facilitate change. This involves letting go of the idea and burden that you have to (or can) make people change. It is, in essence, relinquishing a power that you never had in the first place.

Affirmation

Finally, acceptance as we understand it involves affirmation, to seek and acknowledge the person's strengths and efforts. As with worth, autonomy, and empathy, this is not merely a private experience of appreciation, but an intentional way of being and communicating (Rogers, 1980b). Its opposite is the search for what is wrong with people (which is so often the focus of "assessment"), and having identified what is wrong, to tell them how to fix it.

Taken together, these four person-centered conditions convey what we mean by "acceptance." One honors each person's *absolute worth* and potential as a human being, recognizes and supports the person's irrevocable *autonomy* to choose his or her own way, seeks through *accurate empathy* to understand the other's perspective, and *affirms* the person's strengths and efforts.

COMPASSION

We have chosen in this third edition to add the element of compassion to our description of the underlying spirit of MI. Here again we are not talking about a personal feeling, an emotional experience such as sympathy or identification, for these are neither necessary nor sufficient for the practice of compassion. One need not literally "suffer with" in order to act with compassion, nor is felt sympathy without action of much benefit. To be compassionate is to actively promote the other's welfare, to give priority to the other's needs. Our services are, after all, for our clients' benefit and not primarily for our own. Virtually every major world religion advocates the cultivation and practice of this virtue, to benevolently seek and value the well-being of others. Compassion is a deliberate commitment to pursue the welfare and best interests of the other. This promotion of others' welfare is, of course, one motivation that draws people into helping professions.

> To be compassionate is to actively promote the other's welfare, to give priority to the other's needs.

Why have we added compassion to the other three elements of MI spirit? Because it is possible to practice the other three in pursuit of self-interest. A skillful salesperson establishes a working partnership with potential customers, evokes their own goals and values, and is well aware that the customer ultimately decides whether to buy. We do not mean to disparage the enterprise of sales, which can certainly be practiced in a way that benefits both customer and seller, but only to say that psychological knowledge and techniques, including those described later, *can* be used to exploit, to pursue one's own advantage and gain undeserved trust and compliance (Cialdini, 2007). To work with a spirit of compassion is to have your heart in the right place so that the trust you engender will be deserved.

EVOCATION

So much of what happens in professional consultations about change is based on a deficit model, that the person is lacking something that needs to be installed. The implicit message is "I have what you need, and I'm going to give it to you," be it knowledge, insight, diagnosis, wisdom, reality, rationality, or coping skills. Evaluation is so often focused on detecting deficits to be corrected by professional expertise. Once you have discovered the missing ingredient, what the client lacks, then you will know what to install. This approach is reasonable in automobile repair or in treating infections, but it usually does not work well when personal change is the focus of the conversation.

The spirit of MI starts from a very different strengths-focused premise, that people already have within them much of what is needed, and your task is to evoke it, to call it forth. The implicit message is "*You* have what you need, and together we will find it." From this perspective it is particularly important to focus on and understand the person's strengths and resources rather than probe for deficits. The assumption here is that people truly do have wisdom about themselves and have good reasons for doing what they have been doing. They already have motivation and resources within themselves that can be called on. One of the unexpected outcomes of our early MI research was that once people resolved their ambivalence about change, they often went ahead and did it on their own without additional professional assistance or permission.

Consider two different approaches to education. The first is to lecture, essentially to insert knowledge. Open up the head, install facts, and suture. The corresponding Latin verb is *docere*, which is the etymological root of *doctrine, docent, indoctrinate, docile*, and *doctor*. This perspective starts very much from a deficit model, that the person is lacking what is needed. There is a time and place for this kind of teaching, but usually it is not very effective in helping people change. The contrasting approach is to draw out (literally in Latin, *e ducere*), as in drawing water from a well. From an MI perspective, the assumption is that there is a deep well of wisdom and experience within the person from which the counselor can draw. Much of what is needed is already there, and it's a matter of drawing it out, calling it forth. The MI practitioner is therefore keenly interested in understanding the client's perspective and wisdom.

This spirit of evocation also fits with the conception of ambivalence presented in Chapter 1. People who are ambivalent about change already have *both* arguments within them—those favoring change and those supporting status quo. This means that most clients do already have pro-change voices on their internal committee, their own positive motivations for change. These are likely to be more persuasive than whatever arguments you might be able to provide. Your task, then, is to evoke and strengthen these change motivations that are already present.

The MI spirit emerges at the intersection of these four components (see Box 2.2). This provides the context for our second pragmatic definition of MI—a practitioner's definition that answers the question "Why would I want to learn MI, and how would I use it?"

Motivational interviewing is a person-centered counseling style for addressing the common problem of ambivalence about change.

BOX 2.2. The Underlying Spirit of MI

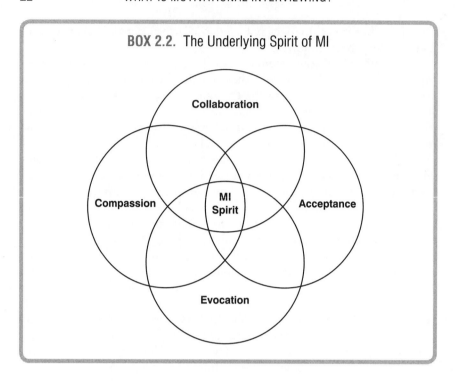

SOME PRINCIPLES
OF PERSON-CENTERED CARE

The underlying spirit we describe here lies squarely within the long-standing tradition of person-centered care. It has also been called client-centered counseling (Rogers, 1965), patient-centered medicine (Laine & Davidoff, 1996) and relationship-centered care (Beach, Inui, & the Relationship-Centered Care Research Network, 2006), but its essence is to place the recipient's perspective at the center of services. In this regard we suggest, in closing, some general principles within a broader person-centered approach to care.

1. Our services exist to benefit the people we serve (and not vice versa). The needs of clients (participants, patients, consumers, customers, etc.) have priority.
2. Change is fundamentally self-change. Services (treatment, therapy, interventions, counseling, etc.) facilitate natural processes of change (Prochaska & DiClemente, 1984).

3. People are the experts on themselves. No one knows more about them than they do.
4. We don't have to *make* change happen. The truth is that we can't do it alone.
5. We don't have to come up with all the good ideas. Chances are that we don't have the best ones.
6. People have their own strengths, motivations, and resources that are vital to activate in order for change to occur.
7. Therefore, change requires a partnership, a collaboration of expertise.
8. It is important to understand the person's own perspective on the situation, what is needed, and how to accomplish it.
9. Change is not a power struggle whereby if change occurs we "win." A conversation about change should feel like dancing, not wrestling.
10. Motivation for change is not installed, but is evoked. It's already there and just needs to be called forth.
11. We cannot revoke people's choice about their own behavior. People make their own decisions about what they will and will not do, and it's not a change goal until the person adopts it.

A DEVELOPMENTAL PROCESS

We have tried in this chapter to describe the set of mind and heart with which one ought to enter into the process of MI. As we said earlier, having fully internalized this state of mind and heart is not a prerequisite for the practice of MI; otherwise, who could ever begin? In a very real sense, practicing MI over time teaches one this underlying spirit. The Dalai Lama offered this description of developing compassion:

> There is a developmental process for cultivating compassion for others. . . . The first step is knowledge. . . . Then you need to constantly reflect and internalize this knowledge . . . to the point where it will become a *conviction*. It becomes integrated into your state of mind. . . . Then you get to a point where it becomes spontaneous. (The Dalai Lama & Ekman, 2008, pp. 156–157)

That is our experience of learning MI. We no longer rehearse before each session what our heart-set should be (although it can be useful to do so). It becomes automatic; practicing this style of being with others evokes it. So do not fret if you think your "spirit" is lagging. Practice will teach and remind you.

BOX 2.3. Personal Reflection: An MI Prayer

Living in the American Southwest, I have often been privileged to talk with Native American providers about motivational interviewing. Some have told me that this respectful way of relating to others is quite compatible with tribal conversational norms. A tribal leader once observed, however, that in order to teach MI to American Indians, it should have a prayer, a song, and a dance. I leave the dance and song to more capable people, but I did craft this prayer with the help of Raymond Daw. This particular version reflects meditative preparation to work with a female client, but the pronouns can easily be changed.

Guide me to be a patient companion,
to listen with a heart as open as the sky.
Grant me vision to see through her eyes
and eager ears to hear her story.
Create a safe and open mesa on which we may walk together.
Make me a clear pool in which she may reflect.
Guide me to find in her your beauty and wisdom,
knowing your desire for her to be in harmony:
healthy, loving, and strong.
Let me honor and respect her choosing of her own path,
and bless her to walk it freely.
May I know once again that although she and I are different,
yet there is a peaceful place where we are one.

—WRM

KEY POINTS

✓ MI is a person-centered counseling style for addressing the common problem of ambivalence about change.

✓ MI is done *for* or *with* someone, not *on* or *to* them.

✓ Four key aspects of the underlying spirit of MI are partnership, acceptance, compassion, and evocation.

✓ Acceptance includes four aspects of *absolute worth*, *accurate empathy*, *autonomy support*, and *affirmation*.

✓ MI is about evoking that which is already present, not installing what is missing.

CHAPTER 3

The Method
of Motivational Interviewing

People are generally better persuaded by the reasons
which they have themselves discovered than by those
which have come into the mind of others.
                                        —BLAISE PASCAL

You are a midwife, assisting at someone else's birth. Do
good without show or fuss. Facilitate what is happening
rather than what you think ought to be happening.
If you must take the lead, lead so that the mother is
helped, yet still free and in charge. When the baby is
born, the mother will rightly say, "We did it ourselves!"
                                        —TAO TE CHING

FOUR PROCESSES IN MOTIVATIONAL INTERVIEWING

In our first two editions we described two phases of MI: building motivation (Phase 1) and consolidating commitment (Phase 2). As a simple guideline it had some merit. For example, "Take care not to talk exclusively
about the *how* of change, more relevant in Phase 2, before talking about the
why of change, mostly a Phase 1 activity." Yet in practice, this simple distinction failed to reflect a decision-making process that often seems more
circular than linear. It also seemed incomplete. For example, clinicians told
us that they sometimes struggled to practice MI because clients seemed
disengaged. Another clinical challenge for some practitioners was the range
of clients' possible change options to consider, and they found it difficult to
narrow down the conversation.

   This led us to think more clearly about processes that comprise MI. We
decided to loosen the sequential thread of "phases" and try to more nearly
approximate what one encounters in practice as four overlapping processes.

As designations for these processes we chose the gerunds "engaging," "focusing," "evoking," and "planning." This book is organized around these four processes.

Our purpose in this chapter is to overview these central processes that form the flow of MI. In one sense these processes do emerge in the order in which we describe them. If you don't engage with a client, you're unlikely to get much further. Evoking as discussed in this book is only possible with a clear focus in mind. Deciding *whether* to change is usually a prerequisite for planning *how* to change. Yet they are also recursive; one does not end as the next begins. They may flow into each other, overlap, and recur. It is the confluence of these four processes that best describes MI.

Because the four processes are both sequential and recursive, we have chosen to represent them as stair steps (see Box 3.1). Each later process builds upon those that were laid down before and continue to run beneath it as a foundation. In the course of a conversation or case one may also dance up and down the staircase, returning to a prior step that requires renewed attention.

Engaging

Every relationship begins with a period of engagement. When people come seeking consultation or services they wonder and often imagine what the provider will be like, how she or he will treat them. First impressions are powerful (Gladwell, 2007), although not irrevocable. In the course of any initial visit people are deciding, among other things, how much they like and trust the provider and whether they plan to come back. In some settings the modal number of visits is one!

Engaging is the process by which both parties establish a helpful connection and a working relationship. Sometimes this can occur within seconds; sometimes its absence can be felt for weeks. Much can be done within the conversation to enhance engagement. Factors outside of the immediate conversation can also facilitate or undermine it: the service system within

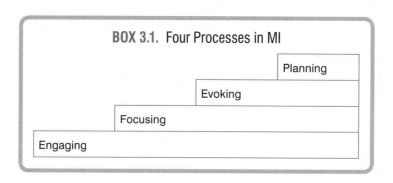

BOX 3.1. Four Processes in MI

			Planning
		Evoking	
	Focusing		
Engaging			

which client and practitioner work, the clinician's emotional state, the client's circumstances and state of mind on entering the room.

Therapeutic engagement is a prerequisite for everything that follows. This is not unique to MI, of course. Developing a working alliance is important in many service settings. Clients' ratings of the quality of this working relationship with a provider tend to predict retention and outcome, although sometimes the providers' ratings do not (Crits-Christoph et al., 2011). Engagement involves more than just being friendly and nice to the client. The chapters in Part II of this book address this challenge of engaging.

> Therapeutic engagement is a prerequisite for everything that follows.

Focusing

The process of engaging leads to a focus on particular agenda: what the person came to talk about. The provider may also have agenda; some of which overlap with the client's whereas others may not. For example, a person might seek health care regarding an upper respiratory infection and shortness of breath, wanting at least symptomatic relief. Recalling that the person is a smoker, the provider wonders about suggesting a change. What will they talk about? Certainly they will address the presenting complaints, but the provider may also raise the topic of smoking. *Focusing* is the process by which you develop and maintain a specific direction in the conversation about change.

In the course of helping relationships, a direction toward one or more change goals usually emerges. These may be formalized in a treatment plan, although we prefer a broader change plan because treatment is often just one of many possible avenues toward change.

These goals may or may not involve behavior change. Often they do. Chronic disease management is very much about health behavior change (Rollnick, Miller, et al., 2008). There are behavioral treatment approaches for eating disorders, exercise and fitness, anxiety disorders, depression, chronic disorganization, shyness, substance use, and chronic pain, to name but a few. As discussed in Chapter 1, other change goals are less about overt behavior than making a choice—whether to forgive someone, whether to stay or leave—or deciding on one's attitude and way of thinking (e.g., to be more compassionate). Some involve reaching resolution or acceptance—working through complicated grief, finding peace about a decision, or developing more tolerance for ambiguity, solitude, or anxiety. A choice for acceptance may involve doing nothing differently.

Within MI, the focusing process helps to clarify direction, the horizon toward which one intends to move. What changes are hoped to arise from this consultation?

Evoking

With one or more change goals as a focus, the third common process in MI is evoking. Evoking involves eliciting the client's own motivations for change, and it has always been at the heart of MI. It occurs when there is a focus on a particular change and you harness the client's own ideas and feelings about why and how they might do it.

This is the mirror opposite of an expert-didactic approach: assess the problem, determine what they are doing wrong, and educate them on how to fix it. Within that model the expert provides both the diagnosis and the solution. That's quite appropriate in acute medicine; for example, in diagnosing and treating infections or broken bones: "Here's the problem. Let's try this." When the goal is personal change, however, this expert directing approach usually breaks down. Personal change requires the individual's active participation in the change process. An antibiotic may be taken for 7 days or a cast kept on for 7 weeks, but personal change is a long-term process.

Most simply put, evoking is having the person voice the arguments for change. Although the righting reflex is to voice these arguments oneself, it can be counterproductive to do so. People talk *themselves* into changing, and are commonly disinclined to be told what to do if it conflicts with their own judgment.

There are exceptions, of course. Some people come for consultation fully prepared for change and asking for best advice on how to proceed.[1] With such people one quickly moves into planning.

Alas, such ready-to-go people are often the minority rather than the norm in many human service settings. One would think:

- That having had a heart attack would be enough to persuade someone to quit smoking, exercise, and eat a more healthy diet.
- That spending any amount of time in the privations of prison would convince people not to go back there.
- That the very real threats of kidney failure, blindness, and amputations would be sufficient to motivate people with diabetes to keep their blood glucose under control.
- And that alcohol-related injury, blackouts, arrest, and damaged

---

[1] An example that comes to mind is a desperate family member who calls for help regarding a loved one who is lost in the world of alcohol or other drugs and yet refuses to get help. These are some of the most motivated people we have ever encountered. They are often willing to do whatever it takes to save their loved one and relieve their own stress and suffering. We saw painful examples of this vulnerability being exploited, such as being persuaded to mortgage their home to pay for an expensive private treatment program. Happily, much can be done to help them and get their loved one on the road to recovery (Meyers & Wolfe, 2004; Smith & Meyers, 2004). These people were definitely ready for change and didn't need much of the evoking process of MI to increase their motivation.

relationships would persuade people to do something about their drinking.

Yet so often it is not enough, and more lecturing and finger wagging is unlikely to boost the odds of change. Something else is needed: the collaborative process of nurturing the person's own inherent motivation for positive change. This process of evoking leads to our last definition of MI, the most technical one that speaks to the question "How does it work?"

> *Motivational interviewing is a collaborative, goal-oriented style of communication with particular attention to the language of change. It is designed to strengthen personal motivation for and commitment to a specific goal by eliciting and exploring the person's own reasons for change within an atmosphere of acceptance and compassion.*

Planning

When people's motivation reaches a threshold of readiness, the balance tips and they begin thinking and talking more about when and how to change and less about whether and why. There is usually not a discrete moment when this happens, although some people can point to the

---

BOX 3.2. Three Definitions of MI

Layperson's definition

> *Motivational interviewing is a collaborative conversation style for strengthening a person's own motivation and commitment to change.*

Practitioner's definition

> *Motivational interviewing is a person-centered counseling style for addressing the common problem of ambivalence about change.*

Technical definition

> *Motivational interviewing is a collaborative, goal-oriented style of communication with particular attention to the language of change. It is designed to strengthen personal motivation for and commitment to a specific goal by eliciting and exploring the person's own reasons for change within an atmosphere of acceptance and compassion.*

particular time or event when the switch flipped and the lights went on. More often people begin thinking about how they might do it, envisioning what it would be like to have made a change. At this point people may seek information and advice about how to proceed, whether from a professional, friends, a bookstore, or the Internet. It also happens that, having reached a decision for change, people may want and need no additional help with planning.

Planning encompasses both developing commitment to change and formulating a specific plan of action. It's a conversation about action that can cover a range of topics, conducted with a sharp ear for eliciting clients' own solutions, promoting their autonomy of decision making and continuing to elicit and strengthen change talk as a plan emerges.

It is important, we think, to recognize when it is time to begin planning and explore the options. Planning is the clutch that engages the engine of change talk. Later we provide some cues to watch for and a way of testing the water to see whether it's time to negotiate a change plan (Chapter 20). All of the previous processes and skills continue as you proceed toward a specific change plan (or at least next step) that the client finds acceptable.

> Planning is the clutch that engages the engine of change talk.

Like the other three processes, planning is something that one often needs to revisit from time to time as change proceeds. Unanticipated challenges and new obstacles arise that may cause a person to rethink plans and commitment. Higher priorities may emerge that compete for attention. Prior plans give way to better ones. Planning is not something done once and then finished. It is an ongoing process that—like engaging, focusing, and evoking—may need to be revisited (see Chapter 22).

We do not intend to provide a comprehensive model of change or an all-encompassing system of treatment. We think of MI as one clinical tool that is used for a particular purpose: to help people move through ambivalence and toward change. We found early on (to our initial surprise) that once people had been through the evoking and planning processes of MI they were often content to proceed with change on their own and did so. The hump for them was really *deciding* to make the change, and having done so they often felt no need for additional help. In two early studies we anticipated that MI would trigger help seeking for alcohol problems, and we provided a menu of local treatment resources. Almost no one sought treatment, but most made substantial and lasting reductions in their drinking (Miller, Benefield, & Tonigan, 1993; Miller, Sovereign, & Krege, 1988). As we discuss in Part VI, the method of MI also blends well with many other treatment approaches to facilitate retention and change (Hettema, Steele, & Miller, 2005).

THE FLOW OF MOTIVATIONAL INTERVIEWING

Unless a working alliance has previously been established, engaging is necessarily the opening process of MI. Without engagement the consultation goes no further. Even when an ongoing therapeutic relationship is established, MI for a particular change often begins with a more open-ended period of engaging that moves toward a clear focus.

Engaging flows into the focusing process, moving toward at least the beginning direction and goal(s) of consultation. The clinical skills of engaging remain important throughout focusing, evoking, and planning. In this sense, engaging does not end when focusing begins. One often needs to re-engage at various points along the way, and similarly it is common to change or enlarge the focus beyond the presenting problem.

Evoking becomes possible only when a change goal has been clarified. In this way, focusing is a logical prerequisite for evoking. Yet evoking often appears in the early minutes of MI if there is a predetermined or quickly emerging direction. There are characteristic counselor strategies and client speech patterns during evoking. Many forms of counseling include an engaging period—otherwise, they would not proceed—and a focusing process to clarify common treatment goals. With strategic evoking, the consultation becomes more distinctly MI. The counselor attends to, evokes, and responds in particular ways to specific types of client language while retaining the person-centered MI style and spirit. There is now reasonable empirical support for a causal chain related to evoking. MI training increases characteristic MI practice behaviors (Madson, Loignon, & Lane, 2009; Miller, Yahne, Moyers, Martinez, & Pirritano, 2004). These affect particular types of client speech (Glynn & Moyers, 2010; Moyers & Martin, 2006; Moyers, Miller, & Hendrickson, 2005; Vader, Walters, Prabhu, Houck, & Field, 2010), the level and strength of which in turn predict behavior change outcomes (Amrhein, Miller, Yahne, Palmer, & Fulcher, 2003; Moyers et al., 2007).

Planning flows naturally from evoking and is carried through in the same collaborative, evocative style. There is a negotiation of change goals and plans, an exchange of information, and usually a specification of next steps for implementation that may or may not involve further treatment. It is common during the planning process to revisit evoking in order to consolidate motivation and confidence. If treatment continues it is common for progress and motivation to fluctuate, inviting a renewal of planning, evoking, refocusing, or even re-engagement.

You might find yourself moving in and out of the four processes of engaging, focusing, evoking, and planning, and even having a conversation that covers more than one process at the same time. Yet their qualities are different. Box 3.3 provides some questions for each process that may help

---

BOX 3.3. Some Questions Regarding Each MI Process

1. **Engaging**
   - *How comfortable is this person in talking to me?*
   - *How supportive and helpful am I being?*
   - *Do I understand this person's perspective and concerns?*
   - *How comfortable do I feel in this conversation?*
   - *Does this feel like a collaborative partnership?*

2. **Focusing**
   - *What goals for change does this person really have?*
   - *Do I have different aspirations for change for this person?*
   - *Are we working together with a common purpose?*
   - *Does it feel like we are moving together, not in different directions?*
   - *Do I have a clear sense of where we are going?*
   - *Does this feel more like dancing or wrestling?*

3. **Evoking**
   - *What are this person's own reasons for change?*
   - *Is the reluctance more about confidence or importance of change?*
   - *What change talk am I hearing?*
   - *Am I steering too far or too fast in a particular direction?*
   - *Is the righting reflex pulling me to be the one arguing for change?*

4. **Planning**
   - *What would be a reasonable next step toward change?*
   - *What would help this person to move forward?*
   - *Am I remembering to evoke rather than prescribe a plan?*
   - *Am I offering needed information or advice with permission?*
   - *Am I retaining a sense of quiet curiosity about what will work best for this person?*

---

you to recognize them and also be useful reminders when actually speaking with clients. They are questions you might ask yourself about the helping process. Some of them you might even ask your client.

CORE SKILLS AND THE FOUR PROCESSES OF MOTIVATIONAL INTERVIEWING

The practice of MI involves the flexible and strategic use of some core communication skills that are shared with many other forms of counseling, particularly with other person-centered approaches (Hill, 2009; Ivey, Ivey,

& Zalaquett, 2009). These skills cut across the four processes described above and are needed throughout MI, although the particular ways in which they are used may vary with each MI process. In subsequent chapters we discuss each of these five skills in more detail, presenting them as they arise in relation to the processes. For present purposes we simply list and briefly describe them.

Asking Open Questions

MI makes particular use of open questions, those that invite the person to reflect and elaborate. Closed questions, in contrast, ask for specific information that can usually be offered as a short answer. In MI, gathering information is not the most important function of questions. In the engaging and focusing processes, open questions help you understand the person's internal frame of reference, strengthening a collaborative relationship and finding a clear direction. Open questions also play a key role in evoking motivation and planning a course toward change.

Affirming

MI relies on clients' own personal strengths, efforts, and resources. It is the client, not the counselor who produces change. Affirmation is both general and specific in MI. The counselor in general respects and honors the client as a person of worth, with the capability for growth and change as well as volitional choice about whether to do so. The interviewer also recognizes and comments on the client's particular strengths, abilities, good intentions, and efforts. Affirmation is also a way of thinking: the clinician consciously is on the lookout for client strengths, good steps, and intentions. This mind-set of "accentuate the positive" is a discipline in itself.

An opposite stance is the peculiar idea that people will change if you can just make them feel bad enough. Gill Woodall and colleagues became interested in the effect of the Mothers Against Drunk Driving Victim Impact Panel (VIP), in which DWI offenders are required to attend a public presentation by people whose lives have been devastated by drunk drivers. Judges agreed to assign offenders randomly to attend or not attend the VIP in addition to the usual sanctions (Woodall, Delaney, Rogers, & Wheeler, 2000). Interviewed as they were leaving the VIP, the offenders felt terrible about themselves—they felt embarrassed, ashamed of what they had done, humiliated, and guilty. When recidivism rates were examined, first offenders who attended the VIP were just as likely to be arrested again as those who did not. For people with one or more prior offenses, however, those who attended the VIP were actually *more* likely to repeat the offense! Lesson: Making people feel terrible doesn't help them to change.

Reflective Listening

Reflective listening is a fundamental skill in MI. Reflective statements that make a guess about the client's meaning have the important function of deepening understanding by clarifying whether one's guess is accurate. Reflective statements also allow people to hear again the thoughts and feelings they are expressing, perhaps in different words, and ponder them. Good reflective listening tends to keep the person talking, exploring, and considering. It is also necessarily selective, in that one chooses which aspects to reflect from all that the person has said. Within the evoking and planning processes of MI there are clear guidelines in selecting what to reflect, where to shine the light of attention.

Summarizing

Summaries are essentially reflections that collect what a person has been saying, offering it back as in a basket. They can be used to pull together what has been said, as at the end of a session. They may suggest links between present material and what has been discussed before. Summaries can also function as a transition from one task to another. In the engaging and focusing processes of MI, summaries promote understanding and show clients that you have been listening carefully, remembering and valuing what they say. They also provide a "What else?" opportunity for the person to fill in what you have missed. In evoking, there are particular guidelines for what to include in a summary in order to collect change talk and move along the process of change. During planning, summaries draw together the person's motivations, intentions, and specific plans for change.

There is overlap among these four skills (see Chapter 6). A summary is essentially a long reflection. The process of reflective listening can in itself be affirming. Good listening encompasses all four of these skills.

Informing and Advising

Because of the person-centered foundation of MI, people sometimes mistakenly conclude that one should never offer clients information or advice. There are definitely occasions within MI when it is appropriate to provide information or offer advice; for example, when a client asks for it. There are at least two important differences, however, from dispensing unsolicited expert opinion in a highly directive style. The first is that, in MI, one offers information or advice *with permission*. The second is not to just unload information on someone, but to understand their perspective and needs carefully and help them reach their own conclusions about the relevance of any information you provide. This is crystallized in the elicit–provide–elicit sequence described in Chapter 11. Whatever the counselor offers, the client is always free to agree or not, heed or not, implement or not, and it is often useful to acknowledge this directly.

These five core skills do not in themselves constitute MI. They are essentially prerequisite skills for the proficient practice of MI. What characterizes MI is the particular way in which these skills are used strategically to help people move in the direction of change.

WHAT MOTIVATIONAL INTERVIEWING IS NOT

Finally, it may be useful to clarify a few things that MI is *not*, ideas and methods with which MI is sometimes confused (Miller & Rollnick, 2009). Some of these, we hope, will already be clear from the foregoing discussion.

First, MI is not just being nice to people, and not identical to the client-centered counseling approach that Carl Rogers described as "nondirective." The focusing, evoking, and planning processes of MI have clear directionality to them. There is intentional, strategic movement toward one or more specific goals.

MI is also not a "technique," an easily learned gimmick to tuck away in one's toolbox. We describe MI as a *style* of being with people, an integration of particular clinical skills to foster motivation for change. It is a complex style in which one can continue to develop proficiency over many years. Asked once, "What is the difference between *doing* MI and *being* MI?" one of us answered, "About 10 years."

At the same time, MI is also not a panacea, a solution to all clinical problems. The spirit and style of MI can certainly be used across a wide range of clinical tasks, but we have never intended to propose a "school" of psychotherapy or counseling to which people would be converted and swear allegiance, forsaking all others. Rather, MI seems to blend well with other evidence-based clinical skills and approaches. MI was developed specifically for the purpose of helping people resolve ambivalence and strengthen motivation for change. Not everyone needs the evoking process of MI. When motivation for change is already strong, move ahead with planning and implementation.

In part because they were developed around the same time (see Chapter 27), MI and the transtheoretical model (TTM) of change have sometimes been confused. MI is not meant to be a comprehensive theory of change, and the popular TTM stages of change are not an essential part of MI. MI and TTM are compatible and complementary (e.g., DiClemente & Velasquez, 2002; Velasquez, Maurer, Crouch, & DiClemente, 2001), and with apologies to our translators we describe them as "kissing cousins who never married." MI is also sometimes confused with a decisional balance technique of equally exploring the pros and cons of change. In this edition we discuss decisional balance as a way of proceeding when you wish to counsel with neutrality rather than move toward a particular change goal (Chapter 17).

MI does not require the use of assessment feedback. The confusion here is related to an adaptation of MI that was tested in Project MATCH (motivational enhancement therapy), combining the clinical style of MI with personal feedback from pretreatment assessment (Longabaugh, Zweben, LoCastro, & Miller, 2005). Although assessment feedback can be useful in enhancing motivation (Agostinelli, Brown, & Miller, 1995; Davis, Baer, Saxon, & Kivlahan, 2003; Juarez, Walters, Daugherty, & Radi, 2006), particularly with those lower in readiness for change (see Chapter 18), it is not a necessary or sufficient component of MI.

Finally, MI is explicitly not a way of manipulating people into doing what you want them to do. MI cannot be used to manufacture motivation that is not already there. MI is a collaborative partnership that honors and respects the other's autonomy, seeking to understand the person's internal frame of reference. We added compassion to our description of the underlying spirit (Chapter 2) precisely to emphasize that MI is to be used to promote others' welfare and best interests, not one's own.

KEY POINTS

✓ Four key processes in MI are engaging, focusing, evoking, and planning.

✓ *Engaging* is the process of establishing a helpful connection and working relationship.

✓ *Focusing* is the process by which you develop and maintain a specific direction in the conversation about change.

✓ The process of *evoking* involves eliciting the client's own motivations for change and lies at the heart of MI.

✓ The *planning* process encompasses both developing commitment to change and formulating a concrete plan of action.

✓ Five key communication skills used throughout MI are asking open questions, affirming, reflecting, summarizing, and providing information and advice with permission.

PART II

ENGAGING
The Relational Foundation

The first of four basic processes in MI is to engage the client in a collaborative working relationship. Engagement can occur within minutes or take much longer to establish and maintain. It is the degree to which someone feels like a comfortable and active participant in the consultation. It is the fuel that drives any good service and is the relational foundation for MI.

Engagement goes both ways. The way you feel can and will affect your connection with the person you are trying to help. So, too, for the client. The forces that undermine engagement often come from pressures outside of your immediate conversation. The culture within a service—its design, procedures, and protocols—can render you overwhelmed and the client passive; unhelpful interviewing is often a natural and predictable consequence. Add to this mix a client who arrives fearful, confused, or angry, and the challenge of establishing a meaningful connection and fostering engagement is clearly the primary one.

One good outcome of engaging is that the client returns, without which your work together ends. In some settings the early dropout rate is high, and often it varies substantially across workers. Some staff seem to retain almost all of their clients, whereas for others dropout happens more frequently. A second important product of good engaging is developing a working alliance, which in turn predicts retention and outcome.

The four chapters of Part II describe the process of engaging and the clinical skills for promoting it with individual clients. Ways to improve engagement systemically through the design and delivery of services more broadly is a topic that we address later, in Chapter 26.

CHAPTER 4

Engagement and Disengagement

Coming together is a beginning; keeping together is progress; working together is success.

—HENRY FORD

The kind of caring that the client-centered therapist desires to achieve is a gullible caring, in which clients are accepted as they say they are, not with a lurking suspicion in the therapist's mind that they may, in fact, be otherwise. This attitude is not stupidity on the therapist's part; it is the kind of attitude that is most likely to lead to trust, to further self-exploration, and to the correction of false statements as trust deepens.

—CARL ROGERS AND RUTH SANFORD

Whatever the particular services being provided, client engagement is a key. In psychotherapy research the quality of the therapeutic alliance between client and therapist (particularly as perceived by the client) directly predicts both retention and outcome. In both psychotherapy (Henry, Strupp, Schacht, & Gaston, 1994; Horvath & Greenberg, 1994) and health care (Fuertes et al., 2007), people who are actively engaged are more likely to stay, adhere to, and benefit from treatment regardless of the particular orientation of the provider. Working alliance may similarly influence outcomes in education (Lacrose, Chaloux, Monaghan, & Tarabulsy, 2010) and rehabilitation (Evans, Sherer, Nakase-Richardson, Mani, & Irby, 2008).

But what *is* this alliance? What constitutes engagement from a therapeutic perspective? One widely used system (Bordin, 1979) highlights three aspects of positive engagement:

1. Establishment of a trusting and mutually respectful working relationship.
2. Agreement on treatment goals.
3. Collaboration on mutually negotiated tasks to reach these goals.

Because in MI we differentiate engaging from the process of establishing goals (focusing; see Part III), we define engaging as *the process of establishing a mutually trusting and respectful helping relationship.*

> Engaging is the process of establishing a mutually trusting and respectful helping relationship.

From the client's perspective (which is the one that better predicts retention and outcome), a person might be asking:

"Do I feel respected by this counselor?"
"Does he/she listen to and understand me?"
"Do I trust this person?"
"Do I have a say in what happens in this consultation?"
"Am I being offered options rather than a one-size-fits-all approach?"
"Does he/she negotiate with rather than dictate to me?"

SOME EARLY TRAPS
THAT PROMOTE DISENGAGEMENT

The basic structure of a working relationship may be communicated quite quickly, even within the first few minutes of a consultation. How much is the client supposed to talk? Is it safe to divulge information and be vulnerable? How much will the counselor direct, guide, or follow? While the counselor is busy getting started, the client is often pondering whether to stay.

Perhaps the largest threat to active engaging as defined above is the communication of nonmutuality. Professional messages that imply, "I'm in charge here; I'll determine what we talk about and decide what you should do" promote client passivity and disengagement when precisely the opposite is needed if personal change is to occur. It is easy to get started in the wrong direction by falling into certain traps early in consultation. It happens with the best of intentions. Here are six such traps.

The Assessment Trap

The first contacts with a provider may not be representative of what is to follow, although this is not always apparent to clients. If "intake" is regarded as a prerequisite to rather than the beginning of treatment, clients may be alienated from the start. Many workers and agencies fall into the assessment trap, as though it were necessary to know a lot of information before being able to help. The structure of an assessment-intensive session is clear: the interviewer asks the questions and the client answers them. This quickly places the client in a passive and one-down role (Rogers, 1942). Furthermore, the usefulness of all this questioning is not necessarily apparent to the client, who already knows the information being conveyed. Rogers (1942) observed:

> The disadvantages of using tests at the outset of a series of therapeutic contacts are the same as the disadvantages of taking a complete case history. If the psychologist begins his work with a complete battery of tests, this fact carries with it the implication that he will provide the solutions to the client's problems. . . . Such "solutions" are not genuine and do not deeply help the individual. (p. 250)

In Chapter 11 we discuss how to integrate MI with an assessment.

Even if there is no preliminary information-gathering hurdle before treatment, it is still possible to fall into the assessment trap with the implicit assumption that "if I just ask enough questions, I will know what to tell the client to do." Asking questions can also be a response to anxiety—either in the counselor, who wants to be in control, or in the client, who is more comfortable with the safe predictability of this passive role. Indeed, counselor anxiety has been associated with less empathic responding, and may favor a structured question–answer format (Rubino, Barker, Roth, & Fearon, 2000). In this trap the counselor controls the session by asking questions, while the client merely responds with short answers. Here is an example.

INTERVIEWER: You're here to talk about your gambling, is that right?

CLIENT: Yes, I am.

INTERVIEWER: Do you think that you gamble too much?

CLIENT: Probably.

INTERVIEWER: What is your favorite game?

CLIENT: Blackjack.

INTERVIEWER: Do you usually drink when you gamble?

CLIENT: Yes, I do usually.

INTERVIEWER: Have you ever gone seriously into debt because of gambling?

CLIENT: Once or twice, yes.

INTERVIEWER: How far into debt?

CLIENT: Once I had to borrow eight thousand to pay off a debt.

INTERVIEWER: Are you married?

CLIENT: No, I'm divorced.

INTERVIEWER: How long ago were you divorced?

CLIENT: Two years ago.

It happens so easily, and there are several problems with this pattern. First, it teaches the person to give short, simple answers, rather than the kind of elaboration needed in MI. Second, it sets the expectation of an active expert and a passive patient. It affords little opportunity for people to explore their own motivation and to offer change talk. The client's part in this relationship is mostly limited to answering the interviewer's questions. During such an exchange, the client has virtually no chance to talk him- or herself into change. It also sets the stage for the next obstacle to a collaborative relationship, the expert trap.

The Expert Trap

Asking a run of questions not only communicates that "I'm in control here," but it also sets up an implicit expectation that once you have collected enough information you will have the answer. As mentioned in Chapter 3, this is sometimes manageable in acute care medicine. You go to your doctor with a sore throat, the doctor goes through a well-rehearsed decision tree of short-answer questions about symptoms, and in 5 minutes you have a prescription or at least advice on what you need to do. Both parties are set up for an uneven power relationship. An "information-in–answer-out" expert role does not work so well, however, when what is needed is personal change, and it sets the stage for both of you to be disappointed. A prescription to "just do this" is seldom effective in itself, and the provider's consequent frustration is that "I tell them and I tell them and I tell them, and *still* they don't change!" Part of MI is knowing that you *don't* have the answers for clients without their collaboration and expertise.

> An expert role does not work so well when what is needed is personal change.

The Premature Focus Trap

A third possible road to early disengagement is the premature focus trap. The basic problem here is focusing before engaging, trying to solve the problem before you have established a working collaboration and negotiated common goals. You want to talk about a particular problem, and the client is concerned about a different topic. This very situation has been one common reason for clinical interest in MI. Counselors often want to identify and home in on what they perceive to be the person's "real" problem. The client, on the other hand, may have more pressing concerns, and may not share the importance placed by the counselor on this "problem."

The trap here is to persist in trying to draw the person back to talk about your own conception of the problem without listening to the client's broader concerns. A struggle may ensue regarding what should be discussed. Indeed, in the person's mind, the counselor's concern may be a relatively small part of the picture, and it may not be clear whether and how this is related to the person's larger life issues. If the counselor presses too quickly to focus the discussion, discord results and the person may be put off, becoming defensive. The point is to avoid becoming engaged in a power struggle about the proper topic for early discussion. Starting with the person's own concerns rather than those of the counselor will ensure that this does not happen. Very often, exploring those things that *are* of concern to the person will lead back to the topic that is of concern to the counselor, particularly when the areas of concern are related. In any event, spending time listening to the person's concerns is useful both in understanding the person and in building rapport that is a basis for engagement and later exploration of other topics.

A women's substance abuse treatment program in New Mexico illustrates this situation. The professional staff found that women who came to the program generally had many more pressing concerns than their use of alcohol and other drugs. They often had health care issues, parenting and child care problems, needed housing, and were traumatized by current or past physical and sexual abuse. These women had much to talk about, and if a counselor tried to home in on substance use too early in treatment, the woman was likely to drop out. If, on the other hand, the counselor listened to and addressed the woman's immediate concerns, conversations invariably came around to the role of alcohol and other drugs in her life.

The point, then, is to avoid focusing prematurely on issues that interest you but are of less concern to the person. When encountering discord around premature focus, start where your clients' own concerns are, listen to their stories, and get a broader understanding of their life situation before coming back around to the topic (see Part III).

The Labeling Trap

The labeling trap is basically a specific form of the premature focus trap. You want to focus on a particular problem, and you call it (or the client) by a name. Counselors and clients can easily be ensnared by the issue of diagnostic labeling. Some believe that it is terribly important for a person to accept (even "admit") the clinician's diagnosis ("You have diabetes," "You're an alcoholic," "You're in denial," etc.). Because such labels often carry a stigma in the public mind, it is not surprising that people with reasonable self-esteem resist them. Even in the field of alcohol problems, where emphasis on labeling has been high (at least in the United States), there is little evidence for any benefit from pressuring people to accept a label like "alcoholic," and the Alcoholics Anonymous (AA) philosophy specifically recommends against such labeling of others.

Often there is an underlying dynamic in a labeling debate. It may be a power struggle in which the counselor seeks to assert control and expertise. Coming from family members the label may be a judgmental communication. For some people, even a seemingly harmless reference to "your problem with . . . " can elicit uncomfortable feelings of being cornered. The danger, of course, is that the labeling struggle evokes discord, which descends into side-taking and hinders progress.

We recommend, therefore, that you de-emphasize labeling in the course of MI. Problems can be fully explored without attaching labels that evoke unnecessary discord. If the issue of labeling never comes up it is not necessary to raise it. Often, however, a person will raise the issue, and how you respond can be quite important. We recommend a combination of reflection and reframing—two techniques we discuss later. Here is a brief example, again from the addiction field, where this issue is often most intense. The counselor here quickly sides with the person's concern, and then offers a reframe.

CLIENT: So are you implying that I'm an addict?

INTERVIEWER: No, I'm really not concerned that much about labels. But it sounds like you are, that it's a worry for you.

CLIENT: Well, I don't like being called an addict.

INTERVIEWER: When that happens, you want to explain that your situation really isn't that bad.

CLIENT: Right! I'm not saying that I don't have any problems.

INTERVIEWER: But you don't like being labeled as "having a problem." It sounds too harsh to you.

CLIENT: Yes, it does.

INTERVIEWER: That's pretty common, as you might imagine. Lots of people I talk to don't like being labeled. There's nothing strange about that. I don't like people labeling me, either.

CLIENT: I feel like I'm being put in a box.

INTERVIEWER: Right. So let me tell you how I see this, and then we'll move on. To me, it doesn't matter what we *call* a problem. We don't have to call it anything. If a label is an important issue for you, we can discuss it, but it's not particularly important to me. What really matters is to understand how your use of cocaine is harming you, and what, if anything, you want to do about it. That's what I care about: you.

We would add that we also see no strong reason to *discourage* people from embracing a label if they are so inclined. Members of AA, for example, often say that it was important for them to recognize and accept their identity as an alcoholic. There is little point in opposing such self-acceptance. The key is to avoid getting into unproductive debates and struggles over labels. When a diagnosis is required for administrative purposes, it is possible to discuss this with the client in a collaborative manner explaining the process and provisional purpose.

The Blaming Trap

Still another obstacle that can be encountered in the first session is a client's concern with and defensiveness about blaming. Whose *fault* is the problem? Who's to blame? If this issue is not dealt with properly, time and energy can be wasted on needless defensiveness. One obvious approach here is to render blame irrelevant within the counseling context. Usually this can be dealt with by reflecting and reframing the person's concerns. If this problem arises, for example, the person may be told: "It sounds like you're worried about who's to blame here. I should explain that counseling is not about deciding who is at fault. That's what judges do, but not good counselors. Counseling has a no-fault policy. I'm not interested in looking for who's to blame, but rather what's troubling you, and what you might be able to do about it."

Concerns about blame may also be averted by offering a brief structuring statement like this at the beginning of counseling. Once the person has a clear understanding of the purpose of counseling, worries about blaming may be allayed.

The Chat Trap

Finally, it is possible to fall into the trap of just chatting, of having insufficient direction to the conversation. Making "small talk" may seem like a friendly opener, and no doubt it can have an ice-breaking function sometimes. In some cultures, a certain amount of chatting is polite and expected before getting down to business. Although off-topic chat can feel comfortable, it's not likely to be very helpful beyond modest doses. In one treatment study, higher levels of in-session informal chat predicted *lower* levels of client motivation for change and retention (Bamatter et al., 2010). In the engaging process, primary attention is devoted to the client's concerns and goals. These in turn lead into the focusing process to be discussed in Part III.

WHAT PROMOTES ENGAGEMENT?

When you visit a new situation for the first time, what influences whether you will return? The new situation might be a health care provider, a club, a congregation, or a regular weekly meeting (e.g., AA, Boy Scouts, or a chess club). What helps you decide whether to return?

We suggest several factors that can influence engagement or disengagement:

1. *Desires or goals.* What did you want or hope for in going? What is it that you're looking for?
2. *Importance.* How important is what you're looking for? How much of a priority is it?
3. *Positivity.* Did you feel good about the experience? Did you feel welcomed, valued, and respected? Were you treated in a warm and friendly manner?
4. *Expectations.* What did you think would happen? How did the experience fit with what you expected? Did it live up to (or even exceed) your expectations?
5. *Hope.* Do you think that this situation helps people like you to get what you're seeking? Do you believe that it would help you?

In essence, you are comparing what you expected (or hoped for) with what you experienced. These five points in turn suggest five basic issues that a counselor or program should attend to with any first visit when engagement is a goal:

1. Why is the person coming to see you now? What does he or she want? Ask and listen.
2. What is your sense of how important the client's goal(s) may be?
3. Be welcoming. Offer a cup of coffee. Look for what you can genuinely appreciate and comment positively about, even something simple, and for other ways to help the client feel welcome.
4. How does the person think you might be able to help? Provide the client with some sense of what to expect.
5. Offer hope. Explain what you do and how it may help. Present a positive and honest picture of changes that others have made and of the efficacy of the services you can offer.

These common-sense factors that any competent businessperson would address so often get lost in the world of human services in the rush to collect assessment information, in efforts to appear objective and professional, and in busyness and routines.

Beyond these basics, the three chapters that follow address professional skills that are important not only in engaging, but in all four processes of MI. They are foundational skills needed by anyone who wishes to understand MI and practice it proficiently. When mastered, they help you to engage people more readily, find clarity of direction, evoke motivation, and facilitate the process of change.

KEY POINTS

✓ Engaging is the process of establishing a mutually trusting and respectful helping relationship.

✓ Beginning consultation with assessment can place the client in a passive role and compromise engagement.

✓ Expert-driven directing does not work well when what is needed is personal change.

✓ The premature focus trap involves trying to focus too early on a goal without sufficient engagement.

✓ Arguments about the appropriateness of a diagnostic label can be counterproductive.

✓ Informal chat is not likely to be very helpful beyond modest doses.

CHAPTER 5

Listening
Understanding the Person's Dilemma

It is astonishing how elements that seem insoluble become soluble
when someone listens, how confusions that seem irremediable
turn into relatively clear flowing streams when one is heard. I
have deeply appreciated the times that I have experienced this
sensitive, empathic, concentrated listening.
—CARL R. ROGERS

So when you are listening to somebody, completely, attentively,
then you are listening not only to the words, but also to the
feeling of what is being conveyed, to the whole of it, not part of it.
—JIDDU KRISHNAMURTI

Good listening is fundamental to MI. The particular skill of reflective listening is one to learn first because it is so basic to all four processes of MI.
It takes a fair amount of practice to become skillful in this way of listening
so that reflections come more naturally and easily. Once you reach that
point of comfort with reflective listening it becomes possible to use it in
guiding. It's a bit like first learning to use a hammer to drive nails—to get
the hang of putting the tool exactly where you want it and hitting nails on
the head—before you move on to the subtleties of using a mallet for sculpt-
ing.

The good news is that reflective listening is a wonderfully useful skill
in its own right. Called "accurate empathy" by Rogers (1965) and "active
listening" by his student Thomas Gordon (Gordon, 1970; Gordon &
Edwards, 1997), it is a cornerstone for client-centered counseling. It is also
a useful skill not only in professional work, but also in one's personal life
and relationships, and yet relatively few people master it. It is fundamental

to good communication. Once you learn reflective listening, you have an invaluable gift to give to those with whom you come into contact. Rogers himself successfully applied his client-centered approach to reach allegedly "unmotivated" patients (Gendlin, 1961).

Behind the discipline of good listening is a trust that it is useful for clients to explore their own experience and perceptions. Healing is not primarily a process of dispensing expertise. The opportunity to follow and reflect on one's own experience is valuable, and it often gets derailed in ordinary conversation. Good listening helps a person keep going, to continue considering and exploring what may be uncomfortable material. Accurate empathy is a very good skill to facilitate such self-exploration.

> Healing is not primarily a process of dispensing expertise.

THOMAS GORDON'S 12 ROADBLOCKS

In popular conception, listening may involve just keeping quiet (at least for a little while) and hearing what someone has to say. The crucial element in reflective listening, however, is what the interviewer says in response to what the speaker offers. That is why Thomas Gordon (1970) called it *active* listening.

In this regard, it helps first to consider what good listening is not. Gordon described 12 kinds of responses that people commonly give to each other, but that are not listening:

1. Ordering, directing, or commanding
2. Warning, cautioning, or threatening
3. Giving advice, making suggestions, or providing solutions
4. Persuading with logic, arguing, or lecturing
5. Telling people what they should do; moralizing
6. Disagreeing, judging, criticizing, or blaming
7. Agreeing, approving, or praising
8. Shaming, ridiculing, or labeling
9. Interpreting or analyzing
10. Reassuring, sympathizing, or consoling
11. Questioning or probing
12. Withdrawing, distracting, humoring, or changing the subject

Gordon called these responses "roadblocks" because they tend to get in the way of self-exploration and they are distractions from listening. They derail the person from staying on the same track of self-exploration. In order to keep moving in the same direction the person must deal with the roadblock, detour around it, and come back to the original line of thought. Roadblocks have the effect of stopping or diverting the person's line of exploration.

Roadblocks also tend to imply an uneven or "one-up" relationship. They are self-centered rather than client centered. The underlying message seems to be "Listen to me; I know best." Instead of continuing to explore the path, the person then has to deal with what the interviewer is throwing out. Consider this well-intentioned but unhelpful counselor talking with a person who feels two ways about an important decision. (The number of each corresponding roadblock from the list above is given in parentheses.)

> Roadblocks are self-centered rather than client centered.

CLIENT: I just don't know whether to leave him or not.

INTERVIEWER: You should do whatever you think is best. (#5)

CLIENT: But that's the point! I don't know what's best!

INTERVIEWER: Yes, you do, in your heart. (#6)

CLIENT: Well, I just feel trapped, stifled in our relationship.

INTERVIEWER: Have you thought about separating for a while to see how you feel? (#3)

CLIENT: But I love him, and it would hurt him so much if I left!

INTERVIEWER: Yet if you don't do it, you could be wasting your life. (#2)

CLIENT: But isn't that kind of selfish?

INTERVIEWER: It's just what you have to do to take care of yourself. (#4)

CLIENT: I just don't know how I could do it, how I'd manage.

INTERVIEWER: I'm sure you'll be fine. (#10)

This person has not been helped to explore ambivalence (see Chapter 17), but instead is prematurely pressed toward one resolution. The counselor in this situation has not really listened, has never given the person a chance to keep on talking and exploring. The client's time has been spent dodging roadblocks.

NONVERBAL LISTENING

We devote most of this chapter to how a counselor responds verbally to what clients say, but there is more to listening than words. Suppose you were to listen to someone intently for 5 minutes without saying a word. How would you let the person know that you are listening and understanding? Chances are that as a helper you take these nonverbal aspects of listening for granted and do them intuitively, but it's worth making a few observations about them before moving on to verbal reflection.

First there is undivided attention. Even if you believe you can listen well while doing something else at the same time, to do so communicates disinterest and disrespect. Shuffling through papers, checking the time, or excessive note-taking all draw you away from good listening and signal inattention. This includes electronic distractions, of course: no texting, checking messages, or playing games while listening. Even if you *can* do two things at once, don't when one of them is listening.

Undivided attention is particularly communicated by the eyes. A good listener normally keeps eye contact with the person who is speaking. For the speaker, in contrast, a normal pattern is to look at the listener periodically but also look away while talking. There are large cultural differences in this. In some cultures is it regarded as disrespectful for someone to make much eye contact while speaking to another person. Nevertheless, the listener's eyes should be readily available for contact, not looking around the room or absentmindedly past the speaker (which can communicate boredom or disrespect). You will know the norms within your own culture, but when working across cultures be sensitive to normative differences.

Comfort with eye contact is affected by spatial arrangement. There are cultural differences in how closely people stand when speaking to each other, but in general eye contact becomes less comfortable as physical proximity increases (except in intimate relationships). When seated it is a good idea for the speaker and listener not to be directly facing each other because this makes it awkward to break eye contact and bespeaks a confrontational (literally: face to face) exchange. Counselors normally angle chairs so that it is easy for the client both to make eye contact and to break it comfortably.

Clues about attention and understanding also come from facial expression. Some people think of a "poker face"—one that does not change in response to different content—as being objective or "professional." A poker face, however, does not offer much emotional support to the speaker and it invites projection, often in the form of imagining that the listener is judging or disapproving. It can cause the speaker to wonder and perhaps worry about what the listener is thinking. In normal conversation people often mirror each other's emotional expression. A verbal statement that bespeaks sadness would likely be reflected nonverbally in a good listener's facial expression. The same would be true with expressions of joy, fear, or surprise. To mirror the client's emotion signals listening, understanding, and joining. A good listener's facial expression would probably mirror the emotion in a speaker's words even if it were not shown on the speaker's own face. A common exception to this mirroring in helping conversations is client anger, which we recommend not reciprocating facially but instead responding with concern and calmness.

FORMING REFLECTIONS

Beyond silence and nonverbal expression, what else is there to good listening? If one avoids all 12 of Gordon's roadblocks described earlier, what is there left to say? We don't mean to imply that it is wrong to use these 12 responses. There is a time and a place for each of them, but reflective listening is something different from any of them.

The essence of a reflective listening response is that it makes a guess about what the person means. Before a person speaks, he or she has a certain meaning to communicate. The meaning is encoded into words, often imperfectly. People don't always say exactly what they mean. The listener has to hear the words accurately and then decode their meaning. Thus there are three steps along the way where communication can go wrong: encoding, hearing, and decoding (see Box 5.1). The reflective listener forms a reasonable guess as to what the original meaning was, and gives voice to this guess in the form of a statement. That closes the circle, as shown at the bottom of Box 5.1.

> The essence of a reflective listening response is that it makes a guess about what the person means.

Why respond with a statement rather than asking a question? After all, the listener is not sure whether the guess is correct. The reason for responding with a statement rather than asking a question is a practical one: a well-formed reflective statement is less likely than a question to evoke defensiveness and more likely to encourage continued exploration. In the dynamics of language, a question requires a response; it places a demand on the other

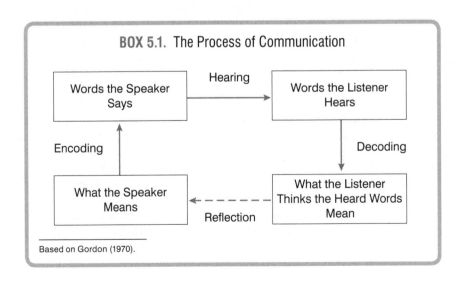

BOX 5.1. The Process of Communication

Based on Gordon (1970).

person. Consider the difference in sound between these pairs of counselor responses. (To hear the difference, you may need to speak them aloud because in speech it is voice inflection that makes them different):

"You're feeling uncomfortable?"
"You're feeling uncomfortable."

"You don't think this is a problem?"
"You don't think this is a problem."

"You're considering a divorce?"
"You're considering a divorce."

Between each of these pairs, can you hear the differing inflections and sense the difference in how someone might respond? In English the voice tone typically goes up at the end of a question, but gently down at the end of a statement. Reflective listening statements should usually turn down at the end. They are statements of understanding. The difference is subtle, and not everyone notices it, but it's real. (Once again, there can be cultural differences in what signals a question.)

But why not just ask people what they mean? Pressing people with questions to explain themselves and their meaning actually seems to distance them from what they are experiencing. They step back to analyze and begin to ask whether they really do or should feel what they have expressed.

In order to practice reflective listening, first train yourself to think reflectively. Keep in mind that what you believe or assume people mean is not necessarily what they really do mean (see Box 5.1). Most statements can have multiple meanings. Emotion words such as "depressed" or "anxious" can have very different meanings to different people. What could it mean for a person to say, "I wish I were more sociable"? Here are some possibilities:

"I feel lonely and I want to have more friends."
"I get very nervous when I have to talk to strangers."
"I should spend more time getting to know people."
"I would like to be popular."
"I can't think of anything to say when I'm with people."
"People don't invite me to their parties."

To think reflectively is to make the decoding process in Box 5.1 more conscious. When hearing any utterance one naturally considers and makes a guess about what it might mean. This decoding process happens quickly and often below consciousness. Many people then act as though this guess were the actual meaning and react to it. Reflective listening is a way of checking your guess rather than assuming that you already understand.

Reflective listening, then, involves responding to the speaker with a statement that is not a roadblock, but rather is one's guess about what the person means. Often, but not always, the subject of the sentence is the pronoun *you*.

Here is an exemplary segment from a counseling session with a man who had had open heart surgery (coronary artery bypass) 3 months prior. The "interviewer" in this case could be most anyone: a nurse, physician, friend, pastor, or physical therapist. For illustrative purposes, every interviewer sentence in this segment is a reflective listening statement. Notice also how the interviewer's reflections move forward rather than just repeating what the person has said. In essence, the interviewer is venturing what might be the next sentence in the person's paragraph instead of merely echoing the last one. This is a skillful form of reflection that we call *continuing the paragraph*.

INTERVIEWER: How have you been feeling lately, since your surgery?

CLIENT: It was quite an ordeal, I can tell you. I'm lucky to be here.

INTERVIEWER: You could easily have died.

CLIENT: They said there was 90% blockage, and at my age that kind of surgery is major, but I made it through.

INTERVIEWER: And you're glad.

CLIENT: Yes, I have plenty to live for.

INTERVIEWER: I know your family is important to you.

CLIENT: I love seeing the grandkids—two boys and two girls, you know, right here in town. I like doing things with them.

INTERVIEWER: You really love them.

CLIENT: I do. And I enjoy singing with the community chorus. They count on me; they're short of tenors. I have a lot of friends there.

INTERVIEWER: You have a lot of reasons to stay healthy.

CLIENT: At least I'm trying. I'm not sure how much to do.

INTERVIEWER: How much activity.

CLIENT: I don't want to overdo it. I played golf last week and I got this pain in my shoulder. The doctor said it was just muscle pain, but it scared me.

INTERVIEWER: You don't want to have another heart attack.

CLIENT: No! One was enough.

INTERVIEWER: And sometimes you wonder how much exercise is good for you.

CLIENT: Well, I know I need to stay active. "Use it or lose it," they say. I want to get my strength back, and they say regular exercise is good for your brain, too.

INTERVIEWER: So that's a puzzle for you—how to be active enough to get your strength back and be healthy, but not so much that would put you in danger of another heart attack.

CLIENT: I think I'm probably being too careful. My last test results were good. It just scares me when I feel pain like that.

INTERVIEWER: It reminds you of your heart attack.

CLIENT: That doesn't make much sense, does it—staying away from activity so I won't have another one?

INTERVIEWER: Like staying away from people so you won't be lonely.

CLIENT: Right. I guess I just need to do it, figure out how to gradually do more so I can stick around for a while.

Notice that the interviewer does not insert any roadblocks throughout this process. It would have been easy enough to substitute some of the roadblocks for these reflections. This is avoided, however, because the purpose is to help the person keep on exploring his own experience and wisdom. Reflective listening involves a certain trust that people are experts on themselves, want to be healthy, and can reach their own conclusions.

Notice also that the skillful dialogue above could plausibly be a client monologue if the pronouns are changed in the counselor's lines:

"The surgery was quite an ordeal, I can tell you. I'm lucky to be here. I could easily have died. They said there was 90% blockage, and at my age that kind of surgery is major, but I made it through and I'm glad. I have plenty to live for. My family is important to me. I love seeing the grandkids—two boys and two girls right here in town. I like doing things with them. I do really love them. And I enjoy singing with the community chorus. They count on me; they're short of tenors. I have a lot of friends there. I have a lot of reasons to stay healthy. At least I'm trying. I'm not sure how much to do, how much activity. I don't want to overdo it. I played golf last week and I got this pain in my shoulder. The doctor said it was just muscle pain, but it scared me. I don't want to have another heart attack. One was enough, and sometimes I wonder how much exercise is good for me. I know I need to stay active. "Use it or lose it," they say. I want to get my strength back, and they say regular exercise is good for your brain, too. So that's a puzzle for me—how to be active enough to get my strength back and be healthy, but not too much that would put me in danger of another heart attack. I think I'm probably being too careful. My last test results were good.

It just scares me when I feel pain like that. It reminds me of my heart attack. That doesn't make much sense, does it—staying away from activity so I won't have another one? It's like staying away from people so you won't be lonely. I guess I just need to do it, figure out how to gradually do more so I can stick around for a while."

That kind of natural flow doesn't happen if the counselor is throwing up roadblocks. Reflective listening focuses on the person's *own* narrative rather than asserting your own understanding of it.

What happens if the counselor guesses wrong and the reflection is not what the speaker intended? Typically, the client simply keeps going,

---

BOX 5.2. Listening Saves Time

The psychiatrist apologized for arriving late at the ongoing afternoon workshop on motivational interviewing. "I'm sorry for being late. I saw 20 patients this morning."

The trainer paused to welcome the newcomer and asked, "Are you able to use MI in your work with such a busy schedule?"

"Do you think that I could actually see 20 patients if I *didn't* use MI?" the psychiatrist replied.

*   *   *

"I don't have *time* to do this," busy practitioners sometimes say about reflective listening in particular and MI in general. "I already have too much to do in the time that I have with patients, and if I open up this door of listening, I'll never get anything done! I just need to tell them and move on."

Yet a few well-chosen words can save many mouthfuls of busy talk, none more so than in the use of a reflective listening statement that captures the essence of what the person is feeling and saying. When you hit the nail on the head with an accurate reflection the person feels understood and there may be little need to explore further. People also tend to repeat themselves when they sense (correctly or not) that they are not being heard, and a good reflection can save time.

Just "telling" people what they need to know or do can feel like having done one's job, and there surely are times when conveying facts is efficient. This is particularly so when the person needs and wants information. When what is needed is behavior change, however, telling and warning often don't help. If you only have a few minutes to talk and your hope is for behavior change, you don't have time *not* to use MI!

clarifying what was meant. There is no penalty for guessing wrong when you reflect. Asking questions is not necessary, nor is it even the best path to understanding. Neither is it necessary to tack words on to preface a reflection, such as "What I hear you saying is that you . . . " *Of course* it's what you heard!

It's possible to turn almost any question into a reflective statement. When you're first practicing, one way to form a reflection is first to *think* the question, "Do you mean that you . . . ?" Then remove the question words at the front ("Do you mean that") and inflect your voice downward at the end to make a statement. Consider a patient who tells the doctor, "I'm getting really discouraged about controlling my diabetes." Here's what might flash through the doctor's mind within a few seconds.

> ["I'm sure you'll do fine." No—that's not listening. I want to make suggestions, but that's my righting reflex and I need to understand. What's discouraging her? "Do you mean that you've been trying hard but your sugar levels are still high?" Now make it a reflection.] (Aloud: "You've been trying hard but your sugar levels are still high.")

That seems like a lot of mental effort for one reflection, and it is. Reflective listening can be hard work at first, more difficult than asking questions. The good news is that, like most skills, it gets easier with practice.

Depth of Reflection

Reflective listening statements can be quite simple. Sometimes the mere repetition of a word or two will keep the person moving. (In the dialogue above, the first reflection could have been "You're lucky.") *Simple* reflections add little or nothing to what the person said. They basically repeat or slightly rephrase the person's content:

CLIENT: I'm feeling pretty depressed today.

> SIMPLE REFLECTIONS:
>   You're feeling depressed.
>   You're feeling kind of down.
>   Pretty depressed . . .

Simple reflections can be useful, but they tend to yield slower progress. If it seems like you're not getting anywhere or just going around in circles, chances are you're relying too much on simple reflections—sticking too close to exactly what the person said.

A *complex* reflection adds some meaning or emphasis to what the person has said, making a guess about the unspoken content or what might come next (continuing the paragraph). An example of inferring meaning in the dialogue above is:

CLIENT: I think I'm probably being too careful. My last test results were good. It just scares me when I feel pain like that.

INTERVIEWER: (*making a guess*) It reminds you of your heart attack.

The client didn't actually say that the pain scares him because it reminds him of his heart attack, but that is a reasonable guess, given what he has said thus far.

Think of an iceberg. A simple reflection is limited to what shows above the water, the content that has actually been expressed, whereas a complex reflection makes a guess about what lies beneath the surface.[1] Sometimes it helps to reflect how the person seems to be *feeling* as he or she speaks.

CLIENT: They said there was 90% blockage, and at my age that kind of surgery is major, but I made it through.

INTERVIEWER: And you're glad.

CLIENT: Yes, I have plenty to live for.

Making a bit of a guess and continuing the paragraph often adds momentum to the exploration process. This is easier, of course, once you have some context and experience with the client.

CLIENT: I'm feeling pretty depressed today.

COMPLEX REFLECTIONS:
Something has happened since we last talked.
Your mood has been up and down in the past few weeks.
You look like you don't have much energy.

More complex reflections tend to move the conversation forward. Making guesses like this in the form of reflective statements can feel uncomfortable at first, but it usually does facilitate communication and understanding. It is important, of course, not to jump *too* far in guessing what the person means. This is a judgment call, and if your guess is too far off you'll see it in the client's response.

Learning Reflective Listening

Although reflective listening can seem challenging at first, it is a learnable skill. What you need in order to learn any complex skill is feedback,

---

[1]Thanks to Marilyn Herie for suggesting this metaphor.

preferably immediate feedback as to whether you are doing it right. When you stand on the driving range of a golf course you can see where each ball goes and adjust your swing and stance accordingly to get the best results—unless, that is, you're golfing in pitch-black darkness, in which case you get little or no feedback and are unlikely to improve your drives much. In reflective listening, you are practicing in daylight. Every time you offer someone a reflection you get immediate feedback as to how accurate it was. As on the practice range, there is no penalty for missing because when you guess wrong, the person simply tells you more about what she or he actually meant! Over the course of years, you'll get thousands of swings and can get pretty good at guessing what people mean from their words, voice tone, context, and nonverbal cues.

Depth of reflection increases with practice. Skillful reflection moves past what the person has already said, but doesn't jump too far ahead. The skill is not unlike the timing of interpretations in psychodynamic psychotherapy. If the person you're listening to balks, you know you have jumped too far too fast.

Overshooting and Undershooting

When using reflection to encourage continued personal exploration, which is the broad goal of reflective listening, it is often useful to understate slightly what the person has offered. This is particularly so when emotional content is involved. There is a rich array of language for describing emotion. Within any particular emotion, such as anger, there are descriptors that vary widely in intensity. There are low-intensity anger words like *annoyed* and *irritated* and high-intensity terms such as *outraged* and *furious*. Intensity can be diminished by adding modifiers like *a little*, *a bit*, or *somewhat*, or increased by adding *quite*, *very*, or *extremely*. As a general principle, if you overstate the intensity of an expressed emotion, the person will tend to deny and minimize it, backing off from the original statement. (This principle is applied strategically in Chapter 15 in the method of amplified reflection for responding to sustain talk and discord.) On the other hand, if you slightly understate the expressed intensity of emotion, the person is more likely to continue exploring and telling you about it. When reflecting emotion, err on the side of undershooting if you want the person to continue exploring it:

Overshooting

CLIENT: I just don't like the way she comments on how I raise my children.

INTERVIEWER: You're really furious with your mother.

CLIENT: Well no, not that angry, really. She's my mother, after all.

Undershooting

CLIENT: I just don't like the way she comments on how I raise my children.

INTERVIEWER: You're a bit annoyed with your mother.

CLIENT: I'll say! It just irritates me how she is always correcting and criticizing me.

Length of Reflection

As a general rule, a reflection should not be longer than the statement it follows. There are exceptions, but briefer is usually better. A reflection doesn't have to be a paragraph elaborating levels and shades of possible meaning. Just make one guess and keep it simple.

If a reflection grows long, remember that the person is most likely to respond to what you said last. Clients, too, continue the paragraph. If you must give a long reflection and you want to put emphasis on particular content and invite comment on it, put it last.

Direction in Reflection

Reflection is not a passive process. Even within 5 or 10 minutes of conversation, a person offers quite a variety of material. Consciously or not, you decide what to reflect and what to ignore, what to emphasize or de-emphasize, and what words to use in capturing meaning. Reflection can therefore be used to shine a light on certain aspects of what a person has said or to reframe its meaning slightly. Carl Rogers maintained that he was nondirective in counseling, but his student Charles Truax (1966) coded audiotapes of Rogers's sessions and found that he was differentially "reinforcing" certain kinds of client statements while letting others pass without reflection or comment. It is truly difficult to respond unconditionally to whatever clients say. It is easy, though, to be unaware of how one is influencing direction.

In the engaging process the primary purpose of reflective listening is to understand the client's dilemma, to see the situation through the client's own perspective. There is no particular direction involved. In the evoking process of MI, however, reflection and other fundamental counseling skills are used strategically to accelerate change (see Part IV). Consciousness of the directional aspect in reflection is a characteristic of MI. Conversely, there are clinical situations in which it is appropriate to avoid even inadvertently influencing a client to choose one direction or another. That scenario of counseling with neutrality can be quite challenging, and is addressed in Chapter 17.

Reflections in Engaging

Reflective listening statements should constitute a substantial proportion of your responses during the engaging process. Reflection is particularly important following open-ended questions. Once you have asked an open question, respond to the person's answers with reflection. These reflections during engagement are designed to clarify your understanding and convey this understanding to the client. You don't need to be clever and complex, just interested and curious. An uncluttered mind helps.

Because questioning is a less demanding skill (for the counselor) than empathic listening it is easy to fall into the question–answer trap, asking a series of questions instead of following and reflecting the person's statements. This pattern may actually evoke defensiveness. Remember, therefore, to follow up a question with reflective listening rather than another question. Counselors skillful in MI offer two to three reflections on average per question asked, and about half of all their responses (not counting the short "uh-huh" type of utterance) are reflections. In coding ordinary counseling sessions, in contrast, we find that questions often outnumber reflections by a ratio of 10 to 1, and reflections constitute a relatively small proportion of all responses. Although it can look easy when done well, reflective listening is actually quite an artful skill that you can continue to refine through decades of practice.

KEY POINTS

✓ The learnable skill of reflective listening ("accurate empathy") is fundamental in all four processes of MI.

✓ The essence of a reflective listening response is a statement that makes a guess as to what the person means.

✓ Reflections vary in depth from simple repetition to complex reflections and "continuing the paragraph."

✓ If it feels like you're going around in circles or getting nowhere, the reflections are probably too simple.

CHAPTER 6

Core Interviewing Skills
OARS

> The curious paradox is that when I accept myself
> just as I am, then I can change.
> —CARL R. ROGERS

> What people really need is a good listening to.
> —MARY LOU CASEY

Reflective listening, as discussed in Chapter 5, is one of the most fundamental skills to develop for client-centered counseling in general and for
MI in particular. In this chapter we address three other core communication skills that are important in engaging and throughout the processes of
MI. Together they form, in English, the mnemonic acronym OARS: asking
Open questions, Affirming, Reflecting, and Summarizing. In the engaging process these are foundational tools for mutual understanding. As we
move later into focusing, evoking, and planning, they become navigational
tools as well for guiding and propelling the course of change. The fifth
core skill mentioned in Chapter 3, informing and advising, is addressed in
Chapter 11.

ASKING OPEN QUESTIONS

An open question is one that invites a person to think a bit before responding and provides plenty of latitude for how to
answer. An open question is like an open
door. You do not know in advance where the
person will go with it.

> An open question is like an
> open door.

"What brings you here today?"
"How has this problem affected your day-to-day life?"
"How do you hope your life might be different 5 years from now?"
"Where do you think this path that you're on is leading you?"
"What would you say are the five things that you most value in life?"
"How do you hope I might be able to help you?"

A simple rhythm in MI is to ask an open question and then to reflect what the person says, perhaps two reflections per question, like a waltz.[1] Even with open questions, though, avoid asking several in a row, or you may set up the question–answer trap.

The opposite of an open question is, of course, a closed question, which typically calls for a short answer and limits the person's options for responding. Closed questions collect a specific bit of information:

"What is your address?"
"How long have you been feeling this way?"
"How many calls have you made?"
"Do you smoke?"
"Do you think you can do this?"
"Who lives with you?"
"When did you have your last drink?"
"Where did that happen?"

There are also closed questions that masquerade as open. One type is the multiple-choice question, which starts out as an open question but then reneges by restricting the options.

"So what are you hoping to do: quit or cut down?"
"What do you think would be the best approach for you: adjust your diet, exercise more, or try medication?"

Then there is the rhetorical question, where even the direction of the answer is prescribed:

"Don't you think it would be better for you to _____?"
"Isn't your family important to you?"
"You don't really expect that to work, do you?"

Chaining together a series of closed questions can be deadly for engagement. It gathers specific information at the cost of a collaborative relationship and

---

[1]Don't treat this like a rigid formula, that you *must* give two reflections after every question! The key is relying more on reflections than on questions.

asserts the expert role. We find that asking open questions often yields more information as well as important things we might have missed had we been going down a checklist. Whether or not time is short, try open questions.

Open questions invite conversation on a topic, focusing attention in a particular direction. The more questions you ask, the more you limit the client's exploration. The more reflections you offer, the more you invite the client to consider and explore. As a style that is both client-centered and directional, MI involves a blend of open questions and reflections.

Yet we hasten to add that closed questions can be quite consistent with an MI style. One might check after a summary—"Did I miss anything?"— or in the planning process—"So is that what you're going to do?" A closed question might pose a challenge: "Wouldn't it be great if there was a way to *want* to quit smoking?" (although this could also be a reflection: "It would be great if there was a way to *want* to quit smoking). Some closed questions are quite close to a reflection: "Does it feel like people are ganging up on you?" Selecting the optimal question type varies with the situation, provider role, and task at hand.

AFFIRMING

In addition to asking open questions and reflecting, a third core skill in MI is affirming: to accentuate the positive. To affirm is to recognize and acknowledge that which is good including the individual's inherent worth as a fellow human being. To affirm is also to support and encourage. Rogers (1967, p. 94) described positive regard as "a kind of love for the client as he is, providing we understand the word love as equivalent to the theologian's term *agape*, and not in its usual romantic and possessive meanings" (cf. C. S. Lewis, 1960; Miller, 2000).

Affirming overlaps in at least two ways with empathy (Linehan, 1997). First, the practice of empathy, of seeking to accurately understand the client's internal frame of reference as a separate individual, is inherently affirming. It communicates, "What you say matters, and I respect you. I want to understand what you think and feel." Second, affirming should be genuine; it should prize what actually is true about the person. In order to do that, you need to listen and understand. You cannot honestly affirm what you do not know and appreciate.

Affirming can serve several positive functions within helping relationships. It is a boon to engagement in that positivity is reciprocal. People are more likely to spend time with, trust, listen to, and be open with people who recognize and affirm their strengths. Affirmation may thus facilitate retention in treatment (Linehan et al., 2002). Affirming also can reduce defensiveness. When confronted with information that threatens their self-image, people are naturally inclined to self-affirm their autonomy and strengths, and doing so seems to diminish the threat to personal integrity (Steele, 1988). Relatedly, affirmation can increase openness to potentially threatening information (Klein & Harris, 2010; Sherman, Nelson, & Steele, 2000), particularly when the affirmation precedes defensive responding (Critcher, Dunning, & Armor, 2010). Affirming the possibilities in others may also directly facilitate change, just as demeaning stereotypes can impede it (Miller, 1985a, 2008).

Not all affirming needs to come from you, nor are you necessarily the most potent source of affirmation. You can ask clients to describe their own strengths, past successes, and good efforts, and such self-affirming has been shown to facilitate openness (Critcher et al., 2010). How readily people will express self-affirmation varies with generational and cultural differences as well as with mood states and contextual factors. Nevertheless, counselor affirmation can also yield surprising therapeutic benefits (Linehan et al., 2002).

So how does one go about affirming? First of all, the focus in affirming is on your client. Affirmation is not the same as praise. To praise is to raise a roadblock (Chapter 5), as it implies at least subtly that the praiser is in a one-up position as the arbiter of praise and blame. In general, avoid affirmations that begin with the word "I," because these focus more on you than on the client. "I am proud of you," for example, may be well intentioned and even well received, but clearly has parental overtones. Like good reflecting, good affirming usually centers on the word "you."

Affirmations comment on something that is good about the person. They involve noticing, recognizing, and acknowledging the positive. An affirming comment can be about something specific such as intentions and actions.

> "You really tried hard this week!"
> "Your intention was good even though it didn't turn out as you would like."
> "Look at this! You did a really good job of keeping records this week."
> "Thanks for coming in today, and even arriving early!"
> "So you made three calls about possible jobs this week. Good for you!"

It is also possible to affirm by reframing the client's actions or situation in a positive light. A classic example is a "glass half full" comment on progress when a client may be discouraged about imperfection:

> "You're feeling really bad that you didn't stick to your plan and instead drank on two days this week, and you're thinking that you blew it. What strikes me, though, is how different this is from where you started. Two months ago you were drinking every day of the week,

and 10 to 12 drinks a day. This week you had a drink one day and two the next, then went back to your plan. In other words, even this week your alcohol use was down by 96%, and you went right back to your goal of not drinking at all. How about that!"

Another way of affirming is to comment on what you perceive to be the person's positive traits or skills. These are framed (or reframed) as general personal attributes, of which more specific positive actions are examples:

"You got really discouraged this week and still you came back. You're persistent!"
"Listening to all you've been through, I'm not sure if I would have been able to come out of that as well as you have. You're a real survivor."

Affirmations may not even be so specific, but can reflect a broader (and genuine) prizing of the person:

"Welcome back! It's good to see you."
"You're amazing."

Living in the United States and the United Kingdom, we are well aware of how culturally relative affirmation is. What in one context will be received as warm appreciation may in another be seen as over-the-top hyperbole or even sarcasm. As with all of MI, the client is your guide. How does this person respond to what you said? If you see a facial reaction, you can reflect or ask about it. Also, affirming does not have to be deadly serious. It can be lighthearted, even teasing if you know the person well. The skill is to discover how best to convey to this person your genuine appreciating, prizing, and positive regard. As with other aspects of MI spirit, there is also an experiential component of affirming for the clinician, whose task is to find what is right rather than what is wrong with the person. This underlying mind-set is at least as important as the behavior of affirming itself.

SUMMARIZING

Summaries are essentially reflections that pull together several things that a person has told you. They can also be affirming because they imply, "I remember what you tell me and want to understand how it fits together." Summaries also help clients to hold and reflect on the various experiences they have expressed. They not only hear themselves describing their experiences, but they also hear you reflect what they have said in a way that encourages them to continue. Then they may hear their own material yet again as you pull it together in summaries.

It is a clinical judgment what to reflect out of all that a client offers and what to include in summaries. To reflect and summarize is to shine a light on the client's experience, inviting further exploration. In Part IV we describe a particular use of reflection and summaries to accelerate change. For now, suffice it to say that it is impossible to reflect and summarize everything that a client tells you. Consciously or not, you are choosing to highlight certain aspects of what people say and to pass over other aspects (Truax, 1966).

Summaries can serve several functions. A *collecting* summary recalls a series of interrelated items as they accumulate. Ask an open question like, "How might you like your life to be different a year from now?" and you are likely to begin accumulating a list. When you have heard two or three items, pull them together in a collecting summary:

> "So one thing you hope will be different a year from now is that you will have a good job, one that you enjoy and brings you in contact with people. You've been relating more positively to your children lately, and you would like that to continue. You also said you might like to quit smoking. What else, as you think of where you'd like your life to be a year from now?"

The "what else" is an invitation to keep adding to the list until the client signals being finished.

One way to combine a collecting summary and affirmation is to ask people about their strengths, the positive attributes that could help them to change.

> "One thing you know about yourself is that you're stubborn. Once you make up your mind to do something, you're pretty good about sticking with it. You said you're also someone who cares about your family. You want to protect them and certainly not hurt them. You're a friendly person, too, which I can see. You're easygoing and can get along with a wide range of people. What other strengths do you have?"

A second and related type is a *linking* summary. Here you reflect what the person has said and link it to something else you remember from prior conversation.

> "You felt really hurt and angry when he didn't bother to call you back— disrespected in a way. I remember you told me about another time when someone just ignored you and it really set you off."

"You're really pleased that you managed to exercise every day this week, and you even started feeling a kind of high from running. I wonder if that's like the way you felt that day when you hiked up to the mountain lake all by yourself."

A third type is the *transitional* summary, to wrap up a task or session by pulling together what seems important or announce a shift to something new. Again you are choosing what to highlight. A transitional summary often begins with an orienting statement that announces you're about to tie things together.

"Well, you remember I told you that I have some specific questions I would need to ask you before we finish today, but before I do that let me see if I understand what you're hoping we can help you with here. You need some emergency help with food and safe housing for you and your children. You also would like legal help in getting a restraining order. You already have a primary care doctor but you'd like to have your children see a dentist. Have I missed anything?"

How are summaries different from reflections? Their special quality is that summaries pull together a number of elements that the person has offered. To hear something immediately reflected back is helpful and invites continued exploring, but to hear a thoughtful pulling together of what one has been saying over a span of time can be more powerful still. A summary allows people to hear various aspects of their own experience *simultaneously*, to hear them juxtaposed in a fairly concise fashion. This might not occur in just thinking about one aspect at a time. There is a "whole picture" quality to a good summary, a putting together of what might seem to be separate pieces. All of the pieces come from the client, but their simultaneous combination in a summary offers something new.

Nowhere is this more evident than in a summary of ambivalence. The person may have been talking about various reasons for and advantages of making a change, while also expressing reluctance and reservations. An ambivalent person often goes back and forth between these poles in thinking or speaking about the dilemma. Reasons for change are salient when the person is voicing them, and this in turn is likely to trigger advantages of the status quo, which are also salient as they are spoken. Stop the process there and it will probably go no further. To offer a reflective summary of the ambivalence, however, adds something more.

"This friendship really evokes some strong feelings for you. On the one hand you're drawn to him. He's interesting. You've never quite known anyone like him, and he's had experiences that are way outside anything that has ever happened to you. You also feel a kind of bond with him. He seems to understand you in uncanny ways. At the same time his perspective sometimes borders on the bizarre, and his insights can creep you out occasionally. He seems needy and lonely, and while that makes your friendship important to him, you also can feel drained by him. You're drawn toward him and drawn away from him simultaneously. Both things are true, and it leaves you feeling confused about this relationship."

Each of the strands in this summary may have been reflected and explored individually as the person spoke them, but in this summary something else happens. The strands are woven together into a fabric, a single piece that contains all their colors. Offered such a summary, a person can really "get" how he or she is stuck, see the whole picture of the forest in a way that wasn't clear from examining one tree at a time. This balanced summary of ambivalence is one useful tool in counseling with neutrality (Chapter 17). We also consider later how an MI summary used in the evoking process can help people move out of the forest in a particular direction (Chapter 14).

ENGAGING: A CLINICAL EXAMPLE

Here is a sample dialogue between a counselor at a community mental health center and Julia,[2] a woman arriving for an initial visit. The interviewer's primary objectives at this point in the conversation are to establish rapport and understand what help Julia is seeking. There is no other direction to this interview; it is an example of person-centered counseling using OARS in the engaging process. No change goal is being addressed because none has yet been identified. This same case example is continued in seven later chapters to illustrate other processes within MI.

INTERVIEWER: Hello, Julia. Thank you for coming in a little early and completing the paperwork our receptionist gave you. [Affirming] I've looked it over, and I'll have some other questions to ask you later, but right now I just want to start fresh and understand what brings you here today. What's happening, and how do you hope we might be able to help? [Open question]

CLIENT: I don't know exactly what you do here, but I feel like I'm falling apart. I don't have any energy. I don't know what's going on with me. Maybe I need some pills.

---

[2] The story of Julia is based on an actual client whom we treated, but the names and all identifying details have been altered to protect her anonymity. The full assembled transcript is available at *www.guilford.com/p/miller2*.

INTERVIEWER: You're feeling upset and confused, and maybe a little surprised, too. [Reflection]

CLIENT: Surprised . . . well, yes. I never thought I'd be acting this way.

INTERVIEWER: One confusing thing, then, is you don't understand why you're doing what you're doing. [Reflection] What's been happening? [Open question]

CLIENT: I just broke up with my boyfriend. I mean we've been living together and I thought he loved me, but he's just so distant. He won't talk to me, and I think maybe he's seeing someone else. Anyhow, he told me I'm crazy.

INTERVIEWER: What you did surprised him, too. [Reflection, making a guess]

CLIENT: I just lost it. I started screaming at him, throwing things at him.

INTERVIEWER: What were you throwing? [Closed question]

CLIENT: Glasses . . . things from the sink. A coffee pot.

INTERVIEWER: You really wanted to hurt him.

CLIENT: I don't know. I just lost it. I don't usually act like that. It's embarrassing even to tell you about it.

INTERVIEWER: You're being really honest! [Affirming] So nothing like that has happened to you before. [Reflection]

CLIENT: Well, it has, actually. That's one reason I decided to come here. Maybe he's right. Maybe I am crazy.

INTERVIEWER: This blowup wasn't the first time that's happened to you. [Reflection]

CLIENT: Men just drive me crazy. This is the third guy I've lived with, and they all kind of ended in the same way. I just seem to fall in love with the wrong guys.

INTERVIEWER: Kind of like a pattern that's repeating itself. [Reflection]

CLIENT: Yes! It's so . . . (*Stops, cries a bit.*) I'm sorry.

INTERVIEWER: These are really strong feelings. It's pretty painful that this has happened once again. [Reflection]

CLIENT: I can't sleep. I can't think. I'm a mess at work. I was waiting on a customer this week and just started crying for no reason. I think I'm losing it.

INTERVIEWER: That frightens you, not understanding what's going on with you. [Reflection]

CLIENT: It's just so discouraging! I was so happy with Ray when we were first together. There's this soft teddy bear inside his tough exterior and that's the man I loved, but then he wouldn't open up to me anymore.

INTERVIEWER: And that annoyed you. [Reflection; continuing the paragraph]

CLIENT: Yes! It's such a waste for him to stay locked up inside there, and I was lonely even though we were living together. Anyhow, he's gone now. He moved out. It's over.

INTERVIEWER: All right. What you've told me so far is that these really strong feelings, and how you've reacted, are scaring you a little. [Understated reflection; starting a collecting summary]

CLIENT: (*interrupting*) A lot, actually.

INTERVIEWER: Scaring you a lot. You're not sure what's going on, and you've wondered whether medication might help. You're having trouble sleeping and with concentrating at work. You really blew up at Ray and felt out of control, and you're also wondering about what seems like a painful pattern that repeats itself in your relationships with men. [Collecting summary] What else? [Open question]

CLIENT: That's most of it, I guess. I just feel like I'm on the edge of losing it. After Ray left, I hated myself and I cut myself. (Pulls up a sleeve to reveal two long cuts running up her arm.) I saw the broken glass on the floor, and I just picked up a piece . . .

INTERVIEWER: You were in that much pain. It seemed like the right thing to do at the time. [Reflection]

CLIENT: I don't know. It's like I wasn't even thinking. I never did that before. I wasn't trying to kill myself or anything.

INTERVIEWER: That was something new, so that's part of what scared you and brought you in today. [Reflection]

CLIENT: Right. Do you think I'm crazy?

INTERVIEWER: That's really worrying you. You keep mentioning that you don't know what's happening to you, and so that's something you hope we can help with—to understand what's going on and what to do about it. [Reflection] I appreciate that it took some courage for you to come here today and talk about this. [Affirming]

CLIENT: Thank you. I do feel a little better, just talking about it to somebody.

INTERVIEWER: Good! It often does help to talk things over. I can see there's a lot that's worrying you. [Continued in Chapter 9]

This engaging process, relying primarily on OARS skills, has already yielded a lot of information. It would be tempting at various points to stop and ask a series of fact-gathering questions. Some of that may be necessary later in the session for agency procedures, for example, to establish a provisional diagnosis that is required for records. There can also be things that you do need to know sooner rather than later, such as whether Julia is at risk for suicide. A primary purpose at the outset, however, is to engage the client, to begin a working relationship. A wealth of specific assessment information is of no use if the client doesn't return.

Engaging the client is a vital process in itself. Those of us who are professional helpers can easily jump right into problem solving, but there is an important role for listening and understanding from the beginning of consultation. Imagine the outcome of this conversation between a couple, one of whom has just returned from work to find the other frazzled at home:

> A wealth of assessment information is of no use if the client doesn't return.

PARTNER 1: You won't believe the day I've had! I had trouble getting the kids out the door on time and they missed the school bus, so I had to drive them. Then on the way back I saw that the car was low on fuel, so I stopped and there was such a line at the gas station—they had a lower price, I guess. I went for groceries for dinner tonight to make something both you and the kids would like, and when I got home I realized I forgot some things and I had to go back. Then the school called and said that Emily was feeling sick and I had to pick her up, but when she got home she seemed fine, and she's been pestering me all afternoon. There are all these bills to pay and I didn't even have time to figure them out.

PARTNER 2: Well, let me tell you how you could organize your time a little better so that you don't get so stressed.

What's called for here is not immediate problem solving, but listening and affirming. In order to help a client, first establish a mutually respectful working relationship. This need not require a long time, just an engaging process of listening to understand the person's dilemma. The OARS are key skills here, and will also prove useful later.

KEY POINTS

✓ OARS is an acronym for four of the core counseling skills in MI: asking Open questions, Affirming, Reflecting, and Summarizing.

✓ An open question invites a person to reflect before responding and provides plenty of latitude for how to answer, whereas a closed question constrains the range of possible replies and usually yields a short answer.

✓ To affirm is to recognize, support, and encourage the client's strengths and efforts.

✓ A *summary* pulls together information that the client has offered and can be *collecting, linking,* or *transitional.*

CHAPTER 7

Exploring Values and Goals

Alike and ever alike we are on all continents in need
of love, food, clothing, work, speech, worship, sleep,
games, dancing, fun. From tropics to arctics humanity
lives with these needs so alike, so inexorably alike.
                                                —CARL SANDBURG

All men are prepared to accomplish the incredible if their
ideals are threatened.
                                                —MAYA ANGELOU

No one is unmotivated. Motivation for change is a continual companion in life. At times it is as simple as finding the next meal or getting some sleep. When basic physical needs are satisfied, people pursue higher goals and values. Perhaps the most familiar catalog of these pursuits is Maslow's (1943) hierarchy of human needs. Most basic are physiological needs for air, food, water, and sleep. Next are fundamental security needs: shelter, health, safety, companions, employment, and property. When these basic needs are met, people seek love and belonging (friendship, intimacy, family, trust) and then esteem (respect, accomplishment, self-confidence). At the highest level in Maslow's pyramid is what he called self-actualization, the pursuit and realization of one's core values—becoming what one is meant to be. That mature *telos* (see Chapter 2) is not uniform, but unique for each person. Both Maslow and Rogers strongly emphasized discovering and actualizing this unique human potential, whatever it may be.

A key in appreciating another's internal frame of reference is to understand their core goals and values. What do they hope for and want? How do they understand their meaning and purpose in life? What do they stand for, live for, and aspire to? Such higher values may not be salient when more basic needs are unmet, yet understanding them is fundamental to knowing someone.

When you understand what people value you have a key to what motivates them. What are this person's longer-term goals? How does this individual hope his or her life will be different a year from now or in 5 years or 10 years? Time horizons vary, of course. When basic needs are pressing, people may have difficulty thinking beyond today or tomorrow. Drug dependence has a way of foreshortening time perspective (Vuchinich & Heather, 2003). Yet exploring potential life goals also has a way of broadening perspective, lifting one's eyes to the farther horizon. We include this chapter here because taking some time to understand a client's own values and goals is another way to promote engagement, providing a solid foundation for a working therapeutic alliance.

Understanding a person's values also can play a key role in MI. An individual's broader life goals represent an important potential source of motivation for change. It is a common human experience for day-to-day behavior to fall short of or even contradict longer-term life values. Such value–behavior discrepancies become apparent precisely through reflection on life values, and perceiving such discrepancy can exert a powerful effect on behavior (Rokeach, 1973). Understanding values can be useful in the processes of focusing (What is most important?), evoking (What motivations does this person have for change?), and planning (What paths toward change would be most compatible with this person's values?).

In any such exploration of values it is important to convey acceptance and respect. This does not mean that you necessarily concur with or approve of the values being expressed; only that you accept that these are the client's stated values as you seek to understand what is important to her or him.

AN OPEN-ENDED VALUES INTERVIEW

One way to learn about a client's values and priorities is simply to ask about them. Here are a few examples of open questions of varying complexity:

> "Tell me what you care most about in life. What matters most to you?"
>
> "How do you hope your life will be different a few years from now?"
>
> "What would you say are the rules you live by? What do you try to live up to?"
>
> "Suppose I asked you to describe the goals that guide your life, the values you try to live by. What would you say are your five most important values, maybe just one word for each to begin with. What would they be?"

"If you were to write a 'mission statement' for your life, describing your goals or purpose in life, what would you write?"

"If I were to ask your closest friends to tell me what you live for, what matters most to you, what do you think they would say?"

Obviously the language used in such open questions should be appropriate to the person's level of cognitive complexity and abstraction. The purpose is to inquire about what larger goals or values people have internalized as guiding principles for their lives.

Having posed an open question like this, follow up with quality reflective listening. When people offer an adjective (*faithful*), noun (*provider*), or verb (*to care*), what do they mean by it? Rather than just asking, make a guess in the form of a reflection.

CLIENT: Well, one thing I want to be is loving.

INTERVIEWER: To care for other people. [Reflection, continuing the paragraph]

CLIENT: I don't mean just having warm feelings. I mean *being* a loving person.

INTERVIEWER: To love in a way that makes a difference. [Reflection]

CLIENT: Yes. I want to make a difference.

INTERVIEWER: For the people you care for, who are close to you. [Reflection]

CLIENT: Not just for them, although I certainly try to be loving to my family and friends, too.

INTERVIEWER: But you mean something beyond your circle of friends. [Reflection]

CLIENT: Yes, to act in a loving way to people I don't even know; the checkout clerk at the market, children, a beggar in the street.

INTERVIEWER: You want to be kind to them, too, to strangers. [Reflection]

CLIENT: Kind—yes, that's a good word.

You can also intersperse open questions to help the person elaborate, exploring more about a value.

"How do you express [value] in your life?"

"In what ways is [value] important to you?"

"Give me some examples of how you might be [value]."

"Why is [value] important to you? How did this come to be a value for you?"

Be conscientious about following up with reflections instead of just asking questions.

INTERVIEWER: So why is it important for you to be loving, even to people you don't know? How did that get to be a value for you? [Open question]

CLIENT: I've been so fortunate myself. I mean, I've had people who have really reached out to me and loved me and made a difference at crucial times in my life. It's so important to do that. Sometimes you don't even know how important what you did was.

INTERVIEWER: It's like passing on what others have given to you. [Complex reflection]

CLIENT: "Pay it forward" some people say, rather than paying it back. Make a deposit—add a little kindness to the world without expecting anything back.

INTERVIEWER: That's really important to you—something you want to do with your life. [Complex reflection]

CLIENT: Yes. There's so much unkindness. That's all you see in the news.

INTERVIEWER: Inhumanity. [Simple reflection]

CLIENT: Right. But there's a lot of kindness out there too, and that's what I want to add to.

INTERVIEWER: Give me some examples of times when you have done that. . . . [Open question]

The net effect of this sequence for engagement—of identifying, then asking more about, then reflecting and exploring values—is manifold. First it yields a deeper, more human, and multidimensional understanding of your clients and their motivations. Second, it promotes engagement and rapport. Third, the voicing of positive values is a form of self-affirmation, as discussed in Chapter 6, with therapeutic benefits of its own. Finally, understanding a person's core values may provide background later for developing discrepancy in the evoking process (see Part IV), if there is a genuine discrepancy between the status quo and the person's own values.

STRUCTURED VALUES EXPLORATION

There are also more structured approaches for exploring values. One common method for doing so is rooted in the Q technique that was originally developed by William Stephenson (1953), a colleague of Carl Rogers at the University of Chicago. Rogers (1954) quickly perceived the usefulness of Q sorting as a tool for understanding personality and adapted it within his client-centered counseling method. A typical approach involves a set of cards, each of which describes a personality characteristic such as "conscientious" or "shy." The cards are shuffled and then the person sorts them into five to nine piles ranging from "very unlike me" to "very much like me." In Rogers's approach the cards were then reshuffled, and the person sorted them again, this time according to how he or she would *like* to be— the "ideal self." The degree of discrepancy between "real" and "ideal" perceptions of self was a measure of interest to Rogers. In his theory of personality, psychological health is reflected in a close correspondence between real and ideal self-perceptions, and a decrease in this discrepancy would be an expected positive outcome of client-centered counseling. Reduced discrepancy can be accomplished, of course, by changing one's actual self, ideals, or both.

Similar methods have been used to study human values. Following on the work of Allport (1961), Milton Rokeach (1973) conceptualized values as beliefs that guide behavior prescriptively or proscriptively. He developed a set of 36 values that could guide behavior, including 18 instrumental (e.g., "pleasure: an enjoyable, leisurely life") and 18 terminal values (e.g., "helpful: working for the welfare of others"). Within each set of 18, the person would rank order the values from lowest to highest priority. A Web search for "values assessment" yields many such sets of values that can be

---

BOX 7.1. Personal Reflection: Her Heart's Desires

In 2007 I was asked to help with the further integration of motivational interviewing into a service for vulnerable pregnant teens run by home visiting nurses, what the U.K. director Kate Billingham called "the intensive care end of prevention." The scale was ambitious. I went to meet the founder of the Nurse Family Partnership Project, Dr. David Olds, who described the potential thus: "Motivational interviewing is a powerful ingredient in the fuel that drives good practice." The easy fit between our work and theirs lay in a number of well-developed practical exercises for exploring teens' values, with a rallying cry among nurses to seek out "her heart's desires." This provided a foundation for approaching sensitive issues such as how these desires relate to alcohol and drug use, promiscuity, unstable accommodation, smoking, or abusive relationships (see *www.familynursepartnership.org*). My training and mentoring role has continued for 4 years, and I am truly moved each time I return to this project. The stories I hear sing of the power of using engagement, values exploration, and MI to celebrate change and the courage of young mothers to make a new start.

—SR

prioritized, used particularly in career and vocational counseling. Box 7.2 provides such a set of 100 items that can be used in values exploration. Paralleling the Q technique, we have printed the values shown in Box 7.2 onto 100 cards, one for each value.[1] For any such a priori set of values, of course, there are reasonable questions about the extent to which it is comprehensive (Braithwaite & Law, 1985) and culturally appropriate (Lee, 1991), and adaptations may be needed for particular applications or populations.

Although the process of sorting the cards into piles is often interesting in itself, the clinical value of this exercise is in the discussion that follows, the purpose of which is to understand what these values mean to the person. This can be done through a combination of open questions and reflective listening.

INTERVIEWER: I see the value that you have put on top is "Protect." How is that important to you? [Open question]

CLIENT: It's my job to protect my family, to provide for them.

INTERVIEWER: So it's a combination of protecting them and providing for them. [Simple reflection]

CLIENT: Yes. I think that's what a man should do.

INTERVIEWER: And it's one of the most important things in your life. What are some ways in which you protect your family? [Reflection and open question]

CLIENT: Well, I bring home a paycheck and put food on the table.

INTERVIEWER: That's something you feel really good about. [Complex reflection]

CLIENT: Yeah. I haven't always been so reliable, if you know what I mean. I'm getting my life together and want my family to be able to count on me.

INTERVIEWER: So you provide for your family by bringing home a paycheck. How else do you protect them? [Reflection and open question]

CLIENT: I make sure they're safe at home. Smoke alarms, good solid doors, and things like that.

INTERVIEWER: So they can be safe even when you're not there. [Complex reflection]

CLIENT: Right. I can't always be there, but I want them to feel safe, to know that I'm there for them.

---

[1] See *www.guilford.com/p/miller2.*

(text resumes on page 84)

BOX 7.2. A Values Card Sort

William R. Miller, Janet C'de Baca, Daniel B. Matthews, and Paula L. Wilbourne

These values are usually printed onto individual cards that people can sort into three to five piles. We have five header cards that read: "Most Important," "Very Important," "Important," "Somewhat Important," and "Not Important." It is wise to provide a few empty cards so people can add values of their own. These items are in the public domain and may be copied, adapted, or used without further permission. A downloadable version sized for printable business cards is available at *www.guilford.com/p/miller2*.

Sample instructions for sorting the cards:

> *These cards each contain words describing values that are important to some people. Sort them into these five different piles depending on how important each one is to you. Some may not be important to you at all, and you would put those in the "Not Important" pile. Others that are just "Somewhat Important" go into this second pile. Those that are "Important" go here in the middle, and this fourth pile is for those that are "Very Important." Finally, this pile is only for those values that are the "Most Important" to you. Go ahead and sort them now into these different piles based on how important each one is to you. When you're done, if there are any other values that are important to you that are not mentioned on these cards, you can use these blank cards to add them. Any questions?*

The starting order of the cards does not matter—simply shuffle them before beginning (except for blank cards). It is also possible to use fewer than five piles for sorting, such as "Not Important," "Important," and "Most Important."

A possible next step is to have the person pick out the 5 or 10 values that are most important and rank-order them from 1 (most important) to 5 or 10. There may already be this many cards or more in the "Most Important" pile, or it may be necessary to add some from the "Very Important" pile. Alternatively, it is possible to skip the first (sorting) step and just have people pick out and rank-order the 10 that seem most important. This could be done just from the list below, but having the values on cards allows people to move them around visually when sorting and rank-ordering.

1. ACCEPTANCE   to be accepted as I am
2. ACCURACY   to be correct in my opinions and beliefs
3. ACHIEVEMENT   to have important accomplishments
4. ADVENTURE   to have new and exciting experiences
5. ART   to appreciate or express myself in art

(cont.)

BOX 7.2. *(cont.)*

6.	ATTRACTIVENESS	to be physically attractive
7.	AUTHORITY	to be in charge of others
8.	AUTONOMY	to be self-determined and independent
9.	BEAUTY	to appreciate beauty around me
10.	BELONGING	to have a sense of belonging, being part of
11.	CARING	to take care of others
12.	CHALLENGE	to take on difficult tasks and problems
13.	COMFORT	to have a pleasant and comfortable life
14.	COMMITMENT	to make enduring, meaningful commitments
15.	COMPASSION	to feel and act on concern for others
16.	COMPLEXITY	to embrace the intricacies of life
17.	COMPROMISE	to be willing to give and take in reaching agreements
18.	CONTRIBUTION	to make a lasting contribution in the world
19.	COOPERATION	to work collaboratively with others
20.	COURAGE	to be brave and strong in the face of adversity
21.	COURTESY	to be considerate and polite toward others
22.	CREATIVITY	to create new things or ideas
23.	CURIOSITY	to seek out, experience, and learn new things
24.	DEPENDABILITY	to be reliable and trustworthy
25.	DILIGENCE	to be thorough and conscientious in whatever I do
26.	DUTY	to carry out my duties and obligations
27.	ECOLOGY	to live in harmony with the environment
28.	EXCITEMENT	to have a life full of thrills and stimulation
29.	FAITHFULNESS	to be loyal and true in relationships
30.	FAME	to be known and recognized
31.	FAMILY	to have a happy, loving family
32.	FITNESS	to be physically fit and strong
33.	FLEXIBILITY	to adjust to new circumstances easily
34.	FORGIVENESS	to be forgiving of others
35.	FREEDOM	to be free from undue restrictions and limitations
36.	FRIENDSHIP	to have close, supportive friends
37.	FUN	to play and have fun
38.	GENEROSITY	to give what I have to others

(cont.)

BOX 7.2. *(cont.)*

39.	GENUINENESS	to act in a manner that is true to who I am
40.	GOD'S WILL	to seek and obey the will of God
41.	GRATITUDE	to be thankful and appreciative
42.	GROWTH	to keep changing and growing
43.	HEALTH	to be physically well and healthy
44.	HONESTY	to be honest and truthful
45.	HOPE	to maintain a positive and optimistic outlook
46.	HUMILITY	to be modest and unassuming
47.	HUMOR	to see the humorous side of myself and the world
48.	IMAGINATION	to have dreams and see possibilities
49.	INDEPENDENCE	to be free from depending on others
50.	INDUSTRY	to work hard and well at my life tasks
51.	INNER PEACE	to experience personal peace
52.	INTEGRITY	to live my daily life in a way that is consistent with my values
53.	INTELLIGENCE	to keep my mind sharp and active
54.	INTIMACY	to share my innermost experiences with others
55.	JUSTICE	to promote fair and equal treatment for all
56.	KNOWLEDGE	to learn and contribute valuable knowledge
57.	LEADERSHIP	to inspire and guide others
58.	LEISURE	to take time to relax and enjoy
59.	LOVED	to be loved by those close to me
60.	LOVING	to give love to others
61.	MASTERY	to be competent in my everyday activities
62.	MINDFULNESS	to live conscious and mindful of the present moment
63.	MODERATION	to avoid excesses and find a middle ground
64.	MONOGAMY	to have one close, loving relationship
65.	MUSIC	to enjoy or express myself in music
66.	NONCONFORMITY	to question and challenge authority and norms
67.	NOVELTY	to have a life full of change and variety
68.	NURTURANCE	to encourage and support others
69.	OPENNESS	to be open to new experiences, ideas, and options
70.	ORDER	to have a life that is well-ordered and organized

(cont.)

BOX 7.2. *(cont.)*

71.	PASSION	to have deep feelings about ideas, activities, or people
72.	PATRIOTISM	to love, serve, and protect my country
74.	POPULARITY	to be well liked by many people
75.	POWER	to have control over others
76.	PRACTICALITY	to focus on what is practical, prudent, and sensible
77.	PROTECT	to protect and keep safe those I love
78.	PROVIDE	to provide for and take care of my family
79.	PURPOSE	to have meaning and direction in my life
80.	RATIONALITY	to be guided by reason, logic, and evidence
81.	REALISM	to see and act realistically and practically
82.	RESPONSIBILITY	to make and carry out responsible decisions
83.	RISK	to take risks and chances
84.	ROMANCE	to have intense, exciting love in my life
85.	SAFETY	to be safe and secure
86.	SELF-ACCEPTANCE	to accept myself as I am
87.	SELF-CONTROL	to be disciplined in my own actions
88.	SELF-ESTEEM	to feel good about myself
89.	SELF-KNOWLEDGE	to have a deep and honest understanding of myself
90.	SERVICE	to be helpful and of service to others
91.	SEXUALITY	to have an active and satisfying sex life
92.	SIMPLICITY	to live life simply, with minimal needs
93.	SOLITUDE	to have time and space where I can be apart from others
94.	SPIRITUALITY	to grow and mature spiritually
95.	STABILITY	to have a life that stays fairly consistent
96.	TOLERANCE	to accept and respect those who differ from me
97.	TRADITION	to follow respected patterns of the past
98.	VIRTUE	to live a morally pure and excellent life
99.	WEALTH	to have plenty of money
100.	WORLD PEACE	to work to promote peace in the world

INTERVIEWER: You have a really strong sense of family. Why is that so important for you? [Complex reflection and open question]

CLIENT: Well, I didn't feel very safe when I was growing up, and I was pretty lonely. I was the only boy, and sometimes I had to protect my mom.

INTERVIEWER: And now that you're a man, you want your own children to know they're protected, and to stick together as a family. [Complex reflection]

CLIENT: If you have strong family, you have everything.

The complex reflections in this conversation also are examples of continuing the paragraph rather than just repeating or rephrasing what the person has said (see Chapter 5).

Exploring people's top 5 or 10 values in this manner is a good way to develop an understanding of what matters to and motivates them, and of the standards that they want to guide their actions. This exploration alone can cause people to reflect on discrepancies between what they value and how they are living their lives. Perceived value–behavior inconsistencies can in themselves trigger behavior change. When a behavior comes into conflict with a deeply held value, it is usually the behavior that changes (Rokeach, 1973). Consider the true story in Box 7.3. How might you explain what happened?

BOX 7.3. Becoming a Nonsmoker

When his children telephoned, the father jumped into his car and drove down to the city library to pick them up. By the time he arrived a thunderstorm had broken and it was pouring down rain. Waiting at the curb with the engine running he began searching for a cigarette—going through his pockets, checking under the seat and in the glove compartment. No cigarettes. He put the car in gear, and as he pulled away from the curb he glanced in his rear view mirror and saw his children coming out of the library into the rain. Nevertheless, he pushed the accelerator and pulled away to a store around the corner, convinced that he could park, rush in, buy the cigarettes, and get back before his children "got seriously wet." Staring past the windshield wipers, he said to himself, "I'm a father who would actually leave his children standing in the rain to chase after a drug!"

He never smoked again.

Based on Premack (1972).

INTEGRITY

Social psychologist Leon Festinger (Festinger, 1957) argued that people have a strong drive to be (or at least to appear to be) consistent, and will change attitudes or behavior to reduce apparent dissonance. Indeed, sales and marketing strategies often exploit this human desire to maintain personal consistency (Cialdini, 2007). Yet value–behavior inconsistency is a common human experience, as reflected in the language of conscience (one's value system) and guilt (a reaction to violating it). A letter from the first century C.E. bemoans the writer's infidelity to core values: "I do not do the good that I want, but the evil I do not want is what I do."[2] Both things are true: people want to be consistent with their core values and also tend to violate them. It is a common source of internal conflict.

To live with integrity is to behave in a manner that is consistent with and fulfills one's core values. Integrity is a goal or desire toward which one moves imperfectly, an intentional process of moving toward adherence to one's professed values. "This ability to look at the self with what Mowrer[3] referred to as a radical honesty with the self, really seeing who one is with all one's frailties, vulnerabilities, and unfulfilled potentialities, is the essence of integrity" (Lander & Nelson, 2005, p. 52).

> To live with integrity is to behave in a manner that is consistent with and fulfills one's core values.

How does one develop integrity? Clues are found in research on the social development of self-regulation (Diaz & Fruhauf, 1991; Diaz, Neal, & Amaya-Williams, 1990). Infants learn first to attend to and interact with people around them and discover that what they do influences others. As language develops they begin to understand instructions from others: "Come here." "Hot! Don't touch." A first step in developing self-control is learning to follow such instructions, to conform behavior to the demands of language when a caregiver is present. Gradually, these external rules are internalized, and the child verbalizes them first overtly and then covertly. A small child might, for example, approach a hot stove and say, "Hot, don't touch!," drawing back from it. As this occurs, the child becomes able to follow instructions even when a caregiver is not present. Yet this is still largely external regulation, following internalized instructions from others. The developmental jump to self-regulation, usually emerging within the

---

[2](Rom. 7:19; *New Revised Standard Version*, 1989).

[3]The reference is to the eminent learning theorist O. Hobart Mowrer, a president of the American Psychological Association, who in later life described an approach that he called "integrity therapy" (Mowrer, 1966; Mowrer, Vattano, & Others, 1974; Mowrer & Vattano, 1976).

first 6 years of life, comes with the ability to develop a plan of one's own and to implement behavior to carry it out. This capacity for self-regulation continues to emerge over the years, can be affected positively or adversely by biological and psychosocial factors in development (Brown, 1998), is strengthened by practice (Baumeister, 2005; Baumeister, Heatherton, & Tice, 1994), and is mediated by private speech (Diaz & Berk, 1992; Diaz, Winsler, Atencio, & Harbors, 1992).

Such private speech (self-talk) includes what we describe in Chapter 12 as change talk and sustain talk, one's own arguments for and against adherence to a plan or value. The relative balance of these verbalized pros and cons is one marker of a person's level of ambivalence and (conversely) readiness for change (Carey, Maisto, Carey, & Purnine, 2001) and predicts posttreatment outcome (Amrhein et al., 2003; Moyers et al., 2007). The pro–con balance is also clearly responsive to MI counseling skills (Glynn & Moyers, 2010; Moyers & Martin, 2006; Moyers, Miller, et al., 2005; Vader et al., 2010).

MI could be used to promote integrity, that is, to help people clarify their core values and consider how to live in greater consistency with them. This is nondirective in the sense that the goals are entirely the person's own from the outset. The counselor first elicits and clarifies the goals that the person chooses as guiding values. Then using client-centered OARS skills, she or he explores how these values are expressed in the person's life and what changes could yield greater consistency with these guiding values. Obstacles to and distractions from value consistency would also be considered.

The magnetism of integrity also operates within MI. As people hear themselves talk they learn what they believe. Evoking change talk creates momentum to retain integrity by acting in accord with verbal statements and commitments. The relationship is imperfect; people do not always do what they say, but the act of saying it is a step toward doing it.

EXPLORING DISCREPANCY

What is the best way to respond when you perceive a discrepancy between a person's stated goals or values and his or her actions? The righting reflex (as discussed in Chapter 1) would be to point it out, perhaps even to confront the person with it:

> "Don't you see how what you're doing is hurting your family?"
> "How can you say you're an honest person when you're so deceptive?"
> "If you keep on as you are, you're going to destroy your health."

Such a direct challenge, however, is likely to evoke self-defense rather than change. Our experience is that when people are invited to reflect on their values and actions within a safe, nonjudgmental atmosphere they are usually well aware of discrepancies. Such self-confrontation of discrepancies can be uncomfortable, of course, and the counselor's task is to help the person continue attending to and reflecting on them without reverting to defensiveness. The OARS tools described in the preceding chapters are excellent tools for doing this.

The potential impact of self-confrontation is illustrated in a classic series of studies by Rokeach (1973) conducted during the height of the U.S. Civil Rights movement with freshmen at three different colleges. Students participating in a study of an educational "method of active participation" identified and rank-ordered their values from a list of 18 options. This was done in a group setting, with each person having private access to his or her own answers.

Rokeach then described to the experimental group a finding from his prior research: that students on average tended to rank *freedom* as very important (#1) but had ranked *equality* as less important (#6), observing that students "in general are much more interested in their own freedom than they are in freedom for other people" (1973, p. 237). He invited them to reflect privately on how their own value rankings compared with those of students in general at the same university. He further described the finding that previous students' rankings had predicted their own attitude toward civil rights: Those who favored and participated in civil rights actions had ranked freedom and equality similarly, whereas students opposed to civil rights had given much higher priority to freedom for themselves than for other people. After some further measures, he dismissed the experimental group saying, "I asked each of you to think about yourself—about the things you value. One result of this may be a change in your conception of the world around you. But that is up to you . . . no teacher can tell students what to think or what to believe" (1973, p. 239). Those in the randomly assigned control group did the same rank-ordering but were not given any of this additional information, without drawing any attention to possible value discrepancies.

Although the experimental and control groups showed no attitudinal differences before the study began, they responded quite differently afterward on several measures. When they repeated the value ranking, the experimental participants significantly increased the ranking of equality at 3 weeks, and still more at 3 months and 15 months after the study, whereas control participants did not. More striking were behavioral changes. Letters were sent to all participants 3 to 5 months later, with no mentioned connection to the study, inviting them to join a civil rights organization (the National Association for the Advancement of Colored People [NAACP]), on NAACP letterhead signed by the organization's president. In three separate studies, students from the experimental group were more than twice as likely to request more information and to join. In one study, students' declared major subject was determined at 21 months. Students in the experimental group were twice as likely (28%) to have enrolled in an ethnic relations major as compared to control group participants (14%). At another college, students who changed their majors were more likely to change from natural sciences to social sciences or education if they had been in the experimental group (55%) rather than the control group (15%).

How could such a small intervention have such ripple effects even years later? These people were simply invited to reflect privately on the relative importance they had given to two items on a value-ranking task. Any confrontation that occurred was self-confrontation; there were no individual interactions. Students did not connect or attribute their long-term behavior change to the freshman-year study, yet the experimental intervention is the only apparent explanation for the group differences. This is not, of course, the only brief intervention to yield long-term behavior change (Bien, Miller, & Tonigan, 1993; Daeppen, Bertholet, & Gaume, 2010; Erickson, Gerstle, & Feldstein, 2005; Miller, 2000), but it is a good example of the potential impact of reflecting on one's values. In this case it did not occur in a therapeutic context, nor were the participants seeking change.

So what is confrontation? In etymology, to "confront" means to come face to face. In MI, the confrontation is not with someone else, but with oneself. Within a supportive and affirming context, without threat or judgment, people are invited to come face to face with themselves, to reflect on their own behaviors, attitudes, and values. They are invited to look in the mirror and let what they see change them. There is no need to "get in their face" to make it happen. In fact, such heavy-handed strategies are more likely to backfire and inspire defensiveness instead of change (White & Miller, 2007). An MI approach honors people's autonomy, trusting in their own natural wisdom and desire to grow in a positive direction.

> An MI approach honors people's autonomy, trusting in their own natural wisdom and desire to grow in a positive direction.

KEY POINTS

✓ A key in appreciating another's internal frame of reference is to understand his or her core goals and values.

✓ Self-actualization involves moving toward one's natural, ideal, mature state, or *telos*.

✓ A values interview explores the person's core goals: why they are important and how they are expressed.

✓ To live with integrity is to behave in a manner that is consistent with and fulfills one's core values.

✓ Discrepancy between current behavior and a core value can be a powerful motivator for change when explored in a safe and supportive atmosphere.

✓ Self-regulation is the capacity to formulate a plan of one's own and implement behavior to carry it out.

✓ To "confront" means to come face to face, and self-confrontation is usually more powerful than being confronted by someone else.

PART III

FOCUSING
The Strategic Direction

In order to be an effective guide you need to know where you're going. With at least the basic groundwork for engagement in place the next process in MI is to clarify the goal toward which you will move together. Focusing is a necessary prerequisite for the subsequent two processes in MI: evoking (Part IV) and planning (Part V).

Part III is about the focusing process in MI and how you use the core skills described in Parts I and II to find direction. MI is a goal-directed activity in which you help someone unravel whether, why, how, and when they might change. Without a focus MI can't get off the ground. Sometimes the focus is immediately clear, but if it becomes blurred there are constructive ways of finding direction for your conversation about change.

CHAPTER 8

Why Focus?

If you don't know where you are going, any
road will get you there.
—LEWIS CARROLL

I would not give a fig for the simplicity this
side of complexity, but I would give my life for
the simplicity on the other side of complexity.
—OLIVER WENDELL HOLMES

Engaging provides a good platform for the second process in MI: focusing. The two are interrelated, yet different processes. It is possible to be well engaged with someone, enjoying an energetic conversation, but without any clear direction. Consider this example of an opening to an interview:

INTERVIEWER: How do you think I might be of help?

CLIENT: Well, at work I get along OK with the job itself, but people have started to notice that I'm fussy about cleanliness no matter how hard I try to hide it. I go into the bathroom a lot, especially before and after lunch.

INTERVIEWER: It's a bit difficult for you sometimes.

CLIENT: Very difficult, actually. I have been calling in sick sometimes to take the pressure off, and now they're noticing that also, and I might lose this job if I'm not careful. I have a meeting next week with my supervisor to talk about it.

INTERVIEWER: Things are coming to a head at work.

CLIENT: I'm just not one of the group, not a mixer, and it seems like they are looking at me all the time, thinking I am weird.

INTERVIEWER: You feel out of place at work.

CLIENT: At home my parents tell me I must "stand on my own feet," as they say, and they also want me to go out more and get my own place to live, and now they are upset with me for taking time off work. My father isn't speaking to me at the moment.

INTERVIEWER: Both at work and at home, it's not easy for you right now.

CLIENT: And also I'm not sleeping well. My girlfriend is saying she's fed up with all of this drama, but I can't let this relationship go after that awful divorce.

What could or should the focus be here? This man could have arrived at the door of a mental health service, a primary care clinic, an employment service, or the office of a teacher or coach. He might be someone on parole following a conviction of some kind or be seeing a social worker connected to a custody issue with his children from an earlier marriage. He's fairly easy to engage with, but what does he want? What might you focus on? Does he have obsessive–compulsive disorder? Does he want a more formal leave of absence from work? In what part of his life might he make the most progress? Going around in circles and being unsure of a productive direction is a familiar experience. Tempting as it might be to blame the client for this, focusing is part of the helper's task. Feeling overwhelmed by life's demands is common. Focusing is the process of becoming clear about goals and direction in MI, providing the foundation for subsequent evoking and planning to help lift this burden.

FOCUSING IN MOTIVATIONAL INTERVIEWING

Most forms of treatment involve some means of identifying intended outcomes. Although goals may not be clear at the outset of consultation there is usually a process of assessment or formulation to arrive at them. Whatever the role of assessment may be (see Chapter 11), the focus in MI is formed through a purposeful conversation that has change at its heart.

Focusing in MI is actually an ongoing process of seeking and maintaining direction. In any helping relationship it's useful for at least one of you to have a clear sense of direction. Ideally, there is a shared sense of direction, just as a guide and traveler have an agreement about where they are going. The focusing process within MI is about finding that direction and within it more specific achievable goals. This naturally blends into evoking (Part IV) and planning (Part V) to explore specific ways for moving in that direction.

> Focusing in MI is an ongoing process of seeking and maintaining direction.

Sometimes the process of clarifying direction and goals seems straightforward. A man calls a problem gambling hotline and asks for help. A woman consults a family planning service requesting assistance in choosing a contraceptive. Even in seemingly simple situations, though, direction and goals can quickly become complicated. With further exploration one may encounter ambivalence, multiple problems, conflicting goals, and higher priorities. The counselor or service may have different goals from those of the client (a situation we address in more depth in Chapter 10). The focusing process involves navigating these often tricky waters to find and maintain a clear direction. It is also common to make course adjustments along the way, which is why focusing tends to be a continuing rather than one-time process. The well-matched alignment of your agenda for change with those of the client does not necessarily fall easily out of the first few minutes of a conversation; neither does it remain static. You might settle into one direction of movement, and then later the focus can shift, alignment is altered, and you have to adjust.

Agenda

We begin this consideration of focusing in MI with the concept of "agenda," by which we mean more than a list of change goals. A client's agenda may include hopes, fears, expectations, and concerns. Imagine parents referred by the court to receive treatment following a domestic violence incident. The court's goal, presumably, would be to prevent recurrence of domestic violence. A parent in this situation, however, may enter treatment with agenda that include:

- Embarrassment and need to preserve self-esteem
- Anger about invasion of privacy
- Expectation of being lectured, scolded, or shamed
- Fear of future violence
- Problems in the parents' relationship more generally
- Consideration of whether to stay in the relationship
- Reluctance to discuss alcohol or drug use in the home
- Concern about legal consequences and loss of freedom
- Desire to protect the children from adverse effects
- Fear of having children taken out of the home

All of this and more is present as the client walks through the door, and that is just one part of the picture. The other parent, the children, the clinician, and a probation officer may all have agenda of their own. It would be easy to drift unproductively among these agenda without a clear sense of direction. Finding and maintaining that direction is the clinician's task.

The challenge of how to understand and work with such agenda has been discussed in many fields including medicine, social work, counseling, and organizational development. In MI this is done through the process of focusing, using particular tasks and skills to harness the agenda specifically to promote change. Without such focus, even long discussions of change can be unproductive.

It is also clearly the case that differing agenda can conflict. A client's aspirations do not necessarily converge with those of the clinician or agency. We discuss ethical navigation of goals in Chapter 10.

Three Sources of Focus

With varying agenda present, there are different possible sources from which to derive focus and direction. We consider three potential sources here: the client, the setting, and the clinician.

The Client

The most common source of direction is from the client him- or herself. People come through the door with presenting problems and concerns.

"I would like to get in better physical shape to stay healthy as I age."
"I need to quit smoking."
"Help me get back custody of my children."
"I've been feeling really depressed."
"My blood sugar is running too high, and I want to adjust my diet."
"Our son struggles with math and we think some tutoring could help him."
"I want to get my driver's license back and get the probation officer off my back."

If the provider is comfortable and competent to provide the help requested then there is a natural match of guide and traveler. This does not mean that the journey is necessarily easy, only that there is a shared beginning agreement about direction.

The Setting

The direction of service can also be focused by the setting itself. The agency is funded to address specific issues and provide certain services. Some examples include:

- A smoking cessation clinic
- A suicide prevention hotline
- A mandated program for people convicted of driving while intoxicated

- An anger management program for domestic violence offenders
- A state employment service

People walking through the doors of such a program need not wonder what the topic of conversation will be. They may be eager to receive its services and are coming for that very purpose. It is also common, however, that people seek targeted services at someone else's behest:

"My wife says I need to quit smoking."
"The judge told me to I have to be here or go to jail."
"I need to go through this program to get my kids back."
"I don't really think you can help me, but my pastor said I should call you."

In a sense, the initial "client" in these situations may be the referring agent, who has agenda as well. The point here is that the focus of service can be predetermined or limited by the context.

Clinical Expertise

A third potential source of focus is the clinician. Quite commonly, people will seek services with one goal in mind, and in the course of consultation the clinician working with them perceives that another kind of change is needed. The client did not come to the clinician with this in mind (at least not in presenting concerns). So a challenge for the clinician is how to raise the subject and explore the client's willingness to entertain this additional goal or direction. It may be that this new potential change would help in achieving the client's stated goal. It may even be essential for doing so in the provider's opinion. A few examples:

- A mother brings a child to the pediatrician for treatment of asthma and yet another upper respiratory infection. The physician wants to talk about the parents' smoking as a contributing factor.
- An unemployed man seeks help in finding a job. The counselor perceives the client's appearance and hygiene to be significant obstacles to hiring.
- A woman has had numerous recurrences of cocaine use despite her strong stated desire to quit. The counselor believes that quitting drinking would help significantly because alcohol seems to precipitate her cocaine use.
- A nurse monitoring antiretroviral medications for a patient with AIDS wants to discuss nutrition and the disclosure of HIV status to sexual partners.

Clients may or may not perceive a relationship between their presenting concern and the counselor's preference for focus. They may recognize a relationship but be reluctant, hoping they can achieve their goal without additional change. The counselor's hope is to help clients recognize the relationship between the suggested focus and their own goals, enhancing their motivation for making this change.

Three Styles of Focusing

With all of these agenda present from client, context, and clinician, how do you identify a focus or direction? In Chapter 1 we presented a continuum of styles with directing at one end, following at the other, and guiding in the middle. This same continuum can describe different approaches for focusing.

Directing

In a directing approach, the provider determines the focus, rooted in his or her own agenda or that of the agency. At least implicitly the message is, "I'm in charge here and I decide what we discuss and do." Or perhaps more gently you make a recommendation about how to proceed and check with the client for a reaction. If one recommendation fails, you try another. You feel responsible for coming up with both the direction and the solution, and depending on the seriousness of the client's dilemma this could feel like quite a burden. There are certainly circumstances in which a directing style is appropriate in establishing a focus, but as a default approach for promoting client change it has serious limitations (Rollnick et al., 2008).

Following

At the opposite extreme the focus is on the client's priorities, whatever they may be: "What would you like to talk about today?" In a following style of focusing you try to understand the client's agenda and do your best to allow the direction, momentum, and content of the conversation to follow accordingly. If the client raises what seems like a pertinent issue, you'll explore it. A following style can enhance engagement, which is itself a therapeutic process.

Sometimes ongoing professional relationships are mostly supportive (using engagement skills) without the clinician offering specific direction for change, at least for a period of time. In a truly nondirective client-centered form of counseling, focus comes entirely from what the client brings, and the counselor follows wherever the client leads. Focusing, if it does occur, involves moving toward clearer goals for change that are raised by the client. This is common in education, where advisement is designed to help students achieve their own identified learning and career goals.

Such open exploration can occur over time within an ongoing professional relationship. A primary care provider, having attended to the medical concern at hand, says: "We have a few minutes here where we might talk about other concerns if you wish. I wonder if there is some area of your health you might like to discuss." In case management for a person with schizophrenia, the counselor might open a visit by asking: "How are things going for you? What concerns do you have?" There is no particular identified concern to begin with; new direction emerges from this open-ended discussion.

Guiding

Midway between directing and following sits a guiding style. Guiding promotes a collaborative search for direction, a meeting of expertise in which the focus of treatment is negotiated. The client's agenda are important, and any limitations inherent in the context are taken into account. The clinician's expertise is also a possible source of goals. The focusing process of MI commonly starts in this middle ground between directing and following, where the focus, momentum, and content are mutually forged. If you start with your two feet firmly placed in this middle ground of guiding, you'll be able to move to either side whenever you feel the need.

> Midway between directing and following sits a guiding style.

Three Focusing Scenarios

Scenario 1. "I know where we're going; the focus is clear."

Sometimes the focus is clear from the outset. This can happen if you work in a service with a narrowly defined focus. An educator who sees patients with newly diagnosed diabetes, for example, will focus on ways to facilitate glycemic control. This does not mean the particular path for pursuing this goal is predetermined. There may be various options, and a change plan emerges though evoking and planning.

In practice, when the focus of consultation is clear you move straight into the evoking and planning processes. The focus is a light on the horizon toward which you keep moving. The client's motivation may fluctuate and discord may emerge from time to time in your working relationship, but you know where you want to go and you keep steering in that direction in an MI-consistent style.

The importance of evoking in this situation depends on the client's initial level of motivation for change. When a client presents with a clear stated goal, having already decided to pursue it and asking for your help in reaching it, there may be little need for evoking. The aim of evoking—motivation and commitment for the change—has apparently been reached, and the most appropriate strategy may be to move directly into planning. If in doing so you encounter reluctance, you can always double back to evoking, or even to a reconsideration of focus.

Scenario 2. "There are several options, and we need to decide."

In this scenario there is a finite number of options for a possible focus. You could talk about A or B or C. In the rough and tumble of everyday practice this scenario is common. The range of possible options may be imposed by the service context or by the clinician's span of professional expertise. Most often, though, a list of possible goals emerges over the course of initial consultation. The client might readily describe a number of possibilities, and indeed you might have one or two in mind yourself. A number of concerns emerge, and it would be possible to begin by focusing on any one of them.

In practice it is well worth your time to choose the starting focus thoughtfully. The technique of *agenda mapping* described in the next chapter might be particularly useful when people present with multiple problems. What's on the list? What should be focused on first? Are there concerns that are most urgent to address? Do you perceive a causal link between any of the concerns that could suggest where to focus first? Is treating one particular problem likely to result in broader improvement in other areas? Here, focusing is the process of enumerating and sorting through the options and deciding where to start.

Scenario 3. "The focus is unclear, and we need to explore."

This scenario is at the other end of the focusing spectrum. The focus is not at all clear to you. What does this client most want and need? Clients themselves may not be clear, and come for your help in sorting out what the dilemma is and how to proceed. A client's presenting concerns may be quite diffuse, not leading to obvious direction or goals for change. "My whole life is just a mess; everything is turned upside down!" Yet you trust that with your support the client will be able to find what's in his or her best interest. You always have a "co-therapist" collaborator within the client.

In practice, the process of *orienting* discussed in the next chapter will be relevant here. This is not just a matter of following clients in whatever direction they happen to go. You are seeking light on the horizon, the right direction in which to move. Orienting is basically a process of using core skills to move from general to specific and arrive at mutually agreed-on goals.

This third scenario can also involve clinical formulation, looking for patterns or relationships among concerns that could suggest a focus for change. The case of Julia, begun in Chapter 6 and continued in the next chapter, provides an example of this more complex process of orienting and formulation. The aim is to arrive at a hypothesis to test, an initial focus to try that is mutually agreeable as a way to begin addressing the client's concerns.

CONVERSATION, NOT TRANSACTION

Focusing in motivational interviewing is not like buying salt or seeing a doctor about an infected toe, where the choices are few, the challenge is clear, and a transaction takes place. Conversations about change are not like this; the relationship is important, aspirations vary and fluctuate, and choices are made about large and small conversation streams that you could go down.

This chapter has reviewed the rationale for focusing in MI and provided a few conceptual maps to aid the process. Chapter 9 turns to *how* you can find the horizon toward which to navigate. Every time you wonder where to go next, which avenue to go down, or notice a disengaging client, it may be time to revisit the focusing process. Avenues for change can appear before you, and blurred focus can become sharp and meaningful.

KEY POINTS

✓ The process of focusing involves finding one or more specific goals or intended outcomes that provide direction for consultation.

✓ Focus can arise from the client, the context, or the clinician.

✓ The general counseling styles of directing, guiding, and following also describe three approaches to focusing.

✓ Sometimes there is a clear single focus, sometimes there are several possible topics, and sometimes the focus is quite unclear and exploration is needed.

CHAPTER 9

Finding the Horizon

We have always held to the hope, the belief,
the conviction that there is a better life,
a better world, beyond the horizon.
— FRANKLIN DELANO ROOSEVELT

You are never too old to set another goal or
to dream a new dream.
— C. S. LEWIS

MI is by definition a conversation about change, and focusing involves establishing the direction of travel. This chapter carries forward three common scenarios that we described in Chapter 8:

1. The focus is clear.
2. There are options to choose from.
3. The focus is unclear.

Here we consider how you might proceed with focusing within each of these three scenarios. Before doing so, however, we step back to consider a few important aspects of the spirit of MI, of the general mind-set behind the focusing process (and all processes) in good practice of MI.

COUNSELOR ISSUES THAT CAN ARISE IN FOCUSING

Tolerating Uncertainty

Resisting the righting reflex (Chapter 1) means that you hold back from solving problems for clients and actively support their efforts to do this for themselves. This stance requires a certain tolerance for uncertainty, an unhurried and uncluttered state of mind. Clinicians vary widely in tolerance for ambiguity. Some are content to wait until clarity arises, perhaps even being too comfortable with slow progress, content to wander about for too long without clear direction. Others feel impatient and eager to move along, particularly during the focusing process, where it may not even be clear yet what the topic of conversation will be. The temptation in the latter case is to come to closure and get moving. There is a risk, though, in premature closure: pushing ahead with a particular focus can create discord and disengagement if the client is not with you.

An unhurried mind-set does not necessarily mean that focusing process will take a long time. In fact, the opposite may be true—that a sense of hurry can promote premature focus that undermines progress. This is what Roberts (2001) meant by the principle "slow is fast": If you act like you have only a few minutes, it may take all day; act as if you have all day, and it may take only a few minutes. The difference is in the interviewer's felt sense of urgency. The capacity to tolerate uncertainty is one of the hallmarks of skillful focusing in MI.

Sharing Control

Uncertainty in turn can fuel concern about losing control of the consultation, a concern that can promote poor practice. The right state of mind here is to share control with clients in the confidence that, despite some uncertainty, clarity can and will emerge. You keep hold of the reins in the flow of the interview, while giving clients space to explore and influence its direction. One medical colleague returned from efforts to practice MI with an observation that captured his pushing through uncertainty and worries about losing control: "The long summary is just brilliant. I allow patients to run free while I listen to their story about their goals, and then the long summary gives me back direction and I can see where to go next." MI is like dancing, moving together, in which you offer gentle guidance. If you try to lead in one direction and sense discord or imbalance, try a different path that flows more smoothly.

Searching for Strengths and Openings for Change

So much of everyday practice is concerned with assessment, risk, problem management, and the completion of tasks that it is easy to miss opportunities for change. MI involves constantly listening for those openings, the avenues toward change. The smallest glimmer of change talk may be a coal that if given some air will start to glow, becoming the fuel of change.

It can help to back a few steps away from a problem focus to listen for your client's strengths, values, and aspirations for change, wondering with curiosity about this person's strengths and the way ahead.

THREE FOCUSING SCENARIOS

We turn now to the three scenarios mentioned earlier, three pictures that may come into focus as you explore the direction your conversation will take. Depending on the setting in which you practice, the first of these may be the most common.

Scenario 1. Clear Direction

Some clients present with clear initial goals and concerns in mind. If the direction for change is already clear to both of you, then there's no need to spend much time on focusing. It does make sense to confirm that you are on the same page about direction, asking permission and acknowledging autonomy: "So is that what we should talk about, then, or is there something else you want to discuss?" If your engagement is adequate, clients usually come alongside or suggest another direction. You might then move on to evoking or, if the client seems quite ready to change, directly into planning.

A second way that Scenario 1 occurs is in contexts where the scope of service has a clear focus. A physical therapist whose referral task is to help patients regain function and balance is likely to keep a fairly tight focus. People may come into specialist services with a broader range of concerns, but there is a clear focus for conversation by virtue of the context. This means that the provider, at least, has a clear direction in mind, although the extent to which presenting clients concur with the focus will vary. In this context your direction for discussion is generally clear, and the task at hand is really that of evoking in order to explore whether the client will share the focus. If you can establish a working relationship to move together in this direction, your work proceeds with evoking and planning. If not, there may be little basis for continuing. A guide who is knowledgeable about oceans and fishing is probably not the right guide for someone who only wants to explore inland botany.

A third way in which a clear focus might emerge is that the appropriate direction for change becomes apparent to you in the course of consultation. Again, the client may or may not concur with your sense of focus. If there is a particular direction in which you want to move the conversation about change, there are two steps involved: permission and evoking. The first of these is raising the topic, gaining the client's permission to explore it. Medical practitioners sometimes ask us: "How do I raise the subject of X without upsetting the patient?" For example, a clinician might think it to be in the client's best interest to consider not just her own eating habits but also those of her children, a topic that feels difficult because it might threaten her sense of being a good mother. The challenge here is to move the focus to a topic that you think is important, but may not be apparent or welcome to the client. We return to this specific task later in this chapter.

Having raised a potential focus and gained at least provisional permission to explore it, the task then becomes one of evoking, of listening for the person's own motivations to move in this direction (a process we discuss in Part IV). Lapsing back into the righting reflex at this point by lecturing clients about why and how they should change is unlikely to yield a happy outcome. When a client is already uncertain about the focus, the hope is to bring the person on board and find some motivation for change. Usually there will be some ambivalence to work with; the person already has some inherent values or other motivations to move forward. Exploring those autonomous motivations for change is the process of evoking (Chapter 13). If none are readily found, the process may be more one of developing discrepancy (Chapter 18).

Scenario 2. Choices in Direction: Agenda Mapping

A second common focusing scenario arises when there is a reasonably clear set of possible topics for conversation. The field of possibilities is not wide open (as in Scenario 3), but neither is there a clear primary focus (Scenario 1). You can encounter this scenario at the beginning of a consultation, but also at other times down the line where there is a reasonably clear set of possible issues you could focus on. For example:

> A mental health client disabled by hallucinations is feeling upset about not finding work, is unhappy about the side effects of medication, and acknowledges that cannabis use has increased recently.

Or:

> She's recently suffered from a stroke. You are concerned about her living alone and using a new walking aid, and she wants to drive again although she's worried that she might have another stroke.

All too often when there are multiple options, focusing takes place rather quickly, without much conscious reflection or mutual agreement, usually driven by the judgment of the practitioner. Engagement can suffer from such haste, and the unilateral determination of focus makes it that much harder to promote change. On the other hand, involving the client in the choice of direction will allow for easier integration of MI into your everyday practice.

The obstacles to smooth and skillful focusing can be substantial. Clients may feel submerged in a sea of problems and discouraged about making changes. From your side there is often no shortage of threats to calm and thoughtful practice, including time pressure and multiple tasks that compete for your attention. If you both feel overwhelmed you may fall into any of several traps: focusing unilaterally or too quickly, going down the wrong path, or just going around in circles of mutual hopelessness.

Agenda mapping is a tool to help you focus faster, and, with a more active client, to avoid unnecessary confusion about direction. We prefer the term "agenda mapping"[1] to our earlier "agenda setting" (Stott, Rollnick, Rees, & Pill, 1995) because it is rather like examining a map at the outset of a journey, knowing that it can be consulted again to adjust direction of travel along the way.

In essence, agenda mapping is a metaconversation. It is a short period of time when you and your client step outside of the conversation to consider the way ahead and what to talk about. Essentially, it is a form of "talk about talk." Agenda mapping can involve identifying one step to focus on within an ongoing process of change. Done well, it can provide relief to clients who feel

| Agenda mapping is a metaconversation. |

ensnared by their problems, giving them a chance to leave some things to one side for a while as they focus on others.

It is possible to signal your own preference for a focus without foreclosing the decision process. Your aspiration just becomes one more piece of information to consider when choosing a direction together.

> "We could go in a number of directions here, and I wonder what makes sense to you. You have mentioned your diet and also the possibility of getting more exercise. I would also like to talk a bit about smoking, but you may have something that concerns you more. What would you like to discuss as a way of improving your health?"

This approach is like looking at a map and seeing the places you might go, perhaps like two people on a sailboat slowing down for a moment to agree on a new course before catching the wind again. Try this method when you want to establish or realign your focus. It can be particularly useful when a client is facing a number of interrelated concerns. It is a curious exploration of options leading to an agreed-upon decision about the way ahead, at least for the time being.

Agenda mapping follows an obvious sequence, starting with a list of options and moving toward an agreed-upon focus, and it consists of a number of elements. These elements are not rigid steps, because everyday practice calls for flexibility. Sometimes a focus is quickly established in a very brief mapping discussion; other times it takes longer. Different elements

---

[1] Thanks to Nina Gobat for suggesting this term and helping to think it through.

may be important depending on whether you are doing initial agenda mapping at the outset of consultation or are returning for a course adjustment. In all cases, the core skills described in Chapters 5 and 6 provide the glue that binds the task together. The nature of agenda mapping also varies depending on the context; for example, whether you are considering topics that might be discussed within a few remaining minutes of a medical visit or over the course of months of anticipated psychotherapy.

Structuring

First, it is a good idea to make clear what you're doing. In essence you are stepping back from the conversation for a moment to talk about its direction, and this is usually initiated with a structuring statement. You can ask the client's permission as you transition into agenda mapping, using prefacing phrases like "*Would you mind if* we consider some topics that we could discuss?" or "*Can we* just take stock for a few minutes here about what we might discuss?" The use of *might* or *could* captures the hypothetical nature of mapping. You are not announcing topics that you *will* discuss, but rather at this stage simply identifying those you might.

Keeping the discussion hypothetical can be a challenge, even during a brief period of agenda mapping. A client raises a topic or problem and you might be tempted to start exploring it right then and there. During agenda mapping the task is not to descend into discussing any one issue in depth, but rather to get an overview of different available directions for your conversation. If the client's life is like a forest, agenda mapping involves soaring over it for a moment with the perspective of an eagle. Later it may be useful to drop down to the forest floor with the perspective of the mouse, but not yet. Here is how a structuring statement might sound to demarcate agenda mapping:

> "I wonder if we could just step back for a few minutes here and consider what's most important to focus on. I've started making a little list of things in my head that you have raised as concerns, and I want to check that list with you. Then we can talk about where you think we might start on the list, and I may have some ideas about that, too. Would that be OK?"

Considering Options

After a preparatory structuring statement agenda mapping begins with listing options. What are the concerns that you *might* focus on together? This can be as simple as inviting the client to list concerns that you might discuss, which is what you might do early in a consultation. If you have already had the benefit of some conversation, you may be developing a list of your own possible topics based on what you have heard. However you proceed in developing a list of candidate topics, we find that these guidelines serve the process well:

1. Allow clients the space to reflect and express their preferences and concerns. Don't feel like you need to start talking immediately if 7 seconds of silence pass. Open the door with an invitation and wait to see what emerges.
2. Include affirmation and support as appropriate. Comment on clients' apparent strengths and aspirations. Emphasize their personal choice and autonomy in decisions about their own life, health, and decisions.
3. Invite the client to raise completely new ideas that haven't been discussed yet.
4. Use hypothetical language like "we might," "you could," and so on. Glide over the landscape and survey it; where you will land is for the next part of agenda mapping. Reflective listening is probably your most useful and efficient route to understanding the client's perspective and finding a useful focus.
5. Include your own opinion. Your suggestions also matter, and clients often value hearing your perspective on what is important to consider. Within MI this is done in a modest way that acknowledges and honors the client's autonomy (see Chapter 11).

> "Another possibility that occurs to me is to discuss your sleeping pattern, since lack of sleep can affect many of the other concerns you've been expressing. We could consider that, or maybe that's for another time."

Zooming In

With the big map and a bird's-eye view of the possible terrain to explore, the next step in agenda mapping is to move from hypothetical to provisional. This is a delicate and productive part of the task, getting to a shared concrete understanding about where the conversation will focus, at least for the time being, and of what topics will be discussed. If you are familiar with digital maps this is a bit like pushing the plus (+) button to zoom in on and get a better look at a particular area. Later, as conditions change, you may zoom back out to get a broader perspective and find a different focus.

As discussed in Chapter 8, various considerations can influence the selection of focus. The client may have clear and strong priorities for where to start. Some topics require more urgent attention. The service context may limit the possible areas of focus. You may also have an opinion about what needs to be addressed first, perhaps because you see possible causal relationships among the client's concerns. Choosing where to focus on the map is a matter of negotiation, always keeping client engagement in mind. It's no use setting off for a clear destination if the client won't go with you.

This zooming in step, then, involves exchanging information with clients about their and your sense of priorities and coming to an agreement about direction. You are seeking a shared sense of direction, which is an important component of a working alliance (Bordin, 1979). That direction may be as simple as one or more topics to explore, or it may include clear goals to be reached.

> It's no use setting off for a clear destination if the client won't go with you.

The core skill of summarizing helps to wrap up agenda mapping before stepping back into the stream of consultation. A good summary could include these elements:

1. The big map: A list of topics or goals that you have considered together. You can include topics that you will or might discuss, as well as any that you won't be addressing together.
2. The focal map: Your starting point for the conversational journey. This may be one topic or a set of high-priority topics to be addressed.
3. A reminder that you can return to this mapping task again as needed later in your consultation. This provides a reference point you can use later to step aside again for agenda mapping.
4. Asking for the client's response. Is this agreeable? Are there additional concerns that need to be addressed soon? Is it all right to proceed?

In some of the examples below you'll notice briefer variations of agenda mapping that can be used throughout the consultation for different reasons, perhaps to change the topic or if you are feeling stuck. Stepping aside for a metaconversation is their singular common element.

Using Visual Aids

One of the earliest forms of agenda mapping in behavior change consultations involved using a visual aid that sat between the practitioner and the client as a prompt (Stott et al., 1995). It consisted of a page with a series of bubble shapes containing possible topics in some bubbles, with additional empty bubbles that could be filled in by the client (see Box 9.1). Such sheets can be targeted to particular applications. For example, a diabetes educator might fill the bubbles with different ways of managing blood glucose: diet, exercise, oral medication, insulin, stress reduction, monitoring, and so on. Another approach is simply to take out a blank sheet of paper and write

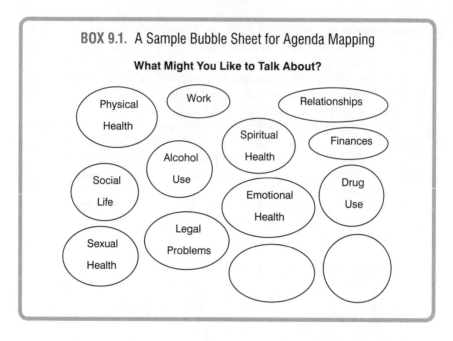

BOX 9.1. A Sample Bubble Sheet for Agenda Mapping

What Might You Like to Talk About?

down topics as they emerge in the discussion. These topics could be written in hand-drawn bubbles, with a few bubbles left empty, thus creating an individualized mapping sheet.

Agenda mapping can also be used across visits, not only within them. You can keep a visual record with the bubble sheet as a reminder of progress and of current and future possible directions. When you next meet, the map may have changed, but it will have some of the old routes on it.

Agenda Mapping in Practice

The heart of agenda mapping and of skillful focusing more generally is to engage an autonomous client in a collaborative direction. Here are some circumstances in which agenda mapping might be helpful.

CHOOSING A CHANGE TOPIC AMONG MANY

Mapping might not be necessary if your focus is really on a single and agreed-upon topic. People working in the addictions field often point this out: "It's obvious. Over the door of the building it says 'Substance Abuse Treatment Program,' so there's no question what we're going to talk about when someone walks through the door." Yet even in a focused service there may be multiple possible conversation streams. If the client drinks alcohol, smokes tobacco, and uses several other drugs, where will the initial focus be? Furthermore, substance use disorders are usually intertwined with other problems, some of which may be of greater concern to the client and which also may be important obstacles in recovery (Miller, Forcehimes, & Zweben, 2011).

In such situations agenda mapping can help identify a place to start, an area where the client is most eager or at least willing to pursue change. Usually it is not productive to try to change everything at once. While there may be many important potential topics on the list, agenda mapping leads to a first step for focusing.

INTERVIEWER: You were referred here to talk about your drinking, but it sounds like you have quite a few other concerns that feel like higher priorities to you. You talked about wanting to reconcile with your wife and move back home. Your son is also having a lot of problems that have been contributing to the conflict between you and your wife. I mentioned that there are also some standard questions that I will need to ask you before we finish today. Where do you think we should start?

CLIENT: I've got to decide whether I can spend money for a lawyer for my son; he's in a lot of trouble.

INTERVIEWER: This might be the most important thing for us to discuss today.

CLIENT: No, probably not. I mean, it's on my mind because if I don't give him the money he'll be screaming abuse at me as soon as I see him.

INTERVIEWER: So that's definitely on your mind right now, and there may be even more important things for us to discuss. Would it be all right to talk about drinking, since that was why you were referred?

CLIENT: Well, it's not as bad as they make out, but I do get into trouble sometimes.

INTERVIEWER: So that's another topic we could focus on today.

CLIENT: Yes.

INTERVIEWER: What else?

CLIENT: I may get kicked out of my apartment, and I don't have another place to live.

INTERVIEWER: How urgent is that?

CLIENT: I still have some time to work that out, but I'd like to get back with my wife.

INTERVIEWER: OK. What else could we discuss?

CLIENT: My supervisor isn't happy with me at work. He wrote me up for being late, and if I lose that job I'm in trouble with my probation officer.

INTERVIEWER: So that's worrying you, too.

CLIENT: Yeah.

INTERVIEWER: All right, well, there are plenty of things that we could talk about today. Before we get to those questions that I need to ask, where would you like to begin?

CLIENT: I guess getting the lawyer for my son. He'll ask me about that today.

INTERVIEWER: Sure, let's start there, and would it be OK if we then turned to your alcohol use?

CLIENT: Sure.

INTERVIEWER: I'll keep an eye on the time, and we'll see whether we can discuss anything else, OK?

CLIENT: Yes, fine.

CHANGING DIRECTION

Although it is common for the topic of conversation to shift from time to time, it is important in MI to keep your eye on the horizon, to know where you're headed. Over the course of consultation, particularly with repeated visits, you may reach a juncture where it is appropriate to consider changing focus and heading in a new direction. Often this will involve a choice between two possible directions. At times like this we recommend a brief metaconversation to be clear together about goals and aspirations, just as a good guide might stop to discuss possibilities for the next destination(s). A counselor might open up such a discussion in this way:

"The two of you came in originally to talk about improving your relationship, and you in particular, Linda, wanted more open communication, to hear more about what Carl is feeling. We've been working together for four sessions now, and you've been spending more time talking with each other at home and using some of the listening skills we've discussed. Something that has become clearer for you, Carl, is that you're really struggling with trust and feeling vulnerable, and you're wondering whether this is linked to your experience in the army. So let's step back here for a minute and talk about where we're headed. One possibility is for us to keep on working together to strengthen your communication and relationship. Another option would be for you, Carl, to work through your combat experiences and how those are affecting you now, and that would probably involve some individual counseling. If you feel like you're hitting a wall here, that might be a priority before we push ahead on your relationship. Or perhaps there is another possible direction that occurs to you. I guess I'd like to hear from each of you what you're thinking about the best next step."

ACTIVATING CLIENTS BEFORE YOU MEET THEM

It is possible to extend the logic of agenda mapping to encourage clients to consider their aspirations even before you meet them. In one of our recent studies (McNamara et al., 2010) children and young people with diabetes used an agenda-mapping kit to explore and write down in the waiting room what they wanted to talk about. One practitioner was surprised when a previously very reticent child came in with just one question on her map: "How long will I live?" Efforts to activate clients early can have an impact on the culture and organization of a service, a topic to be discussed further in Part VI. Giving the client more time and a bit of structure to prepare beforehand not only saves time in the consultation but makes a statement about how you and your service value the aspirations of the client. This preparation is the beginning of agenda mapping, not the end of it. Progress will then depend on the engagement and focusing skills of the practitioners who sometimes receive unexpected client aspirations.

GETTING UNSTUCK

You are proceeding through a consultation and you get a feeling that the discussion is going in circles, covering too many topics, and not getting anywhere. It can be useful to step outside of the conversation in a frank exchange for a few moments rather than carrying the weight of responsibility for solving the impasse yourself. You are, in essence, using your client as a consultant. Under these circumstances, agenda mapping need not proceed through all the phases described above, but can take an abbreviated form, such as:

> "I'd like to pause for a moment [demarcating the metaconversation] and just check in with you on how you are feeling about this discussion so far. I'm wondering where to go next, to be honest, and what's going to be most useful to you. Of all the things you've mentioned, what do you think we should focus on as most important?"

It's possible to be frank about feeling a little lost without losing your credibility. A short period of listening can be quite helpful. Another possibility in this situation is to start or restart the mapping process with a summary that lists the topics that have emerged:

> "It would be helpful to me if we could just step back for a moment and talk about where we're going. We've talked about your getting back to work, some of the obstacles you're encountering, how you feel about this, about your daily routines, some of the problems you're having with your daughter, and even about how you would like your life to be in 10 years' time. How are you feeling about our conversation so far? I wonder whether you would particularly like to focus on one of these topics at this point."

RAISING A DIFFICULT TOPIC

Practitioners sometimes wonder how to ask just the right question to raise a difficult topic. The problem can often be one of poor engagement, which, if rectified, will allow you to be frank about your concerns. However, circumstances are often far from ideal, engagement can feel tenuous despite your best efforts, and agenda mapping can help. You step back, raise the difficult subject among several others, emphasize autonomy, and gauge the client's readiness to go further. Taking the example of possible alcohol abuse in a clearly sensitive person talking about her stomach ailment and stress, one could proceed as follows:

> "Can I ask you where we might take our discussion from this point onward? You've talked about what you call your sensitive stomach, and do let me know if there are any further concerns you have about that. You've also talked about stress, and we could talk about how you might improve things and help you manage this better. I also wonder about alcohol use, and how it might be affecting your stomach. Then there might be other things you'd like to raise. It's up to you."

If you think it is important to discuss a particular topic you can raise it by asking specific permission.

> "Listening to the troubles you've been having with your stomach, I've thought of one thing that might turn out to be important. Would it be all right if we talked a bit about your use of alcohol?"

FITTING IN AN ASSESSMENT

If your service routinely requires a standard assessment, you may struggle with how this affects engagement. Charging right into an inquisition is not the best way to engage with clients. One way to address this problem is to begin with some agenda mapping before undertaking detailed assessment. Your structure for an initial visit can include the necessary assessment, and you can agree with the client when this will be done. For example:

> "This is our first visit together, and there are at least two things for us to do. There are some questions that I will ask you to fill in this form that we complete with everyone who comes here. I also want to hear what concerns you bring today, and how you hope we might be able to help with those. We could start with either, and the questions will take about 15 minutes. What's your preference? Shall I start by listening to your concerns, or do you prefer to get this form out of the way first?"

Some people will want to tell their story first, and others will prefer the structured safety of answering questions for a while. Either way, they get to choose and have the clear expectation of addressing both tasks within the conversation.

CLARIFYING YOUR ROLES IN TOUGH CIRCUMSTANCES

Some practitioners have a duty to inhabit at least two worlds simultaneously: the well-being of the client and the protection of others like vulnerable children, abused partners, and the community at large. In defense of the latter, assessment procedures and policies may be prominent in the consultation. Yet you also want to advocate for and promote change in the client, who can't be blamed for wondering defensively whose side you are on. In truth you're on both sides, and it can be challenging to establish and maintain a collaborative relationship focused on change.

Agenda mapping can also be useful here to clarify roles, thus making it easier to navigate transitions later in the conversation from one topic to another. You step into a metaconversation, clarify roles, and then proceed through agenda mapping as appropriate. A metaphor like changing hats can be useful. If you want to shift topics or roles at a later point, the transition is easier because you have already flagged the distinctions. For example:

> "It might help if I take a moment to tell you about my different roles. You can think of it as me wearing different hats. With my counseling hat on, my job, if you are willing, is to help you meet your own needs and goals in your everyday life. Then, as you know, there's another hat I wear, and that's about protecting others. It's not always easy for me to wear this hat, but I have a responsibility to look after the safety and best interests of your children. I have two jobs, that is, two hats: to help

you, and to help your children be safe. I hope we can work together no matter which hat I'm wearing. So let's begin with your needs and concerns. What changes would you like to see in your own life?"

Scenario 3. Unclear Direction: Orienting

Agenda mapping begins with a menu of possibilities—a list of possible change topics from which to choose. Sometimes, however, there is not a list of discrete concerns. There is no clearly marked map with a choice of destinations. The client's presenting scenario may be quite diffuse. Certain concerns are mentioned, but it's not clear how they fit together, and there isn't an obvious focus for change. The client seems to be "all over the map," and the initial challenge appears to be one of reducing confusion (Gilmore, 1973). Picking any one problem as a focus for change misses the bigger picture.

Here the clinician's task is more complex than compiling a prioritized list. It is a matter of listening to the client's story and puzzling together about a route out of the forest. You may follow various streams for a while in trying to map the terrain. The overall process of orienting is one of moving from general to specific, and solid engagement is all the more important as a foundation for this more involved process.

Often, part of the task in orienting is case formulation, developing a clear shared picture (or at least hypothesis) of what the client's situation is and how it might best be addressed. The client provides pieces of the puzzle and together you explore how to put them together. This orienting process may start at the beginning of consultation, thus being concomitant with the engaging process. In such cases, the OARS skills described in Chapters 5 and 6 are central in both engaging and focusing. This is illustrated in the unfolding case of Julia that we began in Chapter 6 and continue below. This segment of the initial session begins with the interviewer providing a summary of concerns that emerged early in their conversation. If this were simply agenda mapping, one might just decide which of these problems to start with, but there is something more complex going on. The interviewer is keeping the whole picture in focus (eagle view) rather than zooming down to a particular task (mouse view). The task is one of collaboratively trying out different ways of putting the puzzle together.

INTERVIEWER: Well, that's quite a lot that you have on your mind. Let me see if I have a beginning understanding of what's troubling you. You're angry and smarting from the breakup with Ray and wondering if there's a pattern that you will keep repeating in relationships. You're not sleeping very well, and you notice that you have trouble concentrating. You don't have much energy, you feel lonely, and sometimes you just break out crying for no apparent reason. But especially you wonder what's happening. You want to understand what's going on with you and worry that you're "losing it," maybe going crazy. You're feeling out of control sometimes—screaming, throwing, and breaking things. That's happened before when you broke up with boyfriends, but something new this time was cutting yourself, and that frightened you.

CLIENT: Freaked me out. But it was also kind of a relief in a way, and that scares me, too.

INTERVIEWER: Like you might do it again.

CLIENT: I don't know. I just don't know what's wrong with me.

INTERVIEWER: There's so much going on in your life right now that you hardly know where to start, and so you came here to the clinic.

CLIENT: Yes. Do you think you can you help me?

INTERVIEWER: Yes, I do. This all feels pretty strange to you, even coming here, but I've worked with women before who have had concerns like this, and I believe I can help. A good place to start, I think, is to get clearer about our goals in working together. If our work together were really successful from your perspective, what would be different?

CLIENT: I guess I wouldn't feel so bad all the time. Should I be taking medication?

INTERVIEWER: That's one possibility, but let's talk first about where you want to go before we consider how to get there. So one thing you'd like to change is how you're feeling. Tell me a little more about that.

CLIENT: I just feel upset and I'm crying a lot. I'm not sleeping and I feel worn out, run down.

INTERVIEWER: OK, you'd like to get your emotional life settled down some, to be able to sleep better and have more energy. What else?

CLIENT: I want a good relationship.

INTERVIEWER: Tell me about that.

CLIENT: I want to be with a man I can be close to, somebody who's interesting and will talk to me. Sex is good, but I want someone who really loves *me* and doesn't shut me out. Why do men do that?

INTERVIEWER: That's one thing that was so upsetting for you with Ray—feeling shut out.

CLIENT: Yes! I just want to know why I keep screwing up all my relationships. What's wrong with me?

INTERVIEWER: That's another thing that upsets you—not knowing why you feel so bad and why these things happen to you. You want to understand what's going on with relationships and also with cutting yourself.

CLIENT: Isn't that important—to understand?

INTERVIEWER: Clearly, it's important to you. You don't like feeling out of control, and there are some other things that you're clear about. You want to feel better, to have some peace inside, be able to sleep and concentrate. You'd like to be in a relationship where you can love and be loved and feel close. And you think it would help if you could understand what's going on with you and why it's happening. Is that a good start?

CLIENT: Yes. Especially understanding what's happening.

INTERVIEWER: That's a high priority for you, and I do have an idea that puts some of the pieces of the puzzle together—not all of them, mind you, but it makes sense of a lot of what you are experiencing, at least to me. If it's all right with you, we can talk about that next.

CLIENT: Sure. What's your idea? [Continued in Chapter 11]

What is going on here? The interviewer is not asking Julia which problem she would like to start with as one might in agenda mapping, yet her concerns do remain at the center of the picture. There is a movement from general and diffuse to more specific pieces of the puzzle. The interviewer is not just following wherever she happens to go, nor dictating where she should go. It is a collaborative process with the interviewer serving as a knowledgeable guide. Over time the picture comes into focus, and at the end of this segment the interviewer is about to suggest one possible formulation that would point a way forward. The puzzle is not solved yet: a formulation is a guess, a hypothesis about what the picture might be. If they can agree on this as a working hypothesis, they can proceed toward testing it to see whether, in fact, it begins to address Julia's concerns.

We have chosen to describe this more complex process as orienting. It is not as simple as Scenario 1, where a specific focus emerges rather quickly, or as Scenario 2, where there is a list of possible change goals to be prioritized. The task here is more that of puzzling together over how to put the pieces together. It is a true blending of the clinician's expertise and the client's expert knowledge of herself. It still has the hallmarks of the focusing process: moving from general to specific and coming up with a clear direction in which to move. With the horizon in focus it is then possible to begin moving toward it through evoking and planning.

Orienting is quite a good example of the guiding style. Clients in this much turmoil may not do well with a counselor who merely follows along. There is a need for and comfort in having a guide with expertise. In good guiding the counselor also does not simply take charge. There is still a lot of listening happening, and the counselor consults the client's wishes, concerns, and expertise. The clinician contributes expertise in formulating possible paths to pursue, but the process of focusing remains collaborative.

To be sure, these three focusing scenarios are not distinct; there are gray areas in between. They represent a continuum from a clear single focus at one end to a chaotic jigsaw puzzle at the other. One could approach Julia's situation as an agenda-mapping task, to choose which one or more of her emerging list of concerns to address first. The common denominator in the focusing process is to develop a clear sense of direction, a horizon toward which to move. The horizon is provisional, and over time the goals and direction may shift. Often they do, but to move forward with the MI processes of evoking and planning it is essential to have a clear eye on the far horizon.

KEY POINTS

✓ In MI, focusing is a collaborative process of finding mutually agreeable direction.

✓ When there is a reasonably clear set of possible topics for conversation and consultation, the task is agenda mapping to choose and prioritize.

✓ Agenda mapping is a metaconversation by which you step back for a short time to consider with the client the way ahead.

✓ Agenda mapping can also be useful when changing direction, getting unstuck, raising a difficult topic, or clarifying roles.

✓ When the goals of consultation seem more diffuse, a process of orienting is needed that can include formulation—putting puzzle pieces together in a way that generates a provisional hypothesis about where to start.

CHAPTER 10

When Goals Differ

I have not the right to want to change another
if I am not open to be changed.
—MARTIN BUBER

One dimension along which therapies have traditionally differed is the degree to which the counselor engages as an expert in overt directing. To what extent does the clinician seek to move a client toward a particular choice, change, or way of being? In rational-emotive therapy, for example, the therapist specifically seeks out clients' "irrational" beliefs and uses disputation strategies to replace them with what the therapist regards to be rational beliefs (Ellis & MacLaren, 2005). In reality therapy (Glasser, 1975) the clinician is again in an expert role, with the goal of confronting self-deceived clients with how things actually are. In both cases the therapist is the authoritative arbiter of what constitutes rationality and reality. In other words, these treatment approaches rely heavily on expert directing by the counselor.

At the opposite extreme of this spectrum are treatments intended to be nondirective, a term originally associated with Carl Rogers's (1965) client-centered counseling approach. Here in theory it is the client who wholly determines the content, direction, and goals of treatment. The counselor provides a supportive, nonjudgmental, and value-free atmosphere for the safe exploration of personal experience and relies heavily on following with skillful listening. Within this perspective it is anathema for a counselor to steer a client toward any particular outcome. Therapists from a humanistic or existential orientation might object to the directional aspect of MI, whereby clients would be intentionally guided toward what the counselor regards to be appropriate goals. Within a truly nondirective orientation the goals of treatment should be determined solely by the client.

Comfort with directing varies substantially across clinical contexts. Those who work in correctional settings are unlikely to be scandalized by the notion that a counselor would pursue a goal of reducing future offending. Clinicians in these settings work to prevent further incidents of violence, drunk driving, or sexual predation whether or not that goal is currently endorsed by the offender. Those who staff a suicide prevention hotline by definition have a particular outcome in mind from the moment they pick up the telephone. Few would be surprised or appalled that counselors in an addiction treatment program have a general goal of reducing substance use and related suffering, even if that goal is not initially endorsed by the clients they serve, many of whom are coerced into treatment. Such contexts just seem to call for a clinician to have clear goals for change.

How do you decide whether it is proper to be moving toward a particular focus? Our colleague Dr. Theresa Moyers once proposed a common-sense "waitress test" of clinical practice. Imagine a busy waitress who works on her feet all day and who pays a significant proportion of her earnings in taxes that support, among other things, the public services that a clinician is providing. Would she think it reasonable that a clinician counsels in a way that is not moving toward any particular goal (e.g., if the clinician's practice focuses on schizophrenia, addictions, drunk driving, domestic violence, or child abuse)? Would she regard it to be a good use of her hard-earned tax dollars to support treatment that is not intentionally directed toward positive change?

On the other hand, there are clinical situations where it seems obvious that a professional helper should *not* favor a particular direction in which to move people. Chapter 17 discusses such situations and how to counsel when your intention is neutrality. It seems clear to us, for example, that it is inappropriate to use one's clinical skills and influence to persuade people that they should sign a contract or consent form, donate one of their kidneys, or adopt children.

In between these two ethical extremes (a clear need to have direction, and a clear reason to avoid it) is a large gray area where it is less apparent whether a clinician ought to identify and pursue a particular change goal. Consider the admittedly simplistic 2 × 2 goal matrix in Box 10.1. In Cells A

BOX 10.1. The Meeting of Client and Clinician Aspirations

Is this a current goal of the client?

	Yes	No
Is this *your* hope for the client? **Yes**	A	B
No	C	D

and D there is no apparent problem: the client's and clinician's goals agree. Most practitioners spend most of their time working in Cell A. Cell C contains client goals that you do not share, perhaps because they fall outside the scope of treatment or your area of expertise, or because you are ethically uncomfortable or otherwise unwilling to help the client pursue them. Here you would decline to proceed toward this goal in treatment yourself, perhaps making an appropriate referral.

That leaves Cell B, the situation in which you have an aspiration for change that the client does not currently share. As discussed earlier, this is more common in situations where clients are court mandated or otherwise coerced into treatment (e.g., probation, adolescents brought by parents), or are seeking help for entirely different reasons (e.g., emergency room care for an alcohol-related injury). MI was originally developed for Cell B, and in particular for the situation in which the client is *ambivalent* about making a particular change. The client's internal committee contains both pro-change and counter-change voices. If you ask an alcohol-dependent person, "Are you ready to quit drinking?" the answer may be "No." Abstinence is not currently a goal for this person. However, if you explore this person's experience further you will often hear pro-change arguments. (This is a primary topic of Part IV.) Part of the client's internal committee is persuaded that it is time to make a change, and part wants to keep drinking. Both voices are there, and the issue has not been resolved. In the absence of a new decision the status quo prevails.

Also in Cell B is the situation where the client is seemingly unambivalent—has no apparent motivation whatsoever to make a change (the "precontemplation" stage). Yet the professional is concerned and sees clear reason to work toward change. This situation is discussed in Chapter 18, on developing discrepancy.

So what should a helper do in Cell B? One approach in addiction treatment has been to say, "Come back when you're ready to change." This is one choice, but it is abundantly clear that it is not a *necessary* choice—that one doesn't have to wait for clients to "hit bottom" or "get motivated" before intervening in a helpful way (Meyers & Wolfe, 2004; Miller, Meyers, & Tonigan, 1999; Sellman, Sullivan, Dore, Adamson, & MacEwan, 2001). Another possible professional disposition toward client goals is neutrality—to take no position, and favor no choice over others (see Chapter 17). When continuation of the present pattern poses significant risks to the life and well-being of the client or others, however, there is reason for seeking to enhance motivation for change, and it is often possible to do so.

In this regard, we turn to a brief consideration of ethical aspects of influencing people toward a change about which they are ambivalent or even uninterested. This discussion is relevant precisely because it *is* possible to influence human motivation and choice. The psychology of interpersonal influence has been extensively studied (Cialdini, 2007) and is routinely applied in advertising, marketing, politics, coaching, health promotion, and organizational development. Counselors and psychotherapists sometimes aspire to deliver "value-free" or "nondirective" services, although the possibility of actually doing so is debatable (Bergin, 1980; Truax, 1966). We believe it is important to be aware of and navigate these ethical decisions thoughtfully with a clear set of chosen professional values.

FOUR BROAD ETHICAL VALUES

Professional relationships involve uneven power and thereby incur special responsibilities. Each profession develops a set of ethical standards for practice, which in turn tend to reflect a common set of underlying values that have also been extensively considered in the protection of human participants in research (Israel & Hay, 2006; National Research Council, 2009). These include four broad ethical principles: nonmaleficence, beneficence, autonomy, and justice (Beauchamp & Childress, 2001).

Nonmaleficence

"First, do no harm" is an ancient precept of medical practice. In the traditional Hippocratic oath this is placed even before beneficence (doing good). At the very least, clinical interventions should not harm people. It is also possible for nonintervention (doing nothing) to be harmful. A surgeon colleague came to MI because she questioned whether it was ethical for her to be treating people for trauma in the emergency department without also addressing their drinking that had directly contributed to it and placed them at risk for future reinjury (Schermer, 2005; Schermer, Moyers, Miller, & Bloomfield, 2006; Schermer, Qualls, Brown, & Apodaca, 2001).

Beneficence

Beyond the absence of harm, clinical interventions are meant to provide benefit. One common beneficence guideline is to offer evidence-based treatments that have the best likelihood of efficacy for achieving treatment goals. Beyond science-based efficacy, consideration is also given to clear professional consensus as to the best course of action. This principle of beneficence is reflected in compassion as a component of the underlying spirit of MI: that the primary purpose of consultation is to benefit the client's welfare (see Chapter 2).

Autonomy

A third broad ethical principle is autonomy: a respect for human freedom and dignity. When people consent to treatment, it should be with a clear understanding of the nature and potential risks and benefits of the treatment to be provided and of the alternatives available to them. Value is placed here on self-determination and choice. The client decides whether and how to pursue change, and ultimately that choice cannot be taken away (Frankl, 2006). It can happen, of course, that the person's condition (such as drug dependence) is one that that itself impairs self-determination (Miller & Atencio, 2008), in which case support for autonomy could be expressed by pursuing a goal that the person does not immediately endorse. This is a central consideration, for example, in involuntary commitment to treatment.

> The client decides whether and how to pursue change; that choice cannot be taken away.

Justice

Finally, the principle of justice has to do with fairness, with equitable access to the benefits of treatment and protections against risk. The availability and course of treatment should not be influenced by factors that are unrelated to the likelihood of benefit or harm.

GOALS OF TREATMENT

How do the ethical principles that guide research and clinical care apply when clarifying the goals of treatment? Most commonly, these goals are brought by the client as presenting concerns, and the clinician either agrees to pursue them (Cell A in Box 10.1) or declines to do so (Cell C), perhaps in concern for nonmaleficence.

Ethical discussions often have to do with Cell B, where the clinician may identify and pursue a goal not currently endorsed by the client. This can arise in crisis situations, for example, when a clinician intervenes to save a life through involuntary hospitalization or the resuscitation of an unconscious patient who has overdosed. When the goal involves behavior change of autonomous individuals, however, it cannot be achieved without the person's engagement and cooperation. The clinician cannot decide that the client will change. Even highly extrinsic motivators such as paying people money to abstain from alcohol or other drugs (Stitzer & Petry, 2006; Stitzer, Petry, & Peirce, 2010) assume voluntary participation in the exchange. Offenders can be incarcerated to isolate them from society, but behavior change after release is subject to autonomous choice. This means that pursuit of any change goal that the client does not currently share (Cell B) necessarily involves interventions intended to influence the person to adopt and pursue it as a goal. The hope is to make it a shared goal, moving (in Box 10.1) from Cell B to Cell A. That is one function of the evoking process.

So when is it appropriate to use clinical strategies such as MI to influence what a client wants or chooses to do? Concern (as well as efficacy) is inherent in the potential that MI can alter volition and choice, as well as related behavior. This is not of particular concern when the client's aspirations are consonant with those of the counselor. When counselor and client aspirations are at variance, however, ethical consideration should be given to any methods that are effective in changing client aspirations to more closely match those of the counselor. This issue is further complicated when the counselor's actual "client" (the one desiring change) is not the person who is seated in the consultation room but is another party—such as a court system, parent, or school—asking for change in the person.

Key ethical principles here are beneficence (to promote the person's welfare) and nonmaleficence (to prevent harm to the client or others). As discussed earlier, there are situations in which this seems fairly clear, such as efforts to change life-threatening behavior or predatory reoffending despite an apparent present lack of client motivation to do so. More generally there are situations in which the counselor perceives a change that would be in the client's best interest, although this is not immediately apparent to the person. In such cases the clinician has a change aspiration that the client does not currently share, and the clinician hopes to influence the client to want, choose, and pursue the change.

Does this counselor aspiration violate the ethical principle of autonomy? We are persuaded that it does not, because ultimately decisions about any personal change (in behavior, lifestyle, attitude, etc.) necessarily remain with the client. MI is not about persuading people to do something that is against their values, goals, or best interests. Unless the change is in some way consistent with the client's own goals or values, there is no basis for MI to work.

> MI is not about persuading people to do something that is against their values, goals, or best interests.

WHEN NOT TO USE MOTIVATIONAL INTERVIEWING

As discussed earlier, attempts to influence personal choice are commonplace in society. Advertising and marketing seek to affect what people want, political campaigns to sway voting, health promotion to motivate health behavior change. Are such efforts "manipulative"? This term usually implies the skillful use of change strategies in a way that is unfair or designed to serve the user's own interests.

That is precisely why we added *compassion* as an important component of the underlying spirit of MI (Chapter 2): it is to be practiced with beneficence, to advance the client's best interests rather than one's own. Professional helping relationships require a higher standard of conduct than ordinary relationships; clients enter into them with trust that they will be treated ethically. It is when the client's best interests are potentially in conflict with one's own that the use of MI can become ethically problematic (Miller, 1994; Miller & Rollnick, 2002).

Investment

More specifically, the situation becomes ethically murky or manipulative when you have a personal investment in the outcome. The more you would benefit personally or institutionally from the client making one particular choice rather than another, the more inappropriate we believe it is to use MI to influence that choice. This scenario is usually termed "conflict of interest." Consider two examples.

- A clinician is conducting a clinical trial comparing different treatments for a health problem, each of which has potential benefits and risks. The trial is running behind in enrollment, and she encounters a patient who appears to be eligible. Her salary and professional reputation depend in part on her ability to enroll participants in the trial. She believes the treatments being tested are likely to help the patient. Should she use the evoking process of MI to encourage the person to sign the consent form and enroll?

- A counselor is employed as the intake worker for a private residential substance abuse treatment facility. A father calls concerned about his son's drug use. This particular program is quite expensive, and the father would need to take out a large loan in order to pay the cost, using his home as collateral. There are other less expensive treatment options available in the area. Should the counselor use MI to motivate the father to have his son admitted?

These are two clear examples of situations where, in our opinion, personal or institutional investment makes it inappropriate for a professional to use clinical strategies to influence client choice. We intend MI to be used when the practitioner has a lack of significant investment in the client's choice. What we have learned from MI research, however, is quite useful in knowing how *not* to influence choice, even inadvertently, in situations where neutrality is appropriate (see Chapter 17).

By "lack of significant investment" here we do not mean a lack of caring or compassion. Ideally, one always cares about clients' outcomes. Neither do we mean that one necessarily has no opinion about which course could be best for the client. By "investment" we mean a vested personal or institutional interest in the client's direction of choice; one particular choice that the client could make is significantly better *for the counselor or institution.* A counselor can be of the opinion that very different outcomes will result *for the client* from choosing one path versus another and may compassionately wish the best outcomes for the client, yet be disinterested from the perspective of any personal or institutional loss or gain. We find that differentiating three different types of counselor interest in client outcomes—compassion, opinion, and investment—is helpful in sorting out some of the ethical dilemmas that one encounters in relation to MI. These dilemmas are by no means unique to MI; they are important for any helping professional to ponder.

Personal investment can also be psychological or morally principled. A counselor who is recovering from the same problem being presented by a client may overidentify with the person (particularly if it is early in the counselor's own recovery process) and zealously promote particular choices. Professionals who equate client outcomes with their personal worth and competence are likely to be overinvested in the choices that their clients make. By virtue of deeply held moral convictions counselors may press for particular outcomes in consultations regarding unwanted pregnancy, domestic violence, or prenatal use of alcohol and other drugs. Investment can also arise by virtue of relationship. Family members are not disinterested parties; a client's choices and outcomes may affect them directly in many ways. It is for good reason that psychotherapists ordinarily avoid the entanglements of treating people with whom they have some other personal or professional relationship.

Coercive Power

There is variability from one counseling context to another in the degree of power that the counselor holds to influence client behavior and outcomes. At the low extreme, a counselor has just met the client and is offering only consultation with regard to the client's problems. There is always a power differential in counseling, of course, and the counselor will presumably be able to exert some beneficial influence over the client's behavior. If this were not so there would be little reason for the consultation. At the other extreme, consider an officer who works with offenders on parole and probation and who has the power at any time to revoke that status and order incarceration. A professional who holds such power must choose whether and when to use it to persuade the client to move in a desired direction.

The presence of coercive power does not in itself render MI inappropriate. Within a rehabilitative model of corrections, for example, probation officers have at least two roles: one as an agent of the state to protect public safety and another as an advocate for offenders, supporting and promoting positive change. Although these two roles can conflict with each other at times, they are often consistent: promoting positive change in clients increases public safety. MI can be a helpful tool within the client advocacy role. The realities of court contingencies are made clear, as is the officer's obligation to enforce them, and within these conditions they explore together what choices the offender can and will make. The probation officer cannot dictate the changes because of the offender's inherent autonomy to choose his or her own behavior. With MI, however, it is possible to influence those choices in a positive direction. The supportive, collaborative style of MI is in no way inconsistent with the officer's duty to protect public welfare. To the contrary, helping offenders change promotes public safety (McMurran, 2002, 2009).

The relationship becomes more ethically problematic if coercive power to affect the other's behavior and choice is combined with a personal investment in particular outcomes. Coercive power can be positive or negative, involving reward or punishment. Parents typically have coercive power as well as a personal investment in their children's outcomes. It is therefore very difficult for parents to maintain the disinterested (albeit caring) distance needed for the evoking process of MI. Recruiters may have substantial incentives to offer as well as a personal investment in enlistment rates. We believe that MI should not be used when such conflicts of interest are present.

Benefit

Finally, from the ethical principles of nonmaleficence and benevolence it follows that one should not use MI if it is unlikely to be beneficial or would cause harm. There is some evidence, for example, that MI can deter progress with clients in the "action stage" who have already decided to change (Project MATCH Research Group, 1997b; Rohsenow et al., 2004; Stotts, Schmitz, Rhoades, & Grabowski, 2001). This evidence emerged before we had differentiated the four processes of MI. If a client already has a clear goal and is prepared to pursue it, the objectives of the focusing and evoking processes have been accomplished and there is little obvious reason to spend time building motivation. In this situation one would go directly to the planning process after engaging sufficiently to form a working alliance. If ambivalence subsequently emerges, it's always possible to step back to refocusing or evoking.

ETHICS AND THE FOUR PROCESSES
OF MOTIVATIONAL INTERVIEWING

Our thinking on the ethics of MI has evolved with differentiation of four component processes. In several of the situations described above, it is not MI as a whole but rather particular processes that would be contraindicated.

As just discussed, when clients appear to be ready for change (whether they enter the office that way or reach that point through interviewing), further evoking is contraindicated and it is time for planning. Within a parental role, the engaging skills of good listening can be invaluable tools for communicating with one's children (Gordon, 1970). Helping children to focus is also a common process in parenting. The uneasy conflict of roles emerges with evoking—using strategic tools to try to steer a child's volition in a particular direction. We simply don't have the detachment (thank goodness!) to sit with our own children and dispassionately explore the pros and cons of their injecting drugs or engaging in criminal behavior.

The right ethical question, then, seems to regard the propriety of each of the component processes. Good listening is unlikely to do harm and may in itself promote positive change. Focusing is a process that involves the ethical navigation of goals. Evoking presupposes a chosen goal and strategically guides the person toward it. Evoking is rarely controversial when the identified goal is one that the client has brought. Ethical considerations arise when client and counselor aspirations differ. Finally, planning presupposes readiness to move forward (preparation or action stage within the transtheoretical model). There is a right time and a wrong time to engage in each of these four processes.

SOME ETHICAL GUIDELINES FOR THE PRACTICE OF MOTIVATIONAL INTERVIEWING

We conclude this chapter by offering some practical guidelines for the ethical practice of MI.

1. The use of MI component processes is inappropriate when available scientific evidence indicates that doing so would be ineffective or harmful for the client.
2. When you sense ethical discomfort or notice discord in your working relationship, clarify the person's aspirations and your own.
3. When your opinion as to what is in the person's best interest differs from what the person wants, reconsider and negotiate your agenda, making clear your own concerns and aspirations for the person.
4. The greater your personal investment in a particular client outcome, the more inappropriate it is to practice strategic evoking. It is clearly inappropriate when your personal investment may be dissonant with the client's best interests.
5. When coercive power is combined with a personal investment in the person's behavior and outcomes, the use of strategic evoking is inappropriate.

KEY POINTS

✓ An ethical issue within helping relationships is whether the clinician should encourage resolution of ambivalence in a particular direction.

✓ Ethical concerns arise particularly in situations where the clinician or institution has an aspiration for change that the client does not (yet) share.

✓ Four key ethical considerations in such situations include nonmaleficence, beneficence, autonomy, and justice.

✓ It is inappropriate to use MI to influence choice when the practitioner has a personal or institutional investment in a certain outcome, especially when this is combined with coercive power. This pertains in particular to the MI process of evoking.

✓ The use of particular processes in MI should be adapted to the client's needs; for example, evoking may be unnecessary or even detrimental with clients who have already decided to make a change.

CHAPTER 11

Exchanging Information

Unsolicited advice is the junk mail of life.
—BERN WILLIAMS

Advice is what we ask for when we already
know the answer but wish we didn't.
—ERICA JONG

It sounds simple enough: You've acquired knowledge in your area of expertise and you pass it along to your clients as needed. Yet how best to do this receives curiously little attention when practitioners learn their craft. It probably matters less how you do it in some simpler transactions, but when it comes to conversations about change, the exchange is more complex and calls for skillful practice.

The aim of this chapter is to clarify and illustrate good practice in those situations where information from you might help the client to make changes. This includes your own advice, which is a specific type of information. Offering information and advice is actually a two-way exchange of potentially rich complexity. Unless your client is absolutely silent during the process (which would be informative in itself), you are also receiving information to be considered and incorporated in the exchange.

It is easy to overestimate how much information and advice clients need to be given. To be sure, most clients expect you to have expertise to share with them. Yet they come with a wealth of relevant information themselves; no one knows them better than they do. How much do they already know? In general, it's unhelpful to give people information that they already have. What advice do they have for themselves? What have they

> It is easy to overestimate how much information and advice clients need.

already tried? It's not particularly helpful to suggest what they have already considered or tried.

We address this core skill here because providing information and advice can be called for early in consultation. With an engaging foundation (Part II), information exchange can be vital in finding a clear focus for your conversation and consultation (Part III). It also arises during evoking (Part IV), and is a central task in planning (Part V) where it often seems like the fuel that drives efforts to be helpful. So how is offering information and advice an integral part of MI?

This chapter begins with a concrete example that provides a foundation for considering some common traps and principles of good practice. It then turns to a broad framework to guide skillful practice (elicit–provide–elicit), followed by a discussion of how routine assessment can be improved. Finally, we address the tricky challenge of offering advice to people about change. Put simply, a respectful, thoughtful, and reciprocal flow of information that champions the client's own needs and autonomy can be a rich and life-changing experience and an integral part of MI. The one-way alternative to such a reciprocal flow you can probably do in your sleep: ask lots of expert questions and then tell the client what to do. The outcome of this approach can be a disengaged, frustrated, and unmotivated client.

SPOT THE DIFFERENCE

Consider these two brief exchanges with a mother who was found hyperventilating and obviously intoxicated one morning at the entrance to her children's school. She agreed to make an appointment to get some help, and what follows are two possible conversations during the initial meeting. Example A highlights some common pitfalls that may be familiar. The second conversation, Example B, illustrates expert information exchange consistent with MI.

Example A

CLIENT: I just feel so shaky in the morning that I have some wine before I leave the house.

INTERVIEWER: It sounds like you drink quite a bit. How much are you drinking these days?

CLIENT: Well, I'm not an alcoholic, if that's what you mean. It's just that I need it before I leave the house.

INTERVIEWER: How much would you say you drink on a typical day, even if it's just a guess?

CLIENT: Well, I don't know, maybe just a few glasses a day, sometimes more. I use it to calm my nerves, really.

INTERVIEWER: And how about on the weekends?

CLIENT: I'm lucky if I get to go out on Saturday evening, but I might have a few glasses on my own.

INTERVIEWER: So maybe six to eight glasses or more, pretty much every day?

CLIENT: Yes, I guess so. I haven't really thought about it.

INTERVIEWER: And how big a glass are you talking about?

CLIENT: Just a normal water glass.

INTERVIEWER: So maybe 8 ounces. Well, that's 50 to 60 glasses a week, maybe 7 to 8 gallons of wine. Do you also drink when you go to pick up your children in the afternoon?

CLIENT: When I am nervous, then I have some wine, but it's really not very much.

INTERVIEWER: I see. And how often does this happen when you are with the children?

CLIENT: Well, I don't always have wine before I go to get them, but you have no idea how terrified I get. It's just horrible.

INTERVIEWER: And did you have something to drink before you came out here today?

CLIENT: Maybe just a little more than usual.

INTERVIEWER: And when you drink wine, your nervousness decreases for a while. How long has that been happening?

CLIENT: I don't know. Maybe a year or two. Maybe longer.

INTERVIEWER: And what do your children think about your drinking?

CLIENT: They've never really said anything about it.

INTERVIEWER: Do you think that you have a problem with alcohol?

CLIENT: No, not really. It helps me relax and get to sleep.

INTERVIEWER: Well, I need to tell you something that's quite clear from what you've said. The amount that you're drinking is way above medically recommended limits, and far more than the vast majority of women your age drink. The shakiness sounds to me like you're physically addicted to alcohol. It's making your fears worse rather than better. You're putting your children in danger, and I think you need to quit drinking altogether. If you don't, this is just going to keep on getting worse.

CLIENT: Well, I don't agree.

Example B

CLIENT: I just feel so shaky in the morning that I have some wine before I leave the house.

INTERVIEWER: It helps to settle your nerves. [Reflection, continuing the paragraph]

CLIENT: And then I can shop, go get the kids from school and feed them.

INTERVIEWER: You have a busy life. [Reflection]

CLIENT: Yes, those kids keep me going for hours after that, you know: the food, playing, homework, getting them to bed, and they're not easy, shouting all the time.

INTERVIEWER: It sounds like you get quite a lot done in spite of feeling so stressed. [Affirming]

CLIENT: Yes, and a lot of the time I feel like I need a drink, to be honest! I just don't know where this is all going to end, and I feel so nervous all the time, like I'm suffocating.

INTERVIEWER: If we take a step back from it all for a moment, tell me what you already know about alcohol and how it affects people. [Elicit]

CLIENT: Well, it seems to settle me down to begin with, but then I get all shaky again, if you know what I mean.

INTERVIEWER: I think I do. It sounds like you've really thought about this, and you're not sure whether alcohol is making things worse or better. [Reflection]

CLIENT: Right. I mean, it definitely helps settle my nerves enough to get them off to school and I'm so relieved, but then I start feeling scared again.

INTERVIEWER: Something happens to you as the alcohol wears off that you don't like. [Reflection]

CLIENT: Exactly; it calms me down then knocks me over again. I don't like it.

INTERVIEWER: I wonder if I might tell you some things that I've noticed with other people who were struggling with alcohol. [Asking permission]

CLIENT: All right.

INTERVIEWER: [Provide:] When people drink to settle their nerves, the kind of shakiness that you're describing gradually gets worse over time. It feels like alcohol helps in the short run, but it actually causes the shaking and becomes a problem instead of a solution. It's a real trap because it feels like a terrible panic, and then alcohol calms you down for a little while. How does that sound to you? [Elicit]

CLIENT: Familiar. So are you telling me that the wine is making me more panicky?

INTERVIEWER: Yes, I think so. I know it may not feel that way, because it feels like a panic attack and alcohol helps immediately, but then it comes back to bite you. [Provide]

CLIENT: I've got to find a way to deal with this nervousness. I don't know how I'd get through the day.

INTERVIEWER: Alcohol has become that important to you. [Reflection]

CLIENT: But I can see I'm headed in the wrong direction. What else can I do?

Interviewer B's consultation took about the same amount of time as Interviewer A's, yet this time a focus seemed to emerge for the client much more clearly, along with greater openness to consider change. Both clinicians provided information, but something about the way Interviewer B did it was more helpful. Interviewer A mostly asked closed questions and then provided an uninvited judgment. Interviewer B offers plenty of reflective listening and uses a particular rhythm (elicit–provide–elicit, which we will describe shortly) to get across the same information in a way that the client is more likely to receive. This highlights some of the strengths and characteristics of information exchange when integrated into MI: expert information, in this case about alcohol withdrawal, enriches the client's efforts to make sense of her predicament and to express how and why she might change. She recognizes "I've got to find a way to deal with this nervousness" and instead of getting defensive she asks for advice. The focus for their conversation is quickly becoming clearer.

Consider the contrast between Examples A and B in relation to these questions in each scenario:

- Who is voicing the arguments for change?
- How do you imagine the practitioner is feeling?
- What do you think the client is feeling?
- Would you say that engagement is enhanced or diminished?
- Are they arriving at a common goal in this consultation?

The answers to these questions will inform the discussion that follows, which highlights both common traps and principles of good practice.

SOME COMMON TRAPS

If you were to ask Interviewer A about the role of expert information in the helping process, the following common assumptions might emerge:

1. *"I am the expert on why and how clients should change."* In falling into the "expert trap" Practitioner A is soon going to feel frustrated. Well-intentioned efforts by the practitioner to remedy the client's lack of knowledge and argue in favor of change (which we called the righting reflex in Chapter 1) are likely to be met with defensiveness ("I'm not an alcoholic" and "I don't agree") and a sense of not being understood ("You have no idea how terrified I get"). This practitioner might well label the client as "resistant," "in denial," and "unmotivated," when perhaps the ineffective use of a directing style is responsible for undermining engagement and progress. The client's frustration, fear, and defiant preservation of her self-worth are almost palpable. Ironically, chances are that this MI-inconsistent way of providing information and advice will have an effect opposite to what is intended.

2. *"I collect information about problems."* By asking mostly closed questions Interviewer A imposes a focus on the conversation: to assess the alcohol consumption and its impact, even to the point of ignoring other issues (e.g., panic). This gives rise to what we have called the question–answer trap, where repeated questioning leads to the accumulation of evidence, usually about the severity of a problem, with or without an implicit judgment about client weakness, resistance, lack of willpower, or ignorance. This accumulation of evidence tends to lead up to the delivery of a verdict ("The shakiness sounds to me like you're physically addicted to alcohol . . . and I think you need to quit drinking"), like the denouement of a detective novel. This may be appropriate for differential diagnosis in acute care medicine and is the stuff of television doctor dramas, but it's much less effective when the focus is behavior change.

Assessing and gathering information about the key elements of the client's predicament (alcohol, panic, children, etc.) can be done in an MI-consistent way that is less frustrating for the clinician and more useful to clients. Firing a series of questions might not only waste time and foster defensiveness (Carl Rogers once observed that clients already know all this information), but also miss important information and bypass the rich potential of a collaborative exchange that strengthens engagement and motivation to change.

3. *"I rectify gaps in knowledge."* It might well be concern or even fear of dereliction of duty that drives Interviewer A's gathering and dispensing of information about excessive alcohol consumption. This leads to a single-minded focus on fact gathering and little else, with a view to putting something right that is wrong within the client. At worst, and not uncommon in consulting rooms in health and social care, one can almost see the practitioner trying to lift the lid atop the client's head, fill it with information, and close the lid in the hope that something sinks in. There is a way to enrich knowledge without falling into this trap. Building on clients'

information interests and existing knowledge will enhance engagement and produce better outcomes.

4. *"Frightening information is helpful."* When it comes to sharing the outcome of the assessment, Interviewer A seems to assume that fear is a good motivator of change. So widespread is this scare tactic in care environments that if it were true, there would be little interest in or need for MI or any other approaches to motivate change. Warning about adverse outcomes may have a role, but it doesn't warrant the status of a default approach for promoting change. One would think that the horrible diseases and painful ways of dying that are associated with smoking would be sufficient to persuade people to give it up or not start in the first place. Sometimes it is enough, but so often it is not.

5. *"I need to just tell them clearly what to do."* Interviewer A's advice was clear enough: "I think you need to quit drinking altogether," but there is a strong chance that it won't be followed. Engagement is poor, both parties are feeling frustrated, and the hapless client is confronted with advice that leaves little room for autonomy. The purpose is not to deliver the advice, but rather to foster change. Skillful advising can be helpful in this regard, and that is the topic to which we now turn.

> The purpose is not to deliver the advice, but rather to foster change.

PRINCIPLES OF GOOD PRACTICE

If you were to ask Interviewer B about the MI-consistent exchange of information above, a rather different set of underlying assumptions might emerge that are almost mirror opposites to those behind Interviewer A's approach:

1. *"I have some expertise, and clients are the experts on themselves."* Interviewer B views information exchange as a collaborative search to understand the challenges, the client's strengths, and her information needs. Core skills described in Part I, including affirmation ("It sounds like you get quite a lot done in spite of feeling so stressed") and reflection ("You've really thought about this") are used to highlight her strengths. Engagement is thereby enhanced. Then Interviewer B takes time to find out what she already knew, asks permission to provide some information, does so, and encourages her to consider the implications herself. *Both* people are exchanging useful information in a common search for a focus.

2. *"I find out what information clients want and need."* Curiosity drives Interviewer B's efforts to understand the client's information needs ("Tell me what you already know about alcohol and how it affects people").

This not only averts telling clients what they already know, but has the added advantage of having clients themselves voice the reasons for change (the evoking process discussed in Part IV). Good reflective listening also elicited more information ("Something happens to you as the alcohol wears off that you don't like") and led to discussion not of specific quantity, but of withdrawal effects. This brief pinpointing process, narrowing down to the heart of her concern, provided a solid platform for expert information exchange.

3. *"I match information to client needs and strengths."* Having identified an information need, Interviewer B delivers the information gently with reference to "other people," leaving it the client to judge how this might apply to her ("How does that sound to you?"). The interviewer's goal was to empower the client to clarify the problem and seek a solution.

4. *"Clients can tell me what kind of information is helpful."* Interviewer B makes no assumption about the value (or lack thereof) of frightening information, but uses some good guiding and provides information that the client seems to want.

5. *"Advice that champions client needs and autonomy is helpful."* Interviewer B provided no direct advice so far, but now has an invitation to do so ("What else can I do?"). As described later in this chapter, it is possible to do so in a way that addresses clients' needs and enhances autonomy.

Box 11.1 highlights some of the differences between MI-consistent and MI-inconsistent information exchange.

BOX 11.1. MI-Consistent and MI-Inconsistent Assumptions Underlying Information Exchange

MI-inconsistent information exchange	MI-consistent information exchange
I am the expert on why and how clients should change.	I have some expertise, and clients are the experts on themselves.
I collect information about problems.	I find out what information clients want and need.
I rectify gaps in knowledge.	I match information to client needs and strengths.
Frightening information is helpful.	Clients can tell me what kind of information is helpful.
I just need to tell them clearly what to do.	Advice that champions client needs and autonomy can be helpful.

A SIMPLE STRATEGY
FOR INFORMATION EXCHANGE

An easily remembered approach for information exchange is EPE: elicit–provide–elicit (see Box 11.2). When using this approach, whatever meaty information you provide is sandwiched between two slices of wholesome asking. Although EPE suggests a linear progression, in reality it is often a more circular process accompanied by ample reflective listening. This is essentially what Interviewer B was doing in the example above.

Elicit

Elicit before providing information. There are three general functions that eliciting serves: asking permission, exploring clients' prior knowledge, and

---

BOX 11.2. Elicit–Provide–Elicit

	Tasks	In practice
ELICIT	• Ask permission. • Clarify information needs and gaps.	• *May I . . . ? or Would you like to know about . . . ?* • *What do you know about . . . ?* • *What would you like to know about?* • *Is there any information I can help you with?*
PROVIDE	• Prioritize. • Be clear. • Elicit–provide–elicit. • Support autonomy. • Don't prescribe the person's response.	• What does the person most want/need to know? • Avoid jargon; use everyday language. • Offer small amounts with time to reflect. • Acknowledge freedom to disagree or ignore. • Present what you know without interpreting its meaning for the client.
ELICIT	• Ask for the client's interpretation, understanding, or response.	• Ask open questions. • Reflect reactions that you see. • Allow time to process and respond to the information.

querying their interest in whatever information you may be able to provide. This initial question might have any of several forms:

- Asking permission
  - "Would it be all right if I tell you a few things that have worked for other people?"
  - "I wonder if there is anything on this list here that you might like to talk about."
  - "May I . . . ?"
  - "Would you like to know about . . . ?"
  - "What would you like to know about . . . ?"
- Exploring prior knowledge
  - "Tell me what you already know about the effects of high blood pressure on health."
  - "What do you think might be the biggest benefits for you of more regular exercise?"
- Querying interest
  - "What would you be most interested in knowing about treatment for this condition?"
  - "What have you been wondering about that I might be able to clarify for you?"

Why elicit first? Why not just charge into the information that you want to provide? Each of these three initial eliciting functions has a value of its own. Asking clients' permission to provide information is a respectful thing to do, and we believe it increases their willingness to hear what you have to say. Exploring prior knowledge prevents you from telling people what they already know and allows you to fill in any gaps. Querying interest lets you find out what the person would most like to know, which may be quite different from what you were planning to say. Providing information on what interests the person is likely to increase attention and receptiveness. If there is something else that you just *have* to tell the person, there's always a way to come back around to it, which we explain a bit later in this chapter. So eliciting helps you focus on what information is most important and probably increases the likelihood that clients will hear what you have to say.

What were the initial elicit components in Interviewer B's conversation above?

"Tell me what you already know about alcohol and how it affects people."
"I wonder if I might tell you some things that I've noticed with other people who were struggling with alcohol."

Asking Permission

There are at least three ways to obtain permission to provide information or advice. The first is when a client asks *you* for it:

"What do you think I should do?"
"How do people quit smoking?
"What kinds of treatment are available?"

Such client questions constitute permission for you to provide some information. This doesn't mean that you *must* provide the information. Sometimes we explore the client's own knowledge and ideas first before providing our own:

CLIENT: So how do people find a job in this area?

INTERVIEWER: Yes, I was just wondering what ideas you have about this—what has worked for you in the past, or for other people you know? How might you go about it?

Nor is it necessary to be coy and avoid giving information, as in this example:

CLIENT: So how do people find a job in this area?

INTERVIEWER: You're really wondering about that.

CLIENT: Yes.

INTERVIEWER: You're curious how people get jobs.

CLIENT: Yes, I am.

INTERVIEWER: And you wish someone could give you some ideas.

CLIENT: Yes! Do you have any?

INTERVIEWER: You'd like to know if I have any ideas.

When a client asks for information, it is a judgment call as to whether it's better to provide it right away or to explore the client's own experience first. Neither one is always the right approach.

A second way to proceed, when a client hasn't directly requested information, is to ask for permission to provide it:

"Would it be all right if I told you some things that have worked for other people?"
"What would you like to know about treatment options?"
"I could tell you a bit about managing depression if you're interested. May I?"
"We have a few minutes left in your appointment today, and I wonder if you'd be willing to talk a bit about your weight."

Given sufficient engagement in the context of a helping relationship, the person almost always says "Yes" in response to such a respectful request for permission.

But what if you feel ethically obliged to provide certain information or advice, and you would do so anyhow even if the client said "No" when you asked for permission? Here there is a third form of permission that doesn't directly ask for permission with a closed question, but uses autonomy-supportive language to acknowledge the person's right to agree or disagree, to accept your advice or not, to choose what to think and do. This autonomy cannot be taken away, so you might as well acknowledge it, and doing so again tends to increase receptiveness to the information. Some examples:

> "I don't know whether this will concern you. . . . "
> "See which of these you think might apply to you. . . . "
> "This may or may not interest you. . . . "
> "I wonder what you'll think about this."
> "You might disagree with this idea, and of course it's up to you."

Provide

A second step in the EPE cycle is to provide the information or advice. We focus here on providing information, and then later in this chapter we address giving advice. Here are some guidelines for providing information once you have permission to do so.

Prioritize: Focus on What the Person Most Wants or Needs to Know

As mentioned earlier a good general principle is not to tell people what they already know. That's why it's useful to find out what information the person already has and to ask what he or she would most like to know. Then you can fill in any gaps or misunderstandings. Give priority to what the person most wants or needs to know. Particularly when information is likely to evoke emotion, the heart of your message can get lost in extraneous details.

Present Information Clearly and in Manageable Doses

Provide information in language that the person can understand. It is easy to lapse into professional jargon that has become second nature, but that may confuse listeners. Explain information in what is everyday language for the listener.

Clarity also involves providing information in small doses, as when adding seasoning to a stew. Don't launch into a monologue; make sure the person is staying with you. The EPE cycle helps you to do this. Provide a bit of information, then check (elicit) to see whether the person understands or has any questions. When you have more than a small amount of information to present, the sequence is elicit–provide–elicit. For example:

INTERVIEWER: So this diagnosis is new for you. Tell me what you'd most like to know about this kind of diabetes. [Elicit]

CLIENT: Well, what's wrong with my body?

INTERVIEWER: Sugar is a basic fuel for our bodies, and it is broken down by an organ called the pancreas that makes insulin. [Provide] Have you heard of that? [Elicit]

CLIENT: Insulin—that's what diabetics have to take, right?

INTERVIEWER: Sometimes, yes. With diabetes there is a problem with insulin; either the pancreas is not supplying enough of it, or the supply is OK but the body is not able to use the insulin that's there. Either way, what happens is that too much sugar builds up in the bloodstream. [Provide] What more would you like to know about that? [Elicit]

CLIENT: Why is that a problem, too much fuel?

INTERVIEWER: Good question. For one thing, sugar makes the blood thicker and sticky, and your heart has to work harder to pump it. It's poor circulation that causes damage to your organs, your eyes, and your hands and feet if sugar levels in the blood stay high. [Provide] Does that make sense? What else can I tell you? [Elicit]

Use Autonomy-Supportive Language

When your information has implications for client change, then the way in which you preface and present it, the language that you use, and even your tone of voice can make a real difference in whether and how it is received. Your language can either support or undermine the person's autonomy.

What kind of counselor language undermines client autonomy? One type is talking down to clients in a parental manner. Another is giving advice without permission. A third is coercive language: telling people what they "must," "can't," "have to," or "have no choice about." Usually such a statement is false anyhow, and challenges the person to prove it wrong. The phenomenon of reactance has been well documented (Brehm & Brehm, 1981; Dillard & Shen, 2005; Karno & Longabaugh, 2005a, 2005b): that when one's freedom is threatened there is a natural tendency to reassert it. As discussed in Chapter 2, an alcohol-dependent person who is told "You can't drink" is actually quite capable of doing so. Similarly, a probation officer who says "You have to stay within city limits" is understating the person's autonomy. Usually what such statements mean is a probable consequence: "If you . . . then . . . ," but such consequences—even if swift, severe, and sure—do not remove a person's choice in the matter. It is better, we think, to acknowledge and discuss the choices that a person can make.

Consider a touchy situation in counseling with a parent who loses his temper with his children. You have a legal responsibility to report child abuse to the authorities when you learn about it, and also to inform your client in advance about this duty. How might you provide this information? Here's one example.

> "Now listen, the law is very clear here, and you have to understand it. If you ever tell me that you're harming your children, by which I mean that you are physically abusing them, it is my duty to report this to the authorities. This means that you will face a hearing and then decisions get made about what to do next. So you must keep that in mind when you're talking to me."

There is a distinctly parental, coercive, threatening feel to this speech. Notice the frequent "you" statements and the "must" and "have to" language. You just *can't* do that in counseling! (There—see what we mean?)

What would be a more collaborative, autonomy-honoring way of giving the same important information?

> "[Elicit:] There's something that I need to explain to you, and I wonder what you will think about it. [Provide:] As you know, our conversations are confidential, but there is an important exception in the law to protect children that requires me to report any child abuse to the authorities when I learn about it. Sometimes that results in a hearing. I want our work together to be helpful to you, and I also want to be sure you understand this responsibility I have. [Elicit:] I wonder how you think it might be best for us to proceed at this point. Perhaps you'll want to talk to your spouse or to me about this, and also I'll be glad to answer any questions you have about it. What do you think would be most helpful?"

The law is made equally clear here, but the tone is quite different. There is an EPE structure to it ("I wonder what you will think . . . ," "What do you think . . . ?"). The use of "you" is softer and there is more collaborative "our" language. The respectful, autonomy-honoring tone becomes a cocoon that surrounds the information you provide. As in all of MI, the effectiveness of your approach can be seen in how the person responds. You know you are doing well when the client continues discussing and asks you questions rather than becoming defensive.

Don't Prescribe the Client's Response

You can give information but you cannot predetermine how your client will respond to it. We recommend not telling clients how they ought to respond to or interpret the information you provide. Better to ask.

Elicit

By now the third step in elicit–provide–elicit is obvious. It is checking back in to inquire about the person's understanding, interpretation, or response to what you have said. In the EPE sequence this checking-in happens at regular intervals after each piece of information is provided. There are many different ways to word the "elicit" that comes after "provide":

"So what do you make of that?"
"Have I been clear so far?"
"You look puzzled."
"Does that make sense to you?"
"What else would you like to know?"
"What do you think about that?"
"How does that apply to you?"
"I wonder what all this means to you."
"How can I make this clearer for you?"
"Tell me in your own words what I've said."
"What do you think is a next step for you?"

Note also that this "elicit" component may take the form of reflective listening. Reflect what you see and hear in the client's reaction, including the nonverbal aspects such as facial expression. As with other reflections, it doesn't matter whether your initial guess as to what it means is wrong. The point is to provide space for the client to process and respond to the information that you provide.

THE CASE OF JULIA

Continuing the case example of Julia from the focusing discussion in Chapter 9, here is an example of how the EPE process might occur.

INTERVIEWER: You're really struggling to understand what is happening to you, and I wonder if I might ask you what you know about depression. [Elicit]

CLIENT: I guess it's like when you feel really sad and down, maybe don't have energy to do anything. Do you think that's what I have?

INTERVIEWER: Well, if it's all right, let me describe some of what people experience with depression, and you can tell me what parts of this may fit for you. [Asking permission]

CLIENT: Yes, OK.

INTERVIEWER: [Provide:] Depression is really a set of different symptoms, and you don't need to have all of them. You don't even have to feel particularly sad. It's like when people catch a cold, they experience it in different ways. Some cough or sneeze a lot, some get a fever, some people feel really tired. You might or might not have a sore throat or lose your voice. Depression is like that—a set of symptoms that might or might not be present. [Provide] Does that make sense? [Elicit]

CLIENT: Yeah. What are the symptoms?

INTERVIEWER: One of them, as you said, is a sad mood, feeling down, crying. And people often seem to lose interest in the things that they usually enjoy. [Provide]

CLIENT: That sounds like me. I'm not having much fun lately.

INTERVIEWER: All right. Another one is a change in sleeping patterns. Some people have trouble sleeping, and other people sleep a lot more than usual. And appetite can also change; some people gain weight and some lose it. Do you experience that? [Provide–Elicit]

CLIENT: I'm certainly not sleeping well, but my weight hasn't really changed. I think I'm eating about the same.

INTERVIEWER: OK. And as I said, different people have different symptoms. You mentioned having a hard time concentrating, and that's pretty common with depression. Feeling tired most of the time. How about feeling bad about yourself, feeling worthless or guilty?

CLIENT: Definitely. That's me.

INTERVIEWER: And one more thing is that people who are depressed sometimes find themselves thinking about death a lot, or of taking their own lives. What about that?

CLIENT: I don't really think about killing myself. I don't think I'd ever do that, but I do think about dying sometimes, that it would put me out of my misery. Cemeteries give me a creepy feeling lately.

INTERVIEWER: All right—well, those are the common symptoms of depression, and it sounds like you have quite a few of them. Have I been clear? What else can I tell you about depression? [Elicit]

CLIENT: It sounds like me. [Continued in Chapter 13]

THREE SPECIAL TOPICS

Now we turn to three special information exchange topics that commonly arise in practice: (1) advice, (2) counselor self-disclosure, and (3) assessment and feedback.

Offering Advice

Advice is, in a way, just a special type of information. It is conveying what you think and recommend a client should do. In this regard, all of the conditions pertaining to information exchange also apply when offering advice. Get permission first in one of the three ways described above. Be clear and specific, and offer any advice in small doses, checking in regularly on and listening to the client's reactions. Use autonomy-supportive language. Don't assume the person must or will follow your advice.

Yet advice has some additional aspects beyond merely conveying information. Advice has a *do* component, a recommendation about personal change. As such, it has increased potential to trigger reactance. The more emphatic or authoritarian the advice, the more likely it is to evoke a pushback. Most people simply don't like receiving unsolicited advice, although fewer mind giving it.

Solicited or not, advice also poses a risk for the interviewer of falling into the trap of being the expert arguing for change while the client argues against it. Consider this familiar scenario:

CLIENT: I'm just having so much trouble with my kids. They won't do what I tell them.

INTERVIEWER: Remember how we talked about using a time-out procedure . . .

CLIENT: I tried that, but they wouldn't stay in the time-out.

INTERVIEWER: You just put them in their room and close the door.

CLIENT: They love being in their room! That's where their toys and games are, and I don't want them to be spending more time in there. Besides, I can't see what they're doing if I close the door.

INTERVIEWER: Well, you can sit them in a chair facing into a blank corner—not for a long time, just for a short time-out. Then you can keep an eye on them but you're not reinforcing misbehavior.

CLIENT: You told me that before and I tried it, and they just keep turning around and talking.

Suddenly, even if this has been preceded by skillful MI, the interviewer has become the advocate for change who has to come up with the suggestions while the client knocks them down one by one. It is easy to fall into this suggest–refute cycle. The process of developing a change plan is discussed in more detail in Part V. For now, we provide some specific recommendations when offering advice.

Engage First

Advice is more likely to be received well when there is a solid foundation of engagement. When you have a good working alliance with a client, advice can also convey compassion, respect, and hope.

Use Sparingly

Giving advice is not a mainstay in MI, which relies on evoking solutions from clients rather than providing them. Our sense is that advice and a directing style are overused in many service settings. In terms of timing, beware of the righting reflex to offer an immediate solution, and instead really listen to clients. When you do offer advice, pay attention to how your client responds. A glazed-over passive look, defensiveness, or an explanation of why your advice won't work (sustain talk) is a likely sign that you have missed the mark.

Ask Permission

If the client hasn't invited you to provide advice, ask permission before doing so.

Emphasize Personal Choice

Even when clients do ask what you think they should do, it is wise to acknowledge autonomy or even ask for permission again.

CLIENT: Well what do you think I should do?

INTERVIEWER: I could suggest some things that have worked for other people, but the most important thing is to find what will work for you, and you're the best judge of that. Would you like to hear some ideas?

Here are some examples of autonomy-supportive language that can be used in tandem with advice:

"It's really *up to you*, but I can describe some options."
"This advice *may not be right for you.*"

"I don't know *whether this will make sense* to you . . . "
"You *might or might not agree* with my ideas . . . "
"*I can't tell you what to do*, but I can tell you what some other people have done."
"Something you *could try if you wish* is . . . "

In essence, you are giving people permission to disregard your advice, which of course is always their prerogative whether or not you say it. Acknowledging this freedom has the paradoxical effect of making it more likely that the person will listen to and heed the advice.

Offer a Menu of Options

One specific way to avoid the suggest–refute cycle is to provide a variety of options rather than suggesting them one at a time. Making one suggestion (as in the parenting example above) seems to invite sustain talk. A menu of possibilities prompts a different mind-set: Which of these options might be best? Rather than coming up with objections to a single suggestion, the client's task is to consider a range of possibilities and choose among them. When people perceive that they have freely chosen a course of action from among alternatives, they are more likely to commit to and follow through with it.

In summary, suggested advice can be consistent with MI when used sparingly with permission, giving priority to evoking clients' own solutions and recognizing their autonomy to choose among options.

Self-Disclosure

We have not previously addressed the role of counselor self-disclosure in MI. Within client-centered counseling, Rogers (1959, 1965) emphasized "genuineness" or "congruence" as a crucial precondition for change that counselors should provide. He later defined it as "when my experiencing of this moment is present in my awareness and when what is present in my awareness is present in my communication" (Rogers, 1980b, p. 15). In other words, as with the elements of MI spirit described in Chapter 2, there are two levels to genuineness: awareness and expression. At the awareness level, Rogers advocated being attuned to your own reactions, to what is going on in your own experiencing while working with clients. At the expression level, genuineness involves communicating this to your client.

Notice that what Rogers was describing is quite different from telling clients stories from your past. The term "self-disclosure" might suggest telling clients about personal experiences you have had in your own life that seem related to their situation. Rogers was talking about being aware of and relating what you are experiencing in the moment as you talk with clients.

We certainly don't advocate saying to clients everything that comes into your mind during a consultation, and no clinician whom we know does so. MI focuses on the client's experiencing and welfare, not on the counselor's. It is not necessary or helpful to say everything that occurs to you during counseling. Neither do we support the opposite extreme to which Rogers was reacting, of seeking to remain aloof and to reveal nothing of yourself. In classic psychoanalysis the therapist literally sat behind the reclining client so that even nonverbal cues could be concealed (Viscott, 1972).

Between these two extremes is a balance of being willing to share something of yourself when it seems likely to help. How, then, do you decide what to disclose of your own experiences, either from the past or present? Here are some tests.

Is It True?

To be genuine, what you convey about your own experience should be the truth (though not necessarily the whole truth). Although it's possible to make up a story about one's past or present experience, we don't recommend doing so. Furthermore, denying what you are actually experiencing ("No, no, really—it doesn't make me uncomfortable. I'm not disapproving") is likely to be apparent to clients at some level.

Could It Be Harmful?

Within the precept of "First, do no harm," another test is whether a self-disclosure could be harmful. High on this list is criticism (Simon, 1978), commenting adversely on clients' abilities, intentions, efforts, appearance, and so on.

Is There a Clear Reason Why It Would Be Helpful?

In close friendships, self-disclosure is routine and mutual. In professional helping relationships, however, we believe there should be a specific reason for self-disclosure. There is a difference between judicious self-disclosure (with an appropriate level of detail, keeping focus on the client) and excessive self-disclosure that shifts the focus to the counselor (Rachman, 1990). Before describing your own present or past experiences, ask yourself why you believe it would be helpful. Here are some possibilities:

- To promote trust and engagement (Cozby, 1973).
- To model openness and encourage reciprocity of disclosure (Sullivan, 1970).

- To answer a client question ("Do you have children?"; "Have you ever felt like this?").
- To affirm; affirmations are a form of self-disclosure, a genuine in-the-moment appreciation of the client's nature or actions.

Routine Assessment and Feedback

Practicalities of Initial Assessment

Routine assessment takes many forms, from lengthy formal interviews to a few standard questions within a consultation. It tends to be given priority in the consultation and often involves a one-way gathering of information that is useful to the program or practitioner.[1] It is worth considering how clients are likely to respond to a barrage of assessment as their first experience with a service. It is unlikely to promote engagement, and some clients respond by becoming passive and not returning for further service.

Given that MI has been reported to improve client retention in a variety of settings (e.g., Grote, Swartz, & Zuckoff, 2008; Heffner et al., 2010; Klag, O'Callaghan, Creed, & Zimmer-Gembeck, 2009; McMurran, 2009; Secades-Villa, Fernánde-Hermida, & Arnáez-Montaraz, 2004; Sinclair et al., 2010; Wulfert, Blanchard, Freidenberg, & Martell, 2006), it is possible that integrating MI with initial assessment may serve both program and client needs. We recommend preceding assessment with at least 10 minutes of MI. It's as simple as starting with an open question followed by reflective listening:

> "There are a number of questions that I will need to ask you after a while, but first I would just like to know what brings you here today and how you hope we might be able to help you."

This also implies that intake interviews ought not be a clerical task, but should be done by a skillful clinician. Intake assessment is the beginning of engagement and treatment, and it deserves the attention of an experienced professional.

We also encourage gathering the minimal amount of information that will be needed for focusing and for any reporting requirements. In behavioral health services, intake assessment sometimes grows to require one or more long sessions in itself. The content of such assessment may be mandated by someone quite distant from everyday practice. How much information is really essential? Could some of it be completed by the client on

---

[1] One of us met an addiction counselor working in a prison whose job it was to encourage enrollment in treatment of people newly arrested for drunk driving offenses. His average contact time was 20 minutes, and his assessment schedule was 17 pages long. Someone had lost sight of a helpful horizon for the practitioner and client!

a clipboard in the waiting room, or at home between sessions? Can some of it wait until later? Assessment that jeopardizes client engagement can be wasted effort. An impressive function of a good manager is working with staff to clarify how and when essential service data can be collected in order to enhance client engagement. Usually there is room for flexibility. In an addiction treatment program that one of us directed, we found that the absolutely necessary questions in an initial visit required about 20 minutes to ask. We assigned our most experienced counselors to do these intake interviews, beginning with 30 minutes of open-ended MI before starting assessment. The counselors found, incidentally, that by the time they got to the assessment they already knew most of the needed information. The counselors also thought clients were being much more honest, and the percentage of clients who dropped out after assessment decreased substantially.

Sharing the Outcome of Assessment

All too often, initial assessment information is filed away without being of much use to clients or even to treatment staff. How might the information that you have gathered be used to enhance client engagement and motivation for change?

This was actually one of the first experimental applications of MI, the "drinker's check-up" (Miller & Sovereign, 1989; Miller, Sovereign, & Krege, 1988) that eventually developed into motivational enhancement therapy (MET; Miller, Zweben, Diclemente, & Rychtarik, 1992; Project MATCH Research Group, 1993). The central ingredient, which actually provided the inspiration for the EPE framework, was how the counselor shares information about the findings and then uses open questions and listening to evoke the client's personal responses. In essence, the counselor does not tell clients what they should make of the findings but rather elicits their own interpretation and concerns. It is a Socratic way of presenting information in order to help clients reach their own conclusions and motivation for change. This check-up format has been adapted for marijuana use (Swan et al., 2008), recovery management (Rush, Dennis, Scott, Castel, & Funk, 2008; Scott & Dennis, 2009), classroom management (Reinke et al., 2011), marital (Morrill et al., 2011) and family interventions (Slavet et al., 2005; Uebelacker, Hecht, & Miller, 2006), and domestic violence (Roffman, Edleson, Neighbors, Mbilinyi, & Walker, 2008).

This process might be as simple as asking an open question when initial assessment is done, following with reflections and listening for change talk.

"Well, that's all I need to ask about today. Thanks for all this information. Before we move on, what was there that struck you while we were talking, or what are you wondering about? [Better to ask it this way rather than as a closed yes/no question like 'Is there anything you're wondering about?' which is more likely to elicit a 'No' response.]"

MET, however, involves evoking the client's own responses along the way in an EPE fashion, accumulating change talk to be reflected and summarized. When information is presented in this way, clients often reach the same conclusion that the interviewer might have advocated. The difference, of course, is that they have reached the conclusions in their own way and time.

In summary, we caution against imposing assessment as a one-way information collection task that leaves the client in a passive role. Although some information can be needed for practical or administrative purposes, unilateral fact gathering can be quite disengaging from the client's perspective. There is also a risk of communicating, "Once we have enough information, then we will have the answer for you." When client change is the desired outcome, an expert-driven, information-in, answer-out model is seldom effective. Assessment, therefore, is best kept to a necessary minimum and integrated in the service of the larger task of facilitating change.

A CALL FOR ARTFULNESS

This chapter is a call to reverse a pattern that is widespread across care settings of all kinds: the large-scale absorption of data from clients and the delivery of facts to them, bereft of the very human qualities that can bring this process alive. Artless information exchange will produce nonresponsive clients. The core skills of MI, within a framework like EPE, offer the promise of turning information exchange into an artful activity in which your time is used efficiently to merge the information with your client's aspirations. In this sense, it's a subject that deserves elevation in research, the training of practitioners, and meetings with clients.

KEY POINTS

✓ Within MI, information and advice are offered with client permission.

✓ Elicit–provide–elicit is a sequence for information exchange that honors the client's expertise and autonomy.

✓ Regarding advice: engage first, use sparingly, emphasize personal choice, and offer a menu of options.

✓ Self-disclosure involves a willingness to share something of yourself that is true when there is good reason to expect that it will help and not harm the client.

✓ Any necessary assessment should be done in a context that promotes engagement and makes the process useful to the client as well as to the clinician and system.

PART IV

EVOKING
Preparation for Change

With a working relationship under way and a clear focus established, the stage is set for the third process of evoking and strengthening motivation for change. The engaging and focusing processes are common to many therapeutic endeavors, and it is in the process of evoking that counseling becomes distinctly MI. Component skills here include recognizing change talk when you hear it and knowing how to evoke and respond to it when it occurs. Skillful MI significantly strengthens client change talk, which in turn predicts subsequent change. This is a primary focus of Part IV.

We also address in Part IV how to recognize and respond to sustain talk and to signs of discord in the working alliance (Chapter 15). Hope is widely acknowledged to be an important client factor in change, and there is an MI-consistent style for evoking and strengthening it (Chapter 16). With this background in place, we return in Chapter 17 to the topic of how to counsel with neutrality when you do *not* want to influence a client's direction of choice. In the concluding chapter of this section (Chapter 18) we consider how to evoke motivation for change with clients in "precontemplation," to develop ambivalence when it seems to be absent.

CHAPTER 12

Ambivalence
Change Talk and Sustain Talk

Ambivalence is a wonderful tune to dance to. It has
a rhythm all its own.
—ERICA JONG

I was born condemned to be one of those who has
to see all sides of a question. When you're damned
like that, the questions multiply for you until in the
end it's all questions and no answer.
—EUGENE O'NEILL

Ambivalence is a normal step on the road to change. It is, in fact, progress from an earlier state (termed "precontemplation" in the transtheoretical model) of perceiving no reason at all for change. Ambivalence involves simultaneous conflicting motivations and can thus be an uncomfortable place to be. Think of the emotional turmoil of being "torn between two lovers" or of desperately wanting something that you also know is bound to have regrettable consequences. The sheer discomfort of being suspended in such tension can itself be enough to propel one into change.

Yet ambivalence can also be a sticky place where one may remain suspended for a long time. The dynamics of conflict make this dilemma understandable. Conceptually, ambivalent conflict comes in four different varieties (see Box 12.1). All of them involve being simultaneously pushed or pulled in at least two opposite directions. The more you move toward one choice, the clearer its disadvantages become, and the more its opposite appeals. The discomfort of conscious ambivalence can lead one to stop thinking about it or to resolve that the status quo really isn't all that bad after all, or at least that there's nothing that can be done about it. That, of course, perpetuates the status quo.

157

BOX 12.1. Four Flavors of Ambivalence

Approach/Approach   X ⇐ ☺ ⇒ Y

Here the person is torn between positive choices. It is the candy store problem: which of attractive alternatives to choose. Thinking about or moving in the direction of one (X) seems to accentuate the attractiveness of the other (Y) and vice versa. This is, however, the least stressful type of ambivalence, because it's a win–win choice and either way you choose, the outcome is good. Of course there can still be post-decisional regret: "But what if I had chosen the other . . . ?"

Avoidance/Avoidance   X ⇐ ☹ ⇒ Y

Here the choice is between two unpleasant alternatives. It is the choice of the "lesser of two evils," being caught "between a rock and a hard place," or "between the devil and the deep blue sea." Leaning toward one choice (X) accentuates its unpleasantness, but moving away from X means moving closer to Y and contemplating its disadvantages.

Approach/Avoidance   ☺ ⇔ X

In this type of conflict only one possible choice is being considered, and it has both significant positive and important negative aspects. It is well captured in Billy Ray Cyrus's lyric, "I'm so miserable without you, it's almost like you're here." Moving toward X makes the negative more apparent, but moving away from X accentuates the positive.

Double Approach/Avoidance   X ⇔ ☺ ⇔ Y

The double approach/avoidance conflict is generally acknowledged to be the most vexing of all types. Here there are two options, X and Y, each of which has both powerful positive and important negative aspects. Leaning toward X makes the negative aspects of X more salient while enhancing longing for Y. Moving toward Y, however, makes Y's shortcomings more apparent while making X seem more attractive.

Contemplating change involves self-talk, thinking about the pros and cons of available alternatives. This talk can happen aloud and interpersonally, and that is the context of MI. When people are ambivalent they normally express both pro-change and counter-change arguments. Ambivalence means that they have both motivations within them simultaneously. As discussed in Chapter 2, if someone else voices an argument *for* change, people are likely to respond by expressing a counter-change argument from the other side of their ambivalence. By continuing to express the arguments against change, people can literally talk themselves out of changing. Similarly, people can talk themselves into change by continuing to voice pro-change arguments.

CHANGE TALK

In the first edition of this book we described such pro-change arguments as "self-motivational statements." In the second edition we substituted the term "change talk" to refer to any speech that favors change. That is still the overall definition of change talk—any self-expressed language that is an argument for change.

> Change talk is any self-expressed language that is an argument for change.

Subsequently we had the good fortune of meeting and collaborating with Paul Amrhein, a psycholinguist specializing in the language of motivation and commitment. He had been studying the language by which people in natural conversation ask for and commit to certain actions. Knowing how to read these signals is an important social skill. For example, suppose a student asks a professor to review a draft manuscript and give her comments. She will pay close attention to what the professor says in response to the request, because it contains information about the likelihood of receiving comments any time soon. Consider these replies that the professor might give:

> "I'm sorry. I'd like to, but I'm really very busy."
> "I'll try to get to it."
> "I might be able to read it next week."
> "I promise I'll have it for you in the morning."

The social signals in these replies vary from very low to very high commitment. One thing Amrhein had noticed in his observations is that negotiations didn't go well when the requester's language contained a level of demand that was higher than the other's level of willingness. We had noticed the same thing in counseling sessions and medical consultations, and had been advising clinicians to work with people at their current level of motivation and not get ahead of their clients' readiness for change.

Encountering our concept of change talk, Amrhein observed that we were mixing together quite a few different kinds of speech acts, and it might be helpful to differentiate them. Four of the subtypes that he suggested we now refer to as examples of *preparatory change talk*: desire, ability, reasons, and need.

Preparatory Change Talk

Desire

Desire is a semantic universal: Every language on the face of the earth contains words signaling that one wants something (Goddard & Wierzbicka, 1994). Such language often appears in conversations about change.

> "I *want* to lose some weight."
> "I *would like* to get a better job."
> "I *wish* I were more comfortable around people."
> "I *hope* to get better grades next year."

Wanting is one component of motivation for change. It helps to really want the change, although it's not essential. People can still do things even though they don't want to.

Ability

A second component of motivation is the person's self-perceived ability to achieve it. People won't build up much motivation for change if they believe it is impossible for them. "I'd like to run a marathon [desire] but I don't think I could ever do it [ability]." This language turns up in conversations about change: "I can" or "I am able to." It also appears in hypothetical-subjunctive form when a person feels able to make a change but may not be committed to doing it: "I could . . . " or "I would be able to . . . " Ability language only signals that the change seems possible.

Reasons

A third speech act that Amrhein identified is the statement of a specific reason for change. In talking about reasons for beginning a program of physical exercise, someone might say:

> "I would probably have more energy."
> "I might sleep better at night."
> "It would help me control my diabetes."
> "I'd be more attractive and get more dates."
> "I want to be around to see my grandchildren."

Stating such reasons does not imply either ability or desire. Even though there are good reasons to make a change, a person may not want to or may feel incapable of doing it. A decisional balance exercise (see Chapter 17) typically involves compiling specific reasons for and against a change.

These statements have an implicit "if . . . then" structure: If I exercised regularly, then I would be more attractive.

Need

A fourth component of motivation is reflected in imperative language that stresses the general importance or urgency of change. Need statements don't say specifically why change is important (otherwise, it would probably be a reason).

> "I need to . . . "
> "I have to . . . "
> "I must . . . "
> "I've got to . . . "
> "I can't keep on like this."
> "Something has to change."

Once again, such imperative language does not imply desire or ability to change. If you inquire a bit further upon hearing such language, you can probably learn specific reasons behind the imperative, but in themselves these statements do not say why the person must, needs to, or has to change.

These first four types of speech in English can be remembered by the acronym DARN: Desire, Ability, Reasons, and Need. We refer to them as preparatory change talk because none of them, alone or together, indicate that change is going to happen. To say, "I *want* to lose weight" (desire) is not the same as "I *will* lose weight." Saying that one *can* or *could* quit drinking (ability) is not a commitment to quitting. Listing good *reasons* for making a change does not necessarily mean that one actually intends to do it, and even saying "I *have* to" (need) is not the same as "I'm going to." None of these in themselves constitute what we now refer to as mobilizing change talk.

Mobilizing Change Talk

Whereas preparatory change talk reflects the pro-change side of ambivalence, mobilizing change talk signals movement toward resolution of the ambivalence in favor of change. The clearest example of this is commitment language.

Commitment

To say that one must, can, wants to, or has good reasons to change is not to say that one will. Committing language signals the likelihood of action.

The professor and student example earlier in this chapter was about commitment language. It's what all of us listen carefully for when asking someone to do something for us. Is it going to happen?

Commitment language is what people use to make promises to each other. Contracts are written in commitment language. So are marriage vows. In American courts, someone who is about to give testimony is "sworn in" by asking, "Will you tell the truth, the whole truth, and nothing but the truth?" Imagine answering this question by saying:

> To say that one must, can, wants to, or has good reasons to change is not to say that one will.

"I want to."
"I could."
"I have good reasons to."
or
"I need to."

None of these would be a satisfactory answer in court.[1] Why? Because none of them actually says that the person really *will* tell the truth. None of them makes a commitment.

Commitment language can take many forms. Perhaps the clearest is "I will." Emphatic versions include "I promise," "I swear," and "I guarantee." "I give you my word" is a classic way of doing this. "I intend to" reflects a decision to do it, perhaps with a little shade of doubt.

Activation

Then there are words that indicate movement toward action, yet aren't quite a commitment to do it. Such language does not constitute a binding contract, but does signal that the person is leaning in the direction of action.

"I'm willing to . . . "
"I am ready to . . . "
"I am prepared to . . . "

These wouldn't quite be an acceptable answer when a person is asked, "Do you promise to . . . ?" Activation language is "almost there" and implies a commitment without actually stating it. When one receives an answer like this in everyday conversation, the natural next step is to ask for more specifics: When will you do it? What exactly are you prepared to do?

---

[1] We thank Theresa Moyers for this teaching example.

Taking Steps

A third kind of activation language became apparent in listening for change talk in therapy sessions. Taking steps is a form of speech indicating that the person has already done something in the direction of change. This might occur, for example, when people report that since their last consultation they have taken some specific action toward the change goal:

> "I bought some running shoes so I can exercise."
> "This week I didn't snack in the evening."
> "I went to a support group meeting."
> "I called three places about possible jobs."

Someone who, for example, attended an AA meeting is not necessarily making a commitment to quit drinking, but it's a step in that direction.

A mnemonic in English for these types of mobilizing change talk is CATs: Commitment, Activation, and Taking steps. DARN and CATs are not all of the possible forms of change talk, just common examples. The key is to listen for language that signals movement toward change.

TWO SIDES OF THE HILL

Don't be unnecessarily concerned with classifying the change talk you hear. The important thing is to recognize it. Just by virtue of being social animals people already have an intuitive sense of how this works. As another metaphor we suggest that change talk is a bit like walking up one side of a hill and down the other. The uphill side represents preparatory change talk (like DARN), and the downhill side is mobilizing change talk (like CATs). One thing to ask yourself during a consultation is where you are on the hill. For both client and interviewer the process of evoking preparatory change talk can indeed feel like an uphill slog, an effortful and strategic step-by-step climb up the slippery slopes of ambivalence. As preparatory change talk strengthens you are likely to begin hearing mobilizing change talk, and eventually the process feels more like a downhill journey. There are still hazards on the way down, of course, and it takes skill not to stumble or get ahead of your client. On the downhill slope clients can also become anxious and have doubts if they feel like they are moving too fast. We discuss the downhill slope in Part V, on the planning process. Note the suggested parallel in Box 12.2 between the progression of change talk and the stages of readiness that are described in Prochaska and DiClemente's (1984) transtheoretical model of change.

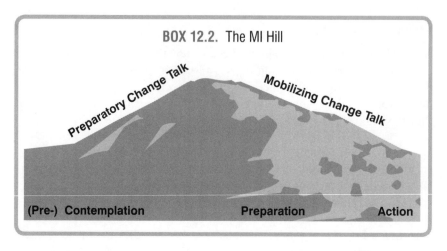

SUSTAIN TALK

Any speech that can be uttered on behalf of change can also be spoken as an equal and opposite reaction on behalf of the status quo. In ambivalence, both arguments are represented in the client's internal committee mentioned in Chapter 1. Using the DARN CATs categories described above, here are some examples of sustain talk:

Desire

"I just love smoking and how it makes me feel."
"I don't want to exercise."
"I'd like to eat whatever I want whenever I want."

Ability

"I've tried, and I don't think I can quit smoking."
"I think my health will be just fine without exercising."
"I can manage on my own without any help."

Reasons

"Smoking helps me to relax."
"I just don't have time to fit in any exercise."
"If I try to lose weight I just gain it back again."

Need

"I have to smoke; I can't get through the day without it."
"I've got to focus my time and energy on other things."
"I just need to accept that this is how I am."

Commitment

"I'm going to keep on smoking."
"I'm just not going to exercise, and that's final."
"I've had it with diets—no more!"

Activation

"I'm prepared to accept the risks of smoking."
"I'm just not ready to consider exercising."
"I'm not willing to do what it takes."

Taking Steps

"I went back to smoking this week."
"I returned those running shoes that I bought."
"I burned the diet sheets that you gave me."

Sustain talk and change talk are conceptually opposite—the person's arguments against and for change—and they predict different outcomes. A predominance of sustain talk or an equal mix of change and sustain talk is associated with maintenance of the status quo, whereas a predominance of change talk predicts subsequent behavior change (Moyers, Martin, Houck, Christopher, & Tonigan, 2009). There is also preliminary evidence for different neural substrates of these two types of speech. In a neuroimaging study, spontaneous sustain talk about drinking was associated with the activation of several key reward (dopaminergic) pathways, whereas spontaneous change talk was not (Feldstein Ewing, Filbey, Sabbineni, Chandler, & Hutchinson, 2011). That is, when expressing sustain talk people may be activating appetitive channels that could be expected to favor continued drinking. Patterns of neural activation are also differentially affected by collaborative versus discordant relational styles (Boyatzis et al., 2012).

> Sustain talk and change talk are conceptually opposite—the person's arguments against and for change.

THE FOREST OF AMBIVALENCE

As discussed in Chapter 1, it is normal to hear change talk and sustain talk intertwined, often within the same sentences. This is the very nature of ambivalence. Both motivations are represented simultaneously on the internal committee.

"I love Christine. At least I think I do. I miss her when I'm not with her and I think about her all the time, but then I think about other women, too. I like being with her, but she's also so jealous that I feel trapped sometimes. I don't know what to do. I want to be with her, but she makes me crazy."

The internal struggle can be a tiring debate with point triggering counterpoint. Beyond the logical arguments, ambivalence can involve passionate emotion as well. Choices about specific behavior may be linked to deeper issues of meaning and identity. Quitting smoking is different from becoming a nonsmoker. Defense of illicit drug use may represent a reluctance to give up the rebellious freedom of adolescence.

How can you help someone out of this morass? When trying to find one's way out of a deep forest, there is a danger of wandering in circles and coming back to the same spot. To avoid this, one needs to keep moving in a straight line. Lacking a compass, a scouting trick is to sight three trees in a straight line: one close at hand, another some length away, and a third off in the distance. One walks from the first tree to the second, keeping the third tree in line of sight. Then, while approaching the second tree one looks past it and the third tree again, spotting a fourth tree in the distance that lies in the same straight line. In this way it is possible to keep moving ahead on a straight path even though one is unable to see past the forest.

The process of MI is like that. Whereas people left to their own devices may think in circles and keep coming back to the same stuck point, MI helps them to keep moving from tree to tree until at last they find their way out of the forest.

KEY POINTS

✓ Ambivalence, the simultaneous presence of conflicting motivations, is a normal human process on the path to change.

✓ In natural language, ambivalence is reflected in a mixture of change talk and sustain talk.

✓ *Preparatory* change talk (e.g., desire, ability, reasons, and need) tends to precede *mobilizing* change talk (e.g., commitment, activation, and taking steps).

✓ The evoking process is intended to help resolve ambivalence in the direction of change.

CHAPTER 13

Evoking the Person's Own Motivation

> It is the truth we ourselves speak rather than
> the treatment we receive that heals us.
> —O. HOBART MOWRER

> A word is dead when it is said, some say.
> I say it just begins to live that day.
> —EMILY DICKINSON

TALKING ONESELF INTO CHANGE

The process of change that occurs in MI is not a unique one. It is how people normally proceed toward change. A period of ambivalence (contemplation) resolves through a tipping of the balance in favor of change. The perceived advantages of changing (pros) begin to outweigh the disadvantages (cons). Sometimes there is a discrete "aha" moment when this occurs, but most often it is a gradual process, moving forward and back. What MI helps people do is to keep moving forward through the forest, through the natural process of resolving ambivalence.

In particular this process occurs in MI by literally talking oneself into change. People tend to become more committed to what they hear themselves saying. Usually ambivalence is debated by the internal committee in a silent thought process that is easily derailed. Among others, Benjamin Franklin advocated listing in writing the reasons for and against as a way of more systematically thinking through

> MI helps people to keep moving forward through the natural process of resolving ambivalence.

a possible change. If one voices the pros and cons equally, however, the expected outcome would be continued ambivalence. MI helps people get out of the forest by continuing to move through language in the direction of change.

There is also something important about speaking one's motivations aloud in the presence of another person. Consider the subjective differences in making a statement like "I am going to go running today" or "I forgive my father" in these ways:

- Thinking it silently to oneself
- Writing it down
- Looking in a mirror while alone and saying the words aloud
- Saying the words to someone else

The interpersonal context also matters. A coercive context can compromise honesty, but when this voicing of one's own motivations occurs within an accepting, affirming, listening, and nonjudgmental relationship it can have particular impact. That is why in MI we pay special attention to evoking and exploring change talk.

This is not to say that one should ignore sustain talk. To do so would violate the spirit of acceptance. When it occurs, sustain talk is listened to, respected, often reflected, and included in the larger picture (see Chapter 15). In MI, however, there is an intentional arranging of the conversation to evoke and explore change talk in particular. A first step is to recognize change talk when you hear it (Chapter 12). In this chapter we discuss strategies for evoking change talk, making it more likely to occur.

In other words, you can substantially influence how much change talk your clients will voice. The frequency and strength of change talk normally increase over the course of an MI session. When we gave the first MI session tapes to psycholinguist Paul Amrhein to analyze, he assumed he was listening to actors rather than actual clients. Why? Because, he said, this amount of increase in commitment language (see Chapter 21) simply does not occur in so short a time within natural conversation. He thought that we had scripted the sessions to represent an ideal scenario. In analyzing a large number of MI sessions, however, he found that this was the normal progression. Box 13.1 shows the increase that he observed in 61 MI interviews with clients who subsequently abstained from illicit drugs (Amrhein et al., 2003). Each point on the horizontal axis represents about 5 minutes (one-tenth) of the session. At the beginning of these sessions the clients, who were entering addiction treatment, on average were expressing commitment to continue using drugs (values lower than zero, which is neutrality). By the end of the session they were voicing stronger commitment to abstain. The slope of the line—the amount of increase in change talk

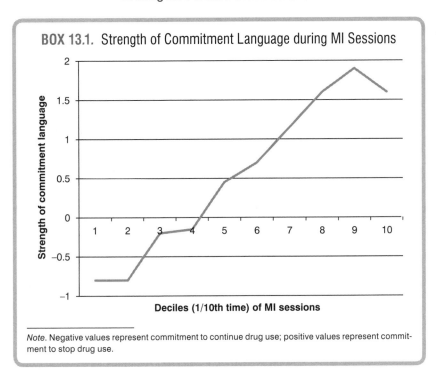

BOX 13.1. Strength of Commitment Language during MI Sessions

Deciles (1/10th time) of MI sessions

Note. Negative values represent commitment to continue drug use; positive values represent commitment to stop drug use.

during the MI session—presaged successful abstinence. In other words, MI produced an unusual shift in change talk that in turn predicted subsequent behavior change.

If such an increase in change talk occurs in naturalistic MI sessions, is it actually caused by something the counselor is doing? To answer this question, Glynn and Moyers (2010) conducted a different type of research. In this study clinicians were instructed, unbeknownst to their clients, to switch their counseling style every 12 minutes within the same session: an ABAB design in which two different conditions (A and B) are alternated (cf. Patterson & Forgatch, 1985). In one condition the counselor was seeking to evoke and strengthen client change talk with regard to alcohol (CT). The other condition was functional analysis (FA), a common component of behavior therapy in which one seeks to understand the antecedents and consequences of drinking. Both involved empathic listening, but only in the former condition did the counselor intentionally try to evoke and strengthen change talk. The order of conditions was varied randomly so that sometimes functional analysis came first and other times the counselor began with the change talk condition. Could counselors influence the amount of change talk that their clients voiced? The result is shown in

Box 13.2. Change talk clearly increased and sustain talk decreased during the expected segments, with a reversal of that pattern during functional analysis segments. Note in particular the changing ratio, the relative proportion of change talk and sustain talk in the CT and FA segments.

In another study Moyers and Martin (2006) examined sequential relationships between counselor responses and client change talk within MI sessions. They found that the probability of change talk uniquely increased following MI-consistent counselor responses but not other counselor behavior.

Yet another research design was implemented in New Zealand by Douglas Sellman and colleagues, who randomly assigned problem drinkers to receive MI or client-centered counseling that offered reflective listening (Chapter 5) without the goal-directed component of MI. Only the MI condition produced significant reduction in heavy drinking in comparison to a control condition (Sellman, MacEwan, Deering, & Adamson, 2007; Sellman et al., 2001).

Taken together, these and other studies indicate that it matters what clients say during treatment: increases in change talk (relative to sustain

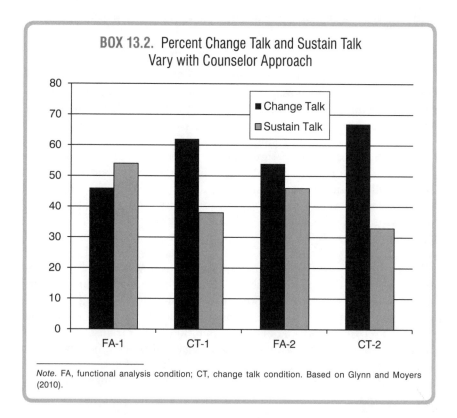

BOX 13.2. Percent Change Talk and Sustain Talk Vary with Counselor Approach

Note. FA, functional analysis condition; CT, change talk condition. Based on Glynn and Moyers (2010).

talk) are associated with subsequent change. Furthermore, it matters what counselors do. Change talk and sustain talk are quite responsive to counseling style, and clinicians can significantly influence how much of each they will hear. This differential effect on change talk and consequent change does not appear to be a function simply of being "nice" to clients or listening well, but results from strategic approaches to evoke change talk.

EVOKING CHANGE TALK

So how, then, does one go about increasing client change talk? Clearly, it is possible, and there is no single strategy for doing so. Your clients will tell you when you are doing it right. If you hear change talk, do more of what you've been doing. If you encounter increasing sustain talk and discord, try something different. An advantage in learning MI is that once you know what to listen for, your clients will provide immediate, ongoing feedback to help you improve your skills.

> In learning MI, once you know what to listen for, your clients will provide immediate feedback to help you improve your skills.

ASKING EVOCATIVE QUESTIONS

Perhaps the simplest and most direct way of evoking change talk is to ask for it. Ask open-ended questions for which change talk is the answer. You are, in essence, inviting the pro-change members of the internal committee to speak.

The DARN CATs acronym can be useful when generating questions to elicit different kinds of change talk. It is not necessary to go through the whole list; just get the process started. Remember that you are usually starting on the near side of the hill in Box 12.2 (preparatory change talk). It is best not to ask mobilizing questions too early in the evoking process. Unless the client comes in already eager for change (in which case you can try bypassing evoking and go right to planning), wait until you develop a nice collection of preparatory change talk and you begin to hear mobilizing change talk occur spontaneously before you do much exploring on the far side of the hill.

So what are some preparatory evocative questions? Use DARN to generate ideas.

Desire

Desire questions most often contain verbs such as *want*, *wish*, and *like*. There are many different ways to ask about desire for change.

"How would you *like* for things to change?"
"What do you *hope* our work together will accomplish?"
"Tell me what you don't *like* about how things are now."
"How do you *want* your life to be different a year from now?"
"What do you *wish* for in your marriage?"
"What are you *looking for* from this program?"

Ability

Ability questions ask about what a person *can* do, is *able* to do, or more gently (in the hypothetical) what they *could* do (which does not commit them to doing it).

"If you did really decide you want to lose weight, how *could* you do it?"
"What do you think you might be *able* to change?"
"What ideas do you have for how you *could* _____."
"How *confident* are you that you could _____ if you made up your mind?"
"Of these various options you've considered, what seems most *possible*?"
"How likely are you to be *able* to _____?"

Reasons

Reason questions ask for specific reasons why. They explore if . . . then reasons for considering or making a change.

"Why would you want to get more exercise?"
"What's the downside of how things are now?"
"What might be the good things about quitting drinking?"
"What would make it worth your while to _____?"
"What could be some advantages of _____?"
"Finish this sentence: 'Things can't go on the way they have been because. . . .'"
"What might be the three best reasons for _____?"

Another direct approach is to ask for change talk in a way that normalizes ambivalence[1]:

"Most people faced with a possible change feel two ways about it. You've probably got several reasons to keep things as they are, and

---

[1]Suggested by Dr. Carolina Yahne.

you probably have considered a few reasons to make a change as well. What are some of the reasons you have considered for making this change?"

Need

Need language expresses an urgency for change without necessarily giving particular reasons. Need questions may well evoke reasons (which is just fine if it happens). Again, there are many ways to ask.

"What *needs* to happen?"
"How *important* is it for you to _____?"
"How *serious* or *urgent* does this feel to you?"
"What do you think *has to* change?"
"Complete this sentence: 'I really *must* _____.'"

As we discuss in Chapter 14 there is more to this than simply asking such questions. There are also specific processes for reflecting and strengthening change talk when it occurs. Nevertheless, it's surprising how much change talk you can evoke just by asking the right questions.

The Wrong Questions

What, then, might be the wrong questions to ask? Even though the following are open questions, they would not be ones we generally recommend in MI.

"Why haven't you changed?"
"What keeps you doing this?"
"Why do you have to smoke?"
"What were you thinking when you messed up?"
"Why aren't you trying harder?"
"What are the three best reasons for you to drop out of this program?"
"What's the matter with you?"
"How could you want to go back to _____?"
"Why can't you _____?"

Why might these questions be ill-advised from an MI perspective? Because if the person answers them literally, the expected result would be sustain talk. There is also a shaming tone to some of these questions that would be likely to damage rapport and create discord.

We are not saying it is *always* improper to ask a question to which the answer is likely to be sustain talk. We do this ourselves sometimes. The point is to think about it before you ask questions like those above and consider, "Is the answer likely to be change talk or sustain talk?" If the latter, what is your reason or strategy for asking it? Some possible reasons might be:

- *To explore obstacles to change during the planning process.* "So what might make it harder for you to do what you want to do?"
- *To side with reluctance in hopes of evoking change talk.* "Do you think, then, that it's just impossible for you to quit smoking?"
- *To get a running head start when change talk is not forthcoming* (see Chapter 15). "Well, tell me this. In what ways is cocaine use good for you? What do you like about it?" [and then] "And what's the downside? What are the not-so-good things about it for you?"

As a general guideline, ask open questions that elicit change talk, recognizing that there can be strategic reasons for asking about the opposite. Remember that the ratio of change talk to sustain talk is a predictor of change actually happening.

> Ask open questions that elicit change talk.

USING THE IMPORTANCE RULER

One of the evocative (need) questions given above is, "How important is it for you to _____?" One version of this asks the person to rate their level of perceived importance on a scale (Butler, Rollnick, Cohen, Russell, Bachmann, & Stott, 1999). We typically use an imaginary scale ranging from 0 to 10:

"On a scale from 0 to 10, where 0 means 'not at all important' and 10 means 'the most important thing for me right now,' how important would you say it is for you to _____?"

The answer will be a number between 0 and 10. In itself, this question is of limited usefulness. The value for change talk comes with the follow-up question about the number that the person chose:

"And why are you at a _____ and not 0 [or a lower number]?"

Note that the righting reflex could prompt one to ask the opposite question, "Why are you at 6 and not 10?" The answer to that question is sustain talk, whereas asking "Why are you at 6 and not 2?" is likely to evoke change talk—the reasons why change *is* important.

What if the person, when asked about importance answers "zero"? It can happen, although it rarely does. Even so, this provides useful information. A true zero would signal no ambivalence at all (at least with regard to current importance) and would suggest exploring other aspects of DARN besides need, or perhaps pursuing strategies to create ambivalence (Chapter 18).

Although this ruler technique has been called a "readiness ruler," we almost never ask "On a scale from 0 to 10, how *ready* are you to change?" Readiness is mobilizing change talk that lies on the far side of the MI hill, and furthermore it is not language that people often use in spontaneous speech (Amrhein et al., 2003). To ask whether a person is *ready* to change is to place a pressure for change. That is why we prefer to ask about perceived need (importance).

It is possible to use the ruler to ask about other aspects of preparatory change talk. In Chapter 16, for example, we discuss using a confidence ruler to strengthen self-efficacy. One could ask, "How much do you *want* to change?," although we seldom do because the numbers are likely to be lower, and it is quite possible to decide to change without wanting to (e.g., for particular reasons or because it is the right thing to do). One ruler is probably sufficient to evoke some change talk, and we do not recommend using more than two in a conversation because it can get tedious.[2]

Another possible follow-up question to evoke change talk is to ask, "What would it take for you to go from a [current number] to, say, a [higher number]?" In other words, what might happen that would make the change more important? You could also ask what number a significant other (such as a spouse) might give (for the client to make this change), and in follow-up ask, "Why do you think his/her number would be so high?"

If numerical ratings don't seem like the best approach with your client or population, develop a scale that is more appropriate. Various points along the scale could be denoted by words, pictures, or even animals. It's also possible to use a visual scale without any marking on it; for example, a simple line with "Extremely important" at one end and "Not at all important" at the other. The person can be asked to make a pencil mark to show where they are, and you can measure it later. Scales with physical manipulation can also be useful, such as a slide that people can move along a line to show their current position. A ruler affixed to the back of such a device would let you quickly assign a number if you need one for data purposes. Amrhein built a small seesaw-like balance that could be tipped anywhere from one extreme to the other, and a protractor on the back yielded a numeric value as the angle of deflection. Whatever type of scale is used, it is possible to ask the follow-up question of why the person chose their point on the scale instead of a lower one.

---

[2]We did develop a paper-and-pencil questionnaire using the ruler to ask about six natural language dimensions of change talk (Miller & Johnson, 2008).

QUERYING EXTREMES

When there seems to be little desire for change at present, another way to elicit change talk is to ask people to describe the extremes of their (or others') concerns, to imagine the extreme of consequences that might ensue:

> "What concerns you the most about your high blood pressure in the long run?"
>
> "Suppose you continue on as you have been, without changing. What do you imagine are the worst things that could happen?"
>
> "How much do you know about some of the things that can happen if you drink during pregnancy, even if you don't imagine this happening to you?"

At the other extreme, it can be useful to imagine the best consequences that might follow from pursuing a change:

> "What do you think could be the best results if you did make this change?"
>
> "If you were completely successful in making the changes you want, how would things be different?"
>
> "Imagine for a minute that you did succeed in _____. What might be some good things that could come of out that?"

LOOKING BACK

Sometimes it is useful, in eliciting change talk, to have the client remember times before the problem emerged and to compare these times with the present situation:

> "Do you remember a time when things were going well for you? What has changed?"
>
> "What were things like before you started using drugs? What were you like back then?"
>
> "Tell me about how you two met, and what attracted you to each other back then."
>
> "What are the differences between the person you were 10 years ago and the person you are today?"
>
> "How has your pain changed you as a person or stopped you from growing, from moving forward?"

Looking back at the past sometimes recalls a time before problems emerged, highlighting both the discrepancy with how things are at present and the possibility of life being better again. If looking back yields a description of a time when problems were worse, you can explore what has happened to yield some improvement to date.

LOOKING FORWARD

Helping people envision a changed future is another approach for eliciting change talk. Here you ask the client to tell you how it might be after a change:

> "If you did decide to make this change, what do you hope would be different in the future?"
>
> "Tell me, how would you like things to turn out for you in 5 years or so?"
>
> "If you were to have a week off from your symptoms/problems, what would you do first?"[3]
>
> "I can see that you're feeling really frustrated right now. How would you like things to be different in the future?"

Similarly, you can invite the person to look ahead in time and anticipate how things might be if no changes are made:

> "Suppose you don't make any changes, but just continue as you have been. What do you think your life will be like 5 years from now?"
>
> "Given what has happened so far, what do you expect might happen if you don't make any changes?"

There is some overlap here with querying extremes. In the looking-ahead method, however, you are asking for either people's realistic appraisal of a future unchanged or their actual hopes for a future changed.

EXPLORING GOALS AND VALUES

An approach that we are using more is to explore the person's broader goals and values. What is most important in this person's life? After all, no one is truly "unmotivated." Their priorities may be quite different from the counselor's, but everyone does have goals and priorities. Exploring what those values are provides some reference points against which to compare the status quo.

---

[3] Suggested by Moria Golan.

As discussed in Chapter 7, exploring what matters most to a person can be a good way to develop rapport and might be undertaken even during the engaging process. That kind of discussion is not limited to benefits that might emerge from a particular change. It is not even necessary to have identified a change focus when exploring values. The process explores what people care most about and what values they choose to guide their lives. Because values are aspirations, there may be a considerable discrepancy between current status and avowed goals. But it is also true that, when discussed in a trusting and respectful counseling relationship, such discrepancy can provide important motivation for change. Values exploration could also be used during the focusing process to identify particular goals for change. In the evoking process, change talk and motivation arise from the discrepancy between current status or behavior and the person's chosen values and goals.

Remember that the goal in evoking is to elicit the person's own motivation for change. The key is to explore and develop themes of discrepancy between important goals or values and the client's current behavior. If such a question evokes discord or defensiveness, don't press it. The client's responses are more important than finishing any particular procedure.

THE BALANCE OF CHANGE TALK AND SUSTAIN TALK

Remember that what shifts over the course of a skillful MI session is the ratio of change talk to sustain talk. Some counselors expect that once they begin to hear some change talk it should be smooth sailing from there on, with little or no more sustain talk. Typically, sustain talk continues to occur but becomes less frequent relative to the change talk with which it is intermixed. Early in an MI session the skill is often to discern a ray of change talk within the sustain talk, like spotting a lighthouse in a storm or detecting a signal within noise. It is not necessary to eliminate the storm or the noise, just follow the signal.[4]

WHAT ABOUT DUBIOUS CHANGE TALK?

Some clinicians are concerned about clients who "just tell you what you want to hear" and thus may be voicing change talk without meaning it. A related concern regards clients whom a counselor perceives to be naïve and unrealistic in their glowing change talk. Does change talk "count" in such cases? How should one respond when sensing that the client's change talk is disingenuous or naïve?

---

[4] Thanks to Theresa Moyers for this analogy.

It will not surprise you that we do not favor confrontation such as responding with statements like these:

"I don't believe you!"
"You're just telling me what I want to hear."
"You're being unrealistic. Get real!"

Such responses are likely to damage rapport and create discord. So what do we do instead?

A problem in both cases (disingenuous or tenuous) is that the change talk focuses on generalities more than specifics. Our inclination is to take people at their word and become very interested in the specifics. Vague and superficial change talk does not (yet) have the necessary depth. Asking for elaboration, for more detail about why and how, is likely to elicit more specific change talk and can actually transform vague generalities into specific intentions. This exploring is done with a mind-set of supportive curiosity, not of cynicism or trying to "catch" the client in deceit or self-deception.

CLIENT: No, I really am going to quit drinking. I want to.

INTERVIEWER: Why would you want to do that? [Evocative question: Reasons]

CLIENT: I just am going to do it, that's all.

INTERVIEWER: Great. And what I'm curious about is why you're so keen to do this when drinking has been pretty important to you.

CLIENT: Well, my family wants me to quit. It gets me when my kid says, "Please Daddy, don't drink tonight!" Really tears me up.

INTERVIEWER: It's pretty hard to say no to your child begging you like that. You care about your kids. [Reflection] What else? Why else would you choose to quit? [Evocative question]

CLIENT: Well, my doctor said that I should.

INTERVIEWER: What do *you* think?

CLIENT: I know she's worried about me, those blood tests and all. She said my liver is crying out for a break.

INTERVIEWER: How important is that? [Evocative question: Need]

CLIENT: Well, I don't know too much about it, but I think if you kill off your liver it's not coming back, and really bad things happen.

INTERVIEWER: You'd like to stay healthy. [Reflection]

CLIENT: Sure. That's why I'm going to quit.

INTERVIEWER: What would a first step be?

The key here is to help clients be more specific about their desire, ability, reasons, need, and plans. Voicing specifics makes change more likely to happen. It is as though your taking clients' change talk at face value makes their change option more credible to them as well. Someone who starts out with vague assurances can end up committing to particular steps toward change. Specifics also increase accountability. General motivations and intentions don't make change happen as readily as specifics do.

The judgment that someone is saying "what they want you to hear" sounds like a signal of discord that the counselor is picking up, an intuition that there is a hollow ring to a client's assurances. In essence, this counselor's perception signals a relational concern. Another possibility when this concern arises, then, is to work on strengthening engagement so that the client feels safe enough to be more honest and does not feel the need to please or deceive you.

JULIA REVISITED

To illustrate the eliciting process we return to the case of Julia previously discussed in Chapters 6, 9, and 11. At this point engagement seems to be progressing well and there is a provisional focus on depression, but what are Julia's motivations for change?

INTERVIEWER: Last time we talked about depression as a common clinical problem. In fact, depression is the most common problem that brings people to our clinic. We went through the signs of depression, and there were quite a few that you recognize in yourself. I guess the next thing I'd like to discuss is how you would like things to be different. [Evocative question: Desire]

CLIENT: I don't want to feel so bad about myself that I'm carving up my arm. [Change talk: Desire]

INTERVIEWER: That really got your attention. You know how you *don't* want to feel. How *do* you want to feel?

CLIENT: Normal, I guess. Happy. To have energy to do things again. [Change talk: Desire] When I broke up with Ray it just made me crazy. I feel like there's something wrong with me, that I always screw up my relationships.

INTERVIEWER: You'd like to feel happy and good about yourself again. [Selectively reflecting the change talk] What else?

CLIENT: I want to be with a man who loves me. [Change talk] I seem to attract guys who are hung up about telling me how they feel. I need a man I can talk to. [Change talk]

INTERVIEWER: How important is that to you, to have a relationship like that? [Evocative question: Need]

CLIENT: Very important. I don't want to be alone. I need to be loved. [Change talk: Need]

INTERVIEWER: You need that.

CLIENT: Yes! I don't want to keep destroying relationships. [Change talk: Desire] I don't know why I do that.

INTERVIEWER: Tell me a little about why you want to feel better. [Evocative question: Reasons]

CLIENT: I just feel like I'm dragging around this heavy weight with me all the time. I like to have fun, but I've really become a drag to be with. I feel like even my friends avoid me. [Change talk: Reasons]

INTERVIEWER: It would be good to feel lighthearted, to enjoy life and being with your friends.

CLIENT: Yes, it would. [Change talk] Do you think it's possible for me?

INTERVIEWER: Well, I was just going to ask you about that. What are some of your personal strengths? What might your friends say that you have going for you? [Evocative question: Ability]

CLIENT: I don't know. They'd probably say that I'm stubborn.

INTERVIEWER: That when you set your mind to doing something, it's going to happen.

CLIENT: Something like that. I don't feel that way now, but I've been pretty persistent in the past. I guess I have it in me. [Change talk: Ability]

INTERVIEWER: Give me an example. When have you done something or made a change in your life that really took some effort, maybe something you weren't sure at first that you could do?

CLIENT: Moving here. I had always lived in Ireland near my father and my sisters, and I moved out here all by myself.

INTERVIEWER: Such a long way. That took some courage.

CLIENT: I just wanted to be on my own for a change, to get away. But now I feel too much on my own.

INTERVIEWER: It takes a lot to move to a new place on your own. How did you do it?

CLIENT: I had to find a job here, and I started going to classes at the university. I had to get used to a different culture, figure out the stores and banking system, and make some friends.

INTERVIEWER: And you did it. That's a lot of change to manage.

CLIENT: I never thought much about it. I guess I can do it when it's important enough. [Change talk: Ability]

INTERVIEWER: So use your imagination here. Suppose that we work together and you are successful in making these changes. How might your life be different, say, 5 years from now? [Looking ahead]

CLIENT: I'd be married, maybe have a family. I'd have a better job that I enjoy more. I just wouldn't be stressing out like this all the time. A calmer life. [Change talk]
[Continued in Chapter 19]

Beneath the wealth of ideas for evoking change talk discussed in this chapter lies something more fundamental. Your task is not to memorize this or that clever technique to use with clients, but rather to listen with curiosity for the person's own inherent motivations for change. Evoking is an emergent process, sensitive to in-the-moment interactions. Eliciting clients' own change statements is powerful "not because they refer to an already formulated inner state (i.e., a pre-existing desire to change) . . . but instead because they prompt and produce the change that they index" (Carr, 2011, p. 236). Evoking is a co-creative process through which the person's potential for change is released. The motivation for change is emerging even as you speak together.

KEY POINTS

✓ A client's balance of change talk and sustain talk predicts change, and is substantially influenced by the interviewer.

✓ Perhaps the simplest method for evoking is to ask open questions that elicit change talk.

✓ A variety of other strategies can be used to evoke the client's own motivations for change.

✓ In MI one would not routinely elicit and explore sustain talk, although there can be strategic reasons for doing so.

CHAPTER 14

Responding to Change Talk

It takes two to speak truth—One to speak,
and another to hear.
——HENRY DAVID THOREAU

After all, when you seek advice from
someone it's certainly not because you
want them to give it. You just want them to
be there while you talk to yourself.
——TERRY PRATCHETT

Whenever you hear change talk, don't just sit there. Within the style of MI there are particular ways of responding to change talk in order to strengthen it. If you only collect change talk ("What else? . . . What else?") you're missing important opportunities to consolidate motivation for change.

A first step, of course, is to recognize change talk when you hear it and not let it pass unnoticed (Chapter 12). There are particular things you can do to evoke change talk (Chapter 13), but how you respond when it occurs can also make a big difference in the amount and quality of change talk you hear.

OARS: FOUR RESPONSES TO CHANGE TALK

In reviewing MI sessions we listen for four particular counselor responses to change talk. The acronym for these is the same one introduced in Chapter 3: OARS

Open question
Affirmation
Reflection
Summary

Responding in one of these ways will often yield additional or more detailed change talk.

Open Question

When responding to change talk, ask a particular kind of open question: one that asks for elaboration or an example. When you hear change talk, ask more about it. Become interested in and

> When you hear change talk, become interested in and curious about it.

curious about it. You want to know more. Ask for more detail or examples. This can apply to both the downside of the status quo and to the advantages of change.

CLIENT: Well, sometimes when I wake up in the morning after drinking I don't feel so good.

ELABORATION: *In what ways* do you feel bad?

EXAMPLE: Tell me about the last time that happened to you.

Whether you are getting more detail or are hearing a specific example, the client is giving you more change talk.

CLIENT: I think my family would be happier if I spent less time at work.

ELABORATION: How do you think it would be better?

EXAMPLE: Tell me about a time when you really enjoyed being with your family.

In essence, ask an open question the answer to which is more change talk.

Affirmation

A second good way to respond to change talk is with affirmation. You recognize and prize what the person is saying about change. It's as simple as commenting positively on what the person has said.

CLIENT: I plan to go to the gym twice this week for some exercise. [Commitment]

AFFIRM: Good for you!

CLIENT: I think my family would be happier if I stayed home more. [Reason]

AFFIRM: You really care about them.

CLIENT: I've got to do something about my weight. [Need]

AFFIRM: Your health is important to you.

CLIENT: I think I could quit smoking if I really decided to. [Ability]

    AFFIRM: Once you make up your mind to do something, you get it done.

Reflection

The mainstay skill of MI, reflective listening, is another good way to strengthen change talk. It can be a simple or a complex reflection.

CLIENT: I wish I didn't feel so anxious all the time. [Desire]

    REFLECT: You'd like that. [Simple]

CLIENT: I could find a better job if I really tried. [Ability]

    REFLECT: And you have some ideas about how to do it. [Complex, continuing the paragraph]

CLIENT: I'm going to stop trying to outdo my brother. [Commitment]

    REFLECT: You've decided. [Simple]

When you reflect change talk, what the client is most likely to say next is more change talk. Here is an example of an interview with a gambler integrating O, A, and R responses to change talk.

INTERVIEWER: What kind of troubles has gambling caused for you?

CLIENT: One obvious place is money.

INTERVIEWER: In what ways is that a concern for you? [O]

CLIENT: Well, I just spend a lot of money on gambling, and I'm not always paying my bills.

INTERVIEWER: Tell me about the last time that happened. [O]

CLIENT: Just last week I went through about $600. I start out setting a limit for myself, but then when I lose that amount I decide to try to win it back.

INTERVIEWER: Over time it really adds up. [R]

CLIENT: I'll say. I've lost about $20,000 over the last 6 months.

INTERVIEWER: And that's a lot for you. [R]

CLIENT: I'll say! We don't have that kind of money. At least we don't now.

INTERVIEWER: You've lost a lot. [R] How much does this money issue concern you? [O]

CLIENT: It's getting to be a big problem, and I worry about it all the time. I've got people knocking on my door, calling on the telephone, sending nasty letters. I've got to do something.

INTERVIEWER: You're a person who wants to be responsible, to pay your bills. [A]

CLIENT: That's how I was brought up.

INTERVIEWER: And in what specific ways does it affect you, to lose so much? [O]

CLIENT: Nobody will give us credit any more, except the casinos. My husband finally noticed all the cash withdrawals, and he's hardly talking to me.

INTERVIEWER: So that's a big stress in your relationship. [R] What else? [O]

CLIENT: He's worried about our retirement, of course. And I can't buy things I want.

INTERVIEWER: Such as . . . [O]

CLIENT: The other day I saw this nice dress in just my size, and I couldn't afford it. My credit cards have all been canceled. Then I get mad and do stupid things.

When you hear change talk, reflect it. It is also possible to reflect change talk that *might* be there but has not quite been spoken. This is a particular form of continuing the paragraph (Chapter 5) that Theresa Moyers calls "lending change talk." Consider this snippet of dialogue with a heavy drinker:

> When you hear change talk, reflect it.

INTERVIEWER: You've been drinking quite a bit. [Reflecting what the client has just said]

CLIENT: I don't really think it's all that much. I can drink a lot and not feel it.

INTERVIEWER: More than most people. [R]

CLIENT: Yes. I can drink most people under the table.

INTERVIEWER: *And that's what worries you.* [R, continuing the paragraph with change talk]

CLIENT: Well, that and how I feel; the next morning I'm usually in bad shape. I feel jittery and I can't think straight through most of the morning.

INTERVIEWER: *That doesn't seem right to you.* [R, continuing the paragraph with change talk]

The italicized responses are reflections that lend change talk. The client hasn't directly voiced it yet, but change talk is one possible guess about what is being said. The client may concur and follow your interpretation with more change talk. If you guess wrong and the client corrects it, you can immediately reflect what the client did mean, or even apologize for missing. As with other reflections in MI, it is vital not to add a tone of skepticism or sarcasm or to try to be too clever. Retaining genuine curiosity and compassion is the raft upon which all else floats.

Another reflective skill is what we call "snatching change talk from the jaws of ambivalence." It is normal to hear change talk embedded in the same sentence or paragraph with sustain talk. Suppose, for example, that you were having a conversation with someone about their inactivity:

> It is normal to hear change talk embedded in the same sentence with sustain talk.

> "By the time I get home from work I'm already tired. I get supper ready and help the kids with their homework, and by the time I get them to bed I'm exhausted. I know I need to get more exercise, but there's just no time to fit it in!"

The helper's righting reflex would be to explain how important physical activity is or to make suggestions about how to fit exercise into the day. The expected response to this would be more sustain talk. But notice that an argument for change is already there in the paragraph. Both pros and cons are already represented on this person's committee. A key is to hear the embedded change talk and reflect it: "Getting more exercise is important for you." It's also possible to ask for elaboration of the change talk ("When you think about needing more exercise, what do you imagine yourself doing?") or to affirm ("Your health is really important to you"). The point is to hear the change talk within the ambivalence and shine a light on it.

Here are some other examples. For each one we give three possible reflections: two that emphasize the sustain talk (ST) and one that highlights change talk (CT).

CLIENT: I was worried there at first, but I don't think I really have diabetes. The doctor said it was "borderline" or something like that, and I feel fine.

ST: You feel fine.

ST: You don't think you really have diabetes.

CT: You don't want to develop diabetes; that worries you.

CLIENT: Well sure, I'd like to be as healthy as I can, but I'm 68, for heaven's sake. I figure I can get away with some bad habits now. They won't have time to catch up with me.

ST: You have nothing to lose at this point.

ST: At 68 it's time to just enjoy life.

CT: You want to stay as healthy as you can.

CLIENT: I wasn't doing anything wrong! I just went along for the ride, and I didn't know they were going to grab that lady's purse. Now they're saying that I violated my probation. I guess it's not smart to be cruising around at 2 in the morning, but it happened so fast, there was nothing I could do about it. I didn't break any laws, and I'm not going back to jail for this.

ST: It wasn't your fault.

ST: You didn't do anything wrong.

CT: Cruising at 2 in the morning wasn't such a good idea.

CLIENT: It's just such a hassle to take all those pills. I'm supposed to remember to take them four times a day, and half the time I don't even have them with me. And I hate how they make me feel. I guess there's a good reason for it, but it's just not possible for me.

ST: There's no way for you to do it.

ST: Having to take all that medicine is a real hassle.

CT: You know it's important to take them.

In general, you will get more of whatever you reflect. If you reflect sustain talk you are likely to hear more sustain talk (although sometimes people do respond with change talk). Reflect change talk and you get more change talk. In a double-sided reflection (on the one hand . . . and on the other hand . . .) you're likely to hear more of whatever element you placed last.

There are times when reflecting sustain talk can be helpful, and in Chapter 15 we explore ways to do this strategically. Sometimes clients respond to the reflection of sustain talk with counterbalancing change talk. Just be sure to *hear* the change talk even when it is surrounded by sustain talk, because it represents the person's own arguments for change. When you hear an ambivalence sandwich (ST/CT/ST) try reflecting the change talk.

Summaries

One of the core counseling skills in MI is providing reflective summaries of what the person has said. In client-centered counseling, however, there is often very little guidance about what to include in summaries and what to leave out. Obviously you can't recount everything your client has said. In forming a summary you necessarily choose, from among all that the person has said, what specific content to include.

Bear with us through a longer discussion here, for there is a lot of technique and art to MI-consistent summaries. We first provide some dialogue from an initial MI session and consider several different ways in which it might be summarized.

Dr. Clark's Referral

Here is an example of a clinical consultation in an MI style, based on an actual case.[1] Following a routine physical examination, Dr. Clark referred Sylvia to a behavioral health counselor to discuss her drinking. The referral indicates that the physician smelled alcohol on her breath during the examination and added an alcohol screen to the panel of lab tests ordered. The lab report indicated a blood alcohol level of 90 mg%, and also a slightly elevated liver enzyme. After you read the transcript we will consider different possible summaries of the same dialogue.

INTERVIEWER: There's not much information on this referral, Sylvia. Perhaps you could tell me how you understand why Dr. Clark wanted you to talk with me.

CLIENT: I was surprised to hear from her. She called me on the phone after my physical, and said she wanted me to see you because she was concerned about me.

INTERVIEWER: Dr. Clark called you personally.

CLIENT: Uh-huh. Actually it kind of scared me. I thought maybe it was bad news from my tests.

INTERVIEWER: So what did she tell you?

CLIENT: Well, that morning, when I went in for my physical, while she was examining me she mentioned that she smelled alcohol. I thought it was probably the mouthwash that I use, and that's what I told her. She didn't say anything more about it.

INTERVIEWER: But then she called you back.

CLIENT: I guess she had them test me for alcohol. I didn't know she was going to do that. Anyhow she told me that I was over the legal limit for driving. But I swear I didn't have anything to drink.

INTERVIEWER: That took you by surprise.

CLIENT: Yes. I never drink in the morning. She also told me that one of the other tests was abnormal—for liver, I think—and that's why she wanted me to talk to you.

INTERVIEWER: I'm sure this has been on your mind in the meantime. What are you thinking at this point about what she told you?

---

[1] As with other case examples in this book, the client's name and identifying details have been altered to protect anonymity and confidentiality, and some details represent composites from many cases.

CLIENT: Well, frankly, I don't like being here. I didn't like her checking up on me like that, and I feel like this is none of her business, or yours either, for that matter. I didn't really want to come.

INTERVIEWER: And yet you did.

CLIENT: It did scare me a little. She didn't really explain the lab test to me, except that it might mean I was drinking too much. Did she explain it to you?

INTERVIEWER: She did send me the result, and the one she mentioned is called GGT. It's a liver function test—you're right about that—and it is one that goes up when a person drinks a fair amount. It's like a warning light going on in your car. What do you make of that?

CLIENT: I don't like it. I guess that's what she was worried about. I know she means well.

INTERVIEWER: She cares about you. And she must have been concerned about the alcohol in your system, too. What time did you go in for your physical?

CLIENT: It was first thing in the morning, on my way to work. I just got up, showered, got ready, and went in. I didn't even have breakfast because of the blood tests.

INTERVIEWER: So that's a puzzle for you, how the alcohol got there in the morning.

CLIENT: I guess it must have been left over. Can that happen? I don't really drink all that much.

INTERVIEWER: Sure. It takes some time for the liver to break down alcohol, so it can stay in the body for a while.

CLIENT: But she said I was legally drunk! I live way over on the west side and I work downtown, so I drive in that awful traffic every morning. I felt perfectly fine.

INTERVIEWER: Nothing out of the ordinary.

CLIENT: No. But she said if I had been pulled over, I could have been arrested.

INTERVIEWER: That kind of shocked you.

CLIENT: I work for the city, for the mayor's office, and if that happened— well, I could lose my job.

INTERVIEWER: All right. Well, I can see why you came in, and I'm glad that you did. All of this is new to you, and you're not happy to be here, but Dr. Clark got your attention. So shall we talk about this a bit?

CLIENT: OK, but I don't want to be lectured about drinking.

INTERVIEWER: I won't lecture you, I promise. Now if it's all right with you, perhaps you could tell me some about how alcohol fits into your life, into an ordinary day.

CLIENT: An ordinary day. I work a long day, and by the time I get home I'm exhausted and ready to relax. I'll usually have some wine while I'm making dinner. If I don't have the kids, I just fix something quick, and then kick back.

INTERVIEWER: It makes a difference if the kids are there or not.

CLIENT: Well, I'll usually have wine with dinner anyhow, and while I'm cooking, but I mean I make something a little nicer when they are there. I'm divorced. Most of the time he has the kids. That's not how it's supposed to be, but he's always been a control freak.

INTERVIEWER: And then after dinner you kick back and relax.

CLIENT: Right. I usually just watch television. I don't have energy for much more than that.

INTERVIEWER: And how does alcohol fit in there?

CLIENT: It helps me relax and just kind of turn off. I'll have some more wine, maybe a martini while I'm watching programs. Then I get tired, go to bed, get up, and do it all over again. That's when the kids aren't with me.

INTERVIEWER: And when they are . . .

CLIENT: We'll watch TV together unless they have some homework, and then I help them with that. I guess I don't drink as much when they're there. Then in the morning I have to get them to school before work, and it gets pretty hectic. I like it when they're with me, though.

INTERVIEWER: You have an arrangement with your ex.

CLIENT: We have joint custody, and I'm supposed to have them Monday through Wednesday and every other weekend, but it doesn't happen. Like I said, he's a control freak. He always dominates me—has to have it his way. If he says they don't come over, they don't. So a lot of the time I don't get them.

INTERVIEWER: It's not happening the way the court ordered it.

CLIENT: Right. But I can't take him to court. I can't afford a good lawyer, and he says if I complain he'll say I'm a drunk and file for sole custody. I can't afford to fight him. (*pause, some tearfulness*) I love my kids, and I feel so much better when they're with me. They belong with me.

INTERVIEWER: In what ways do you feel better when they're there?

CLIENT: I just feel more cheerful. I have something to do. Usually when I wake up in the morning I feel terrible, nervous, exhausted, like I don't want to get out of bed, but I still do. When the kids are there, it's like I have a reason to get up.

INTERVIEWER: And those are also days on which you drink somewhat less, when they are with you.

CLIENT: Oh, I see what you're getting at. You think one reason I feel worse on other mornings is that I'm drinking too much.

INTERVIEWER: Just a possibility.

CLIENT: Well, there's probably something to that, but I also miss my kids.

INTERVIEWER: It hurts you, too, when they're not with you. And at the same time, you wonder if maybe you feel worse some mornings because of drinking the night before.

CLIENT: I don't think I'm really hung over or anything, but I do feel pretty bad. Headache and so forth. Maybe so. But I'm not an alcoholic or anything like that.

Because forming MI-consistent summaries is challenging to do well, here is something to try. Before reading any further, consider how you might summarize what has happened thus far in this interview. If you were to offer Sylvia a collecting summary, what would you choose to include, and why? Write no more than seven sentences, and then end your summary with a question to move the process forward. Then after you have constructed your own summary, read the examples below.

Summary 1

This is the first of four example summaries of the above dialogue, all intended to be helpful to Sylvia. As you read each one, consider what is being emphasized. What seems to have guided the interviewer in choosing what to include and not include? How consistent is each summary with the spirit and style of MI? Why? Consider also how the client is likely to feel and respond to each summary.

> "Well, it sounds like your life is pretty stressful. When you wake up in the morning you often feel bad. You have a stressful commute in traffic in the morning, and you put in a lot of time at work. By the time you get home, you're exhausted. You're a single mom now, and there's a constant battle with your ex about getting time with your kids. You really miss them when they're not with you, but you also feel kind of helpless to do anything about it. Mostly what you do in the evening is watch TV, and alcohol helps you to relax. Have I got it right?"

From a client-centered perspective this is a good summary that focuses on the feelings Sylvia has expressed. Counselors are often trained to focus on the client's emotions. This summary emphasizes her (predominantly negative) feelings, perhaps with a goal of helping her to become more aware and accepting of her current experience. This kind of summary also has a function of joining with the client, communicating understanding and acceptance. For these reasons, this summary is compatible with the engaging process in MI, but it lacks the important goal-oriented component of the evoking process and is not likely to create movement in the direction of change. Our guess is that at the end of this summary, Sylvia would still be feeling discouraged.

Summary 2

> "Let me tell you what I hear so far. Because of some lab tests, Dr. Clark is concerned that you are drinking too much, and asked you to talk to me. You're wondering what the lab test means, and you don't understand how you could still have been legally drunk that morning. Some mornings you do feel pretty bad, though. On the other hand, alcohol helps you to relax, and you don't think you really drink all that much. You don't drink in the morning, and you certainly don't think you're an alcoholic. You weren't too happy to come here, and you don't want to be lectured about drinking. Is that about right?"

Here is another very reasonable client-centered summary. In this case rather than focusing primarily on feelings the counselor seems to be trying to capture both sides of Sylvia's ambivalence in the manner of a decisional balance, beginning with the change talk and ending with the sustain talk. The counselor seeks to summarize both the pros and the cons of change that Sylvia has expressed, giving them approximately equal emphasis. Placing the sustain talk last gives it the greater emphasis of recency, leaving the client to respond to that thought. The underlying mental model is that people need to see clearly and explore both sides of their dilemma. This is an appropriate type of summary when the counselor is not seeking to move the client in a particular direction; for example, when the client is trying to make a choice and the counselor wishes to maintain neutrality, not advocating for one side or the other (see Chapter 17). Like Summary 1, it lacks the directional movement of MI that is needed in the evoking process. The expected outcome of such a summary would be continued ambivalence.

Summary 3

> "Well, I'd say you have a serious problem with alcohol. You say you don't drink that much, but you're drinking enough at night that you're still legally intoxicated in the morning when you're driving to work or taking your kids to school. The way you're feeling bad in the morning

sounds a lot like alcohol withdrawal to me. You're using alcohol like a drug to relax you and help you forget about the stresses in your life. Your ex-husband thinks you have a problem and doesn't want the children to be with you. So you watch television and drink, and deny that you have a problem. Sure sounds like alcoholism to me! How about you?"

A client-centered counselor would be unlikely to offer a summary like this, although it is characteristic of how many people with alcohol problems were counseled for decades (White & Miller, 2007). It is a confrontational summary and is inconsistent with MI. The apparent assumption is a deficit model, that the client is not perceiving reality and needs to be strongly persuaded. The predictable client response to this summary would be defensiveness, sustain talk, and discord.

Summary 4

"So here's what you've told me so far. Dr. Clark noticed a blood test elevated that often is a warning about drinking too much, and she was concerned enough to call you personally. That scared you a little. You were also surprised that there was still enough alcohol in your bloodstream for you to be arrested for drunk driving if you had been stopped, even though you had not had anything to drink in the morning. If that happened, you could lose your job. When you wake up in the morning you often feel pretty bad—headache, tired, nervous. That seems to happen more when the kids aren't with you, and you drink more at night. What else have you noticed?"

This is a quintessential MI summary. It pulls together most of the change talk that Sylvia has offered. There is something powerful about hearing all of one's change talk collected, and such a summary is strategic, consciously directed toward change. This collecting summary ends with an open question intended to elicit further change talk. The normal client response to this summary would be to continue exploring change talk.

All four of these summaries are seven sentences long and end with a question, but what different impacts they are likely to have! Within the evoking process of MI there is a strategic rationale for what to include in a summary. Each bit of change talk is like a flower, and the interviewer collects them into a growing bouquet. With a few flowers in hand, the counselor offers the bouquet to the client and asks for more flowers. A collecting summary like this can be offered periodically throughout the evoking process, and the final big bouquet has a special function in the transition to planning (see Chapter 19).

KEY POINTS

✓ When a client offers change talk, the interviewer's next response should be one that recognizes and strengthens it, such as asking for elaboration, affirming, reflecting, or summarizing.

✓ A summary tends to reinforce what it contains, whether that be demoralization, ambivalence, defensiveness, or motivation for change.

✓ The normal structure of an MI-consistent summary is a "bouquet" of the client's own change talk.

CHAPTER 15

Responding to Sustain Talk and Discord

Where did all the sages get the idea that a man's desires must be normal and virtuous? Why did they imagine that he must inevitably will what is reasonable and profitable? What a man needs simply and solely is *independent* volition, whatever that independence may cost and wherever it may lead.
—FYODOR DOSTOYEVSKY

Out of clutter, find simplicity. From discord, find harmony. In the middle of difficulty lies opportunity.
—ALBERT EINSTEIN

Difficulties do arise, of course, in consultations about change. People may minimize concerns: "I really don't think it's that bad." Disagreements can arise. Sometimes the clinician's credibility is questioned: "Who are you to tell me what to do?" A conversation can start to feel like a polarized power struggle: "I'm not going to do it, and no one can make me!"

We have found that such tensions are far less likely to arise when the interviewer follows the spirit and practices of MI as described in preceding chapters. Nevertheless, they do happen naturally when discussing difficult change issues, and it is helpful to respond to them in an MI-consistent manner. That is the focus of this chapter.

DECONSTRUCTING "RESISTANCE"

When writing the first edition of this book we chose the term *resistance* to characterize any apparent client movement away from change. By the time of our second edition we were already uncomfortable with this term, but were not fully clear why, nor did we find a reasonable synonym to substitute.

In the intervening decade our discomfort with the concept of resistance has continued to grow, particularly because it seems to place the locus and responsibility for the phenomenon within the client. It is as though one were blaming the client for "being difficult." Even if it is not seen as intentional but rather as arising from unconscious defenses, the concept of resistance nevertheless focuses on client pathology, underemphasizing interpersonal determinants. The phenomena we were trying to describe are a product of, or at least highly responsive to, counseling style. They rise and fall in reaction to what the counselor is doing.

A helpful distinction emerged from Theresa Moyers's research examining interactive processes within MI. She pointed out that we had lumped within "resistance" what we now call sustain talk—the client's own motivations and verbalizations favoring the status quo. There is nothing inherently pathological or oppositional about sustain talk. It is simply one side of ambivalence. Listen to an ambivalent person and you are likely to hear both change talk and sustain talk intermingled. When ambivalent, people *naturally* voice sustain talk in response to their own or others' arguments for change. To call this "resistance" is to pathologize what is a perfectly natural part of the process of change.

If we subtract sustain talk from what we were previously calling resistance, what is left? The remainder has a different quality from sustain talk and it more resembles disagreement, not being "on the same wavelength," talking at cross-purposes, or a disturbance in the relationship. This phenomenon we decided to call *discord*. You can experience discord, for example, when a client is arguing with you, interrupting you, ignoring, or discounting you.

Note the presence of the word "you" here. Sustain talk is about the target behavior or change. Discord is about you or more precisely about your relationship with the client—signals of discord in your working alliance. In music as in relationships, discord requires at least two participants. A single voice cannot yield dissonance. Discord is like a fire (or at least smoke) in the therapeutic relationship. So with this edition we intentionally take leave of the concept of resistance and propose instead two important but different phenomena: sustain talk and discord.

> Sustain talk is about the target behavior or change. Discord is about your relationship with the client.

SUSTAIN TALK

Sustain talk is about the target behavior or change and reflects one side of ambivalence. This means that, like change talk, sustain talk cannot be recognized as such unless you know the change target(s). By definition, then, sustain talk cannot occur without first identifying a focus.

In itself, sustain talk is not discordant, although the counselor's response can quickly make it so. Nevertheless, sustain talk matters. The more people verbalize and explore sustain talk, the more they talk themselves out of changing. Because it's a normal part of ambivalence, don't expect an absence of sustain talk or be unnecessarily alarmed by it. What typically happens over the course of an MI session is that the ratio of change talk (pros) to sustain talk (cons) increases. Early on, pros and cons may be evenly balanced in a 1-to-1 ratio, which is one working definition of ambivalence. The cons of change may even outweigh the pros. As MI proceeds, pros typically increase and cons diminish, so that later in the session change talk statements may counterbalance sustain talk by a 2- or 3-to-1 ratio. That is the trajectory associated with subsequent behavior change.

So how, then, should one respond to sustain talk? First of all, don't go fishing for it. It is not necessary or even desirable in MI to evoke and explore all of the client's possible reasons for persisting in the present course. If reasons for reluctance are important the client will tell you so. The likely outcome if you were to thoroughly and equally explore both pros and cons of change would be continued or even reinforced ambivalence. A "decisional balance" strategy is a reasonable approach when you *don't* want to promote change in a particular direction (see Chapter 17), but it is logically contraindicated in MI.

> It is not necessary or even desirable in MI to evoke and explore all of the client's possible reasons for persisting in the present course.

Reflective Responses to Sustain Talk

One type of MI response to sustain talk involves reflective listening (Chapter 5). We consider here straightforward reflection and two variations: amplified and double-sided reflection.

Straight Reflection

Within MI the most common response to sustain talk is to reflect it in one of three ways. The first of these is to offer a simple or complex reflection of what the person has said. Sometimes this in itself will evoke change talk, the other side of the client's ambivalence. Expect and wait for change talk to follow, and it will often come.

CLIENT: I don't think that anger is really my problem.

INTERVIEWER: Your anger hasn't caused any real difficulties for you.

CLIENT: Well, sure it has. Anyone who gets into scraps as much as I do is bound to have some consequences.

Amplified Reflection

A second reflective response to sustain talk is to offer an amplified reflection. This essentially turns up the volume a bit on the client's statement. It accurately reflects what the person has said, adding to its intensity or certitude. The intent behind such overstatement is to evoke the other side of ambivalence: change talk.

CLIENT: I think things are just fine in our marriage the way they are.

INTERVIEWER: There's really no room for improvement.

CLIENT: Well, I mean things aren't *perfect*, but I'm happy enough as it is.

INTERVIEWER: Things just couldn't possibly be any better in your marriage than they are right now.

CLIENT: I'm pretty satisfied, but I guess both of us aren't.

An amplified reflection not only acknowledges what the person is saying, but also takes it up a notch in search of the other side of ambivalence.

Double-Sided Reflection

A third way for responding is with a double-sided reflection. This type acknowledges the sustain talk and integrates it with previously expressed change talk.

There are two artful subtleties to suggest here. The first has to do with the conjunction between the two elements of a double-sided reflection. Should it be *but* or *and*, which serve different functions? *And* highlights ambivalence, giving equal credence to both elements. *But* is more like an eraser, diminishing what has gone before. Have you ever had a work performance evaluation that began like this?

"You've generally done a good job this year. You've been fairly productive, and the quality of your work has been pretty good, *but* ... "

Or imagine a lover who told you:

"I really care about you and I think you're a terrific person and all, *but* ... "

Somehow the *but* says "Never mind what I just told you. Here comes the important information." For this reason we recommend *and* as the default conjunction in double-sided reflections, acknowledging the both/and nature of ambivalence. The person thinks or feels X *and* Y simultaneously. The person wants it and doesn't want it at the same time, and that's normal. Use *but* if you intend strategically to deemphasize the first element of a double-sided reflection.

Second, in either case (*but* or *and*), we think it is better to state the sustain talk first before the conjunction (thus immediately acknowledging it), and then the change talk, giving it the salience of recency and thus inviting the person to respond to it.

> "You think it's going to be a real challenge to change the way you cook and eat, and you also know how important it is to keep your blood sugar level regulated."
>
> "It's so easy and comfortable to sit on the couch and watch television, especially the programs you really like, and at the same time you want to figure out how to be more active and fit in some exercise."

Don't fret too much about these subtleties. You can use either "but" or "and" and put the sustain talk either first or second and still have a good double-sided reflection. The client will tell you whether you did it well. If the client's response happens to head off into more sustain talk or discord you can always recover. Just avoid falling into continued evoking and exploring of sustain talk, as happened in this example:

CLIENT: I really don't want to make any big changes in how I eat.

INTERVIEWER: You like the freedom of eating whatever you want. What do you like to eat?

CLIENT: Ice cream. McDonald's burgers and fries. Fresh bread with lots of butter. All the things that I'm not supposed to eat with diabetes.

INTERVIEWER: Those foods are really important to you.

CLIENT: Yes! They taste so good, and they're easy. I don't like to cook.

INTERVIEWER: It's a lot of hassle, cooking for yourself; not worth it. What else do you like about your current diet?

CLIENT: It's not a diet at all. Like you said, I feel free to have whatever I want whenever I want.

It seems obvious that in focusing on sustain talk this conversation is not headed in the direction of change, at least not so far.

Strategic Responses

There are other helpful ways of responding to sustain talk besides the three types of reflection. The intent is the same as with reflective responses: to acknowledge clearly what the person is saying and not push against it in a way that is likely to entrench sustain talk. Reflection itself will go a long way in this regard, but here are some other options.

Emphasizing Autonomy

CLIENT: I really don't want to exercise.

INTERVIEWER: And it's certainly your choice. No one can make you do it.

What's going on here? The counselor is simply telling the truth. It really *is* up to the person whether or not to make a change. Nobody else gets to decide that. This response specifically acknowledges and honors personal autonomy.

> "It's really up to you."
> "I wonder what you'll decide to do!"
> "You're right. What you choose to do is your business. You could quit, cut back, keep on as you are, or do it even more if you want to."
> "Even if I wanted to decide for you, I can't."

These are spoken with no sarcasm. Add a little cynical attitude in your tone and you'll get a whole different response. A paternalistic or dismissive lilt can instantly turn one of these into a confrontation. Try saying one of them with various inflections that convey different attitudes and meaning, and hear how different it can sound, even though on a transcript the words might be the same.

Emphasizing that people do have a choice seems to make it more possible for them to choose change. As discussed in Chapter 11 in relation to coercive language, telling people (inaccurately) that they "must" or "have to" or "can't" is a recipe for reactance.

Reframing

Familiar to cognitive therapists is the idea of reframing: suggesting a different meaning or perspective for what the person is describing.

CLIENT: I don't know if I can do it.

INTERVIEWER: It would be quite a challenge for you—hard work!

CLIENT: My wife is always nagging me about this.

INTERVIEWER: She must really care about you.

CLIENT: Everybody I know drinks as much as I do.

INTERVIEWER: You really drink with the champions!

CLIENT: I've been through so much lately. I don't know if I want to take this on, too.

INTERVIEWER: You're quite a survivor.

What is the common theme in such offerings? They invite another way of perceiving the situation. Uncertainty becomes a challenge, almost a dare. Nagging bespeaks love. The normal becomes the exceptional. Adversity reflects strength. Reframing is not a matter of arguing about the correct perception—just inviting the person to consider a different angle of view.

Agreeing with a Twist

The impact of a reframe may be increased by prefacing it with a reflection that acknowledges and essentially sides with what the person is saying. It's hard to argue with someone who is agreeing with you. The twist, the suggested reframe, is mentioned without particular emphasis, almost in passing, and again without any hint of sarcasm.

CLIENT: I can't imagine myself not smoking. It's part of who I am, part of everything I do.

INTERVIEWER: You just wouldn't be you without it! It's so important that you may just have to keep on smoking no matter what the cost.

CLIENT: I can really hold my liquor. It just doesn't affect me the way it does other people. I'm still standing when everyone else is passed out.

INTERVIEWER: You don't show or feel the effects of alcohol the way other people do. I can see how that would be a concern. What else?

The balance of language is very sensitive here. We sympathize with our translators because the subtleties differ so much across languages and cultures. The center is truth-telling. The smoker or drinker really can persist in defiance of the consequences. High tolerance truly is a risk factor for alcohol dependence. Agreeing with a twist contains the benefits of reflection and of inviting the person to consider things in a different light.

Running Head Start

What if you're having a hard time finding any change talk and all you hear is sustain talk? One strategy here is to get a running head start toward the pros of change by listening to the cons. If this sounds a bit like decisional balance, it is, but the strategy is to gain access to the change talk by first hearing out the motivations for status quo. This is specifically for the situation in which change talk seems to be scarce. If you already have good change talk to explore, there's no point in going fishing for sustain talk like this:

CLIENT: I really need to get a job. It's time.

INTERVIEWER: Yes, but what have you enjoyed about being unemployed?

It just doesn't make sense to go asking for trouble. The essence of a running head start is to hear out the main motivations for reluctance when change talk seems hard to come by, and *then* to ask about the downside of the status quo and the advantages of change:

INTERVIEWER: I hear loud and clear that you really don't want to be here.

CLIENT: I just want my kids back. The judge had no right to take them away.

INTERVIEWER: It's a puzzle to you why the judge did that.

CLIENT: We got into a fight, but it wasn't a big deal. It was all blown out of proportion.

INTERVIEWER: Nothing serious from your perspective.

CLIENT: We were doing fine. How I run my family is my business.

INTERVIEWER: You certainly don't like anyone else in your business. And now you're supposed to come here and talk to me, when there's nothing wrong as far as you can see.

CLIENT: That's right. It's not fair.

INTERVIEWER: So the things you don't like about this situation are being ordered around, talking to people about your family matters, things being blown all out of proportion, and other people making decisions for you. Anything else?

CLIENT: That's about it, I guess.

INTERVIEWER: And on the other hand, how might coming here be useful to you?

CLIENT: I'm here to get my kids back. I want my family together again.

INTERVIEWER: That's really important to you. What else?

CLIENT: I want to get the judge off my back, to get her out of my private life.

INTERVIEWER: Being here might also help get things back to normal. Maybe even a little better than normal?

CLIENT: Maybe.

In case we haven't been clear enough, we do not recommend the running head start as a routine procedure in MI. It is useful when someone seems reluctant to discuss reasons for change. It is also possible that the absence of change talk indicates that the client truly is *not* ambivalent about change. Chapter 18 addresses the situation where your task is to create ambivalence.

Coming Alongside

When all else fails to yield change talk, try coming alongside. This is essentially agreement without a twist. Joining with the person's sustain talk, even with a bit of amplification, will sometimes trigger some change talk.

CLIENT: I've tried this "exposure" stuff myself, and it doesn't work for me. I just get too anxious. I start to confront my fear, and then I feel like I'm going to die and I back off. It's not for me.

INTERVIEWER: It really may be too difficult for you. It's not everyone's cup of tea, even though it's effective. Exposure means experiencing and getting through the fear, and it may not be worth the discomfort. Perhaps it's better to stay as you are.

DISCORD

> Tune your ear to hear signals of dissonance and recognize them as important.

Now we turn to the phenomenon of discord, signals of disharmony in your collaborative relationship. What are the signs of a fire in your working alliance?

Smoke Alarms

Just as a smoke alarm alerts you to a change in the air, tune your ear to hear signals of dissonance and recognize them as important.

Defending

One sign that something is amiss is when clients appear to feel the need to defend themselves. This can take many forms such as:

- Blaming—"It's not my fault."
- Minimizing—"It's not that bad."
- Justifying—"What I'm doing makes sense."

These may be about "it"—the change target, and thus overlap with sustain talk—but they also have a definite overlay of defending one's integrity, autonomy, or self-esteem. People defend, of course, in response to perceived attack or threat. A more than passing presence of signs such as these is information that the client is feeling personally threatened at present.

Squaring Off

A sure sign of fire in the working alliance is an oppositional stance, which signals that you are perceived as an adversary rather than an advocate. These have more of a "you" quality to them:

> "You don't care about me."
> "Who are you to tell me what to do?"
> "You don't know what you're talking about."
> "You have no idea what it's like for me."
> "You're wrong about that."

Here is an invitation to a power struggle, to argue or persuade. Because the topic of conversation is personal change, however, the client holds most of the power.

Interrupting

Another sign of discord is when a client talks over you, interrupting while you are speaking. It's not necessarily the content but the fact of interrupting that is a signal. What might this communicate? Interrupting might mean:

> "You don't understand."
> "You're not hearing me."
> "You're talking too much. Listen to me."
> "I don't agree."

Some people do this frequently as a characteristic style: to listen (if at all) just long enough to decide what to say next and then start talking; but consider the possibility that it's a signal of discord, particularly if it's a change from the prior rhythm of the conversation.

Disengagement

A fourth smoke alarm is apparent disengagement from your conversation. The person seems to be inattentive, distracted, or ignoring you. Perhaps the client changes the subject and goes off on a tangent. The eyes glaze over or glance at a clock.

Don't worry about which particular signal of discord something is. A client statement might convey two, three, or even all four of these themes. Attend to the smoke that signals a fire in your relationship.

Why is discord a concern? Some might even regard signals like this to be a good sign that you are "getting to them." Discord is a concern because it signals a breakdown in working alliance and is inversely related to subsequent change (Miller et al., 1993; Patterson & Chamberlain, 1994; Safran, Crocker, McMain, & Murray, 1990).

We also hasten to add that signs of discord are culturally relative. What signals a breakdown of collaboration in one culture or subculture may not be important in another. This can be a problem when counseling across cultural differences, where reflection is a particularly good tool to check on meaning.

Your Own Contribution

Discord can also arise from the clinician's mood or approach. It may be more likely to occur when you are feeling tired, under stress or distracted, or even just very concerned to help someone solve an urgent problem. Perhaps you stop listening or your righting reflex twitches. You begin arguing for change and providing solutions, elicit the complementary reaction from the client, and the rapport between you is in jeopardy.

INTERVIEWER: I think it's time for you to take this seriously and do something about it.

CLIENT: It's just not a priority for me right now. I think I'll be all right.

INTERVIEWER: It's difficult for me to see how you're going to be all right if you don't change anything. You keep on doing the same thing and expect a different result!

CLIENT: Look, I'm just fine. I can take care of myself, OK? Can I go now?

Notice how the discord in this instance also takes the form of sustain talk, and it's clearly not the result of the refined listening that lies at the heart of MI. The clinician has become restless to push on and has left the client behind.

You may also experience some signals of discord within yourself. Perhaps it's physical: a tight feeling in the stomach or a flushing in the face. Perhaps it's silent self-talk: "I can't believe she is sitting here and telling me this isn't a problem. What's the matter with her? How many times have we talked about this?" The inner chatter can also arise from anxiety: "What will happen to her if she doesn't change? Will it be my fault?" Of course, when you're attending to this internal monologue you have probably stopped listening to the client.

Sources of Discord

Discord can occur for different reasons across the four processes of MI. Here is a brief discussion of different contexts in which it may be manifest.

Discord in Engaging

Some people come in the door angry and defensive even before the counselor speaks a word. Discord can thus emerge quite early as an obstacle to initial engagement. This can be the product of prior experience such as coercion, expectations, or how the person was treated by others previously. The good news is that in MI, change is predicted not by the client's level of commitment at the start, but rather by the pattern of change in motivation over the course of the session (Amrhein et al., 2003). You're not responsible for the client's starting point, but you do have considerable influence over what happens next. MI has been found to be a particularly effective approach for working with people who are angry and defensive at the outset (Karno & Longabaugh, 2004; Waldron, Miller, & Tonigan, 2001).

There are many factors within treatment contexts that can promote client disengagement. One of us, about to receive a painful medical procedure and potentially a fearful diagnosis, was greeted by a practitioner who fell right into the assessment trap: "Good morning. I need to ask you some questions and you just tell me 'yes' or 'no,'" and into the litany of closed questions we plunged. Disengagement and passivity were assured.

One can unwittingly contribute to discord in more subtle ways than this. Labeling and blaming (see Chapter 4) are likely to promote alienation. When initially interviewing someone who drinks too much, using the term *alcoholic* may generate discord almost immediately, and it can be a challenge to reengage. Even the language of having "a problem" can quickly evoke defensiveness.

Discord in Focusing

Discord can also arise in the focusing process as disagreement about what to discuss and targets for change. Someone walking through the door of a specialty clinic may have multiple concerns, and what is on the practitioner's mind may not be the person's highest priority. The premature focus trap has to do with pushing too soon for a change target that the client does not yet share. In an addiction treatment program for women the staff found that clients had some concerns about their alcohol or other drug use, but these might be fourth or fifth in priority below problems like finding a job, housing, child care, and personal safety. A single-minded focus on one problem is likely to undermine a good working alliance.

Discord in Evoking

There's no simple dividing line between sustain talk and discord. If you have successfully engaged well with a client and have an agreed focus, sustain talk still emerges quite naturally. This need not be viewed as a problem or signal of discord because sustain talk is a normal part of ambivalence. However, you'll notice that if you push the conversation in a direction or at a pace that the client is not ready for, discord can emerge. Discord is a common consequence of the righting reflex. A clinician pushing for change elicits a complementary client response, and if this pattern continues it can escalate in a way that damages rapport.

During the evoking process discord can also arise from trying to move prematurely into planning. Pushing for a change plan before the client is ready can reverse whatever progress has been made with evoking:

INTERVIEWER: You've told me some reasons why making this change would be a good idea. So what are you actually going to *do* about it?

CLIENT: I don't know. I wish I could do something, but it's not so easy.

INTERVIEWER: Well, let's just talk about how you could do it. What ideas do you have?

CLIENT: That's just it. I'm not sure I'm ready for this.

INTERVIEWER: How can I help you be more ready? Don't you see the benefits it will bring?

CLIENT: That's not the point, really. I can see that there could be some benefits, but to be honest I feel like I'm being pushed into this.

This client is indeed feeling pushed. There is still more evoking work to do, and the signals are clear: it's just too early to push ahead toward commitment to a plan. If the interviewer doesn't ease off soon there will be some reengaging to do as well.

Discord in Planning

Finally, discord can arise during the planning process. After successful navigation through engaging, focusing, and evoking it is tempting for a clinician to think, "OK, I can take it from here. Now let me tell you what to do." Planning also needs to be a collaborative process, and directing instead of guiding can lead to a breakdown in the dance. Although client and counselor may agree on the change goal and its importance, discord can arise over the best way to proceed.

What all of these potential sources of discord have in common is a breakdown in the dance. Instead of moving and working together, it begins to feel like a struggle and toes get stepped on. Usually it is the result of a clash between the counselor's righting reflex and the client's ambivalence.

Responding to Discord

In many ways, MI-consistent responses to discord resemble how one responds to sustain talk. Reflection remains a key tool for understanding and for restoring a working alliance.

CLIENT: How old are you? How can you possibly understand me?

> REFLECTION: You're wondering if I'll really be able to help you.
>
> AMPLIFIED REFLECTION: It seems like there's no chance at all that I could help you.
>
> DOUBLE-SIDED REFLECTION: You're looking for some help, and you're not really sure if I'm the right person to provide it.

The strategic approaches discussed above can also be useful in responding to discord. Consider these three examples:

CLIENT: I don't listen to anybody who's not in recovery.

INTERVIEWER: You definitely want to be understood, so let me listen to you instead. [Agreeing with a twist]

CLIENT: I'm not going to quit [Sustain talk], and you can't make me. [Discord]

INTERVIEWER: That's right. I know I can't make that decision for you even if I wanted to. [Emphasizing autonomy]

CLIENT: I hate being told I can't eat whatever I want.

INTERVIEWER: It's tough having to make food choices all the time. [Reframing]

In addition to these, there are some other possible ways of responding to discord that can be helpful. Here are three examples.

Apologizing

When you've stepped on someone's toes it's polite to say "Sorry." This costs you nothing and immediately acknowledges that this is a collaborative relationship.

"Oh, sorry. I must have misunderstood you."
"It sounds like I must have insulted you there."
"I didn't mean to lecture you."

Affirming

An affirmation can also help to heal tension in your working alliance. Sincere affirming tends to diminish defensiveness and reflects a respectful relationship.

CLIENT: I can do this on my own without your help!

INTERVIEWER: Once you make your mind up about something you can get it done.

CLIENT: You don't know what you're talking about.

INTERVIEWER: You've really thought this through.

Shifting Focus

Another possible response to discord is to shift the focus away from the hot topic or sore spot rather than continuing to exacerbate it.

CLIENT: Are you saying that this is my fault, that I'm not a good husband?

INTERVIEWER: Not at all. I'm not interested in placing blame or name-calling. What matters to me is how you would like your relationship to be better, and how you might get there.

CLIENT: Do you think I have a drinking problem?

INTERVIEWER: I really don't care about labels. What I do care about is you.

In summary, there is no single formula for responding to sustain talk and discord. The key is to respond in a collaborative, accepting way that honors autonomy and does not invite defense of the status quo. There are literally hundreds of ways to do this well.

THE DRAMA OF CHANGE

Responding well to sustain talk and discord is a key to successful treatment if you can recognize it for what it is: an opportunity. In arguing for the status quo or expressing discord, the client is probably rehearsing a script that has been played out many times before. There is an expected role for you to play—one that has been acted out by others in the past. Your lines are predictable. If you speak these same lines as others have done, the script will come to the same conclusion as before.

But you can rewrite your own role. Your part in the play need not be the dry, predictable lines that the client is expecting. In a way, MI is like improvisational theater. No two sessions run exactly the same way. If one actor changes roles, the plot heads off in a new direction. Tension is often the life of a play. It is the twist that adds drama and excitement to the plot. Viewing sustain talk or discord as a perverse character flaw is a sad mistake, for these lie at the very heart of human change. They arise from the motives and struggles of the actors and foreshadow certain ends to which the play may or may not lead. The true art of a counselor is tested in recognizing and handling these tensions. It is on this stage that the drama of change unfolds.

KEY POINTS

✓ Sustain talk is a normal part of ambivalence and should not be misinterpreted as "resistance."

✓ The phenomenon of discord signals dissonance in your working alliance.

✓ Both sustain talk and discord can be significantly increased or decreased depending on how the interviewer responds.

✓ Discord can arise for different reasons across the four processes of MI.

CHAPTER 16

Evoking Hope and Confidence

There is no such thing as false hope.
—MARY PIPER

Hope is the thing with feathers that perches in the soul,
and sings the tune without words, and never stops at all.
—EMILY DICKINSON

Motivational interviewing was originally conceived as a method for evoking motivation to change in situations where the importance of change was more apparent to the counselor than to the client. Much of our discussion thus far has focused on how to enhance clients' perceived importance of change, but there is another clinical problem that any counselor will encounter and in which MI can be helpful. This is the situation in which the client clearly recognizes and acknowledges the importance of change but lacks confidence that it is possible.

> "I could get a better job if I got a college degree, but it's been a long time since I was in school and I don't think I could keep up."
> "I know that smoking is bad for me, but I've tried to quit several times and I just can't seem to do it."
> "We definitely need to communicate better, but I don't think my family is really committed to trying."
> "I would like to be healthier, but it hurts too much to exercise."

Notice the "but" in the middle of each of these sentences. They begin with a statement of desire, reason, or need, and then comes the problem: "But I don't believe I can do it."

Hope is the belief that change is possible. A skillful counselor can lend hope when clients are short of their own. Confidence goes one step further: that not only is change possible, but I can contribute to making it happen. One can hope for change from beyond one's own influence—from luck (a windfall) or from God or changed circumstances—without believing that it's possible to do anything about it. MI is about activating personal change, with a particular focus on confidence.

People are unlikely to commit to making a change unless they have some confidence that it is possible. In fact, lack of confidence can be an obstacle even to acknowledging the importance of change. Who would want the experience of "I really have to change, but I can't"? You have not done people any favor if you cause them to believe that change is urgent but beyond their reach. The result would be anxiety or despair, and a normal human response would be to reduce the distress in some way (e.g., to stop thinking about it or minimize the problem). Both importance and confidence are key components of motivation for change (R. W. Rogers, 1975; Rollnick, Miller, & Heather, 1998), and successful MI supports both of these.

> You have not done people any favor if you cause them to believe that change is urgent but beyond their reach.

WHAT IS THE PROBLEM?

A simple way to think about what is needed is the four-celled figure shown in Box 16.1. How important does this person think it is to address this concern (or opportunity), and how confident is the person about being able to do it? This creates four possible situations.

BOX 16.1. Importance and Confidence

	Importance	
	High	Low
Confidence High	1	2
Confidence Low	3	4

Situation 1 is the counselor's dream. The person knows that change is important and also is confident in being able to accomplish it. This is the intended outcome of MI. It is also the situation in which professional help is least likely to be needed. In Situation 2 the person believes that change is possible (I *could* do it) and does not perceive it to be important (but why would I want to?). That is where MI began. Situation 3 is at least temporarily a demoralizing one. The perceived importance of change is high but confidence is low. "I'll try" is one sign of being in this cell. It signals high enough importance to make an effort, but low confidence in success. Of course, confidence can be so low that the person is not even willing to try. Finally, Situation 4 is the clinician's least favorite scenario: the client perceives change to be neither important nor possible.

Note that this applies not only to situations that involve escaping from a problematic status quo but also to those where the contemplated change is a positive opportunity that could further improve a satisfactory status quo. The dilemma can be an approach rather than an avoidance conflict (see Chapter 12).

Situations 2 and 3 pose different challenges for the clinician. In Situation 2 the focus is on enhancing the client's perceived importance of change. In Situation 3, the importance of change seems to be sufficient and the motivational problem is a lack of confidence. In Situation 4 both importance and confidence are low. It is possible that acknowledged importance is low precisely because of a lack of confidence.

STRENGTHENING CONFIDENCE

Of all the client factors predicting change, hope is one of the most potent (Bohart & Tallman, 1999; Hubble, Duncan, & Miller, 1999; Snyder, 1994; Yahne & Miller, 1999). At the level of a specific behavior, confidence has been termed "self-efficacy" and is a good predictor of successful enactment (Bandura, 1982, 1997). Impact on client self-efficacy may be one channel by which MI effects change (Chariyeva et al., in press). At a broader level, hope is an antidote to demoralization (Frank & Frank, 1993). Fortunately, a client's hope is something that can be strengthened within a therapeutic relationship. A cognitive-behavioral strategy is to help clients learn new skills or strengthen old ones for coping with situations that have stymied them (e.g., Linehan, 1993; Monti, Kadden, Rohsenow, Cooney, & Abrams, 2002). Another is to activate change skills that are already present (DeShazer et al., 2007; Hibbard et al., 2007; Lewis & Osborn, 2004). This chapter focuses on how MI can be used to strengthen hope when low confidence is an obstacle to change. As with motivation more generally, hope is evoked from within the client. The seeds of hope are already there, waiting to be uncovered and brought into the light.

Confidence Talk

Recall that one of four examples of preparatory change talk (DARN) given in Chapter 12 has to do with ability. Evoking such language—confidence talk—would be one approach for strengthening hope. It is drawing on resources that are already there. Hope is not installed but rather called forth. The client is the first source of ideas about how change could be accomplished. Ask open questions the answer to which is confidence talk, and then follow with reflective listening.

> "How might you go about making this change?"
> "What might be a good first step?"
> "Given what you know about yourself, how could you make this change successfully?"
> "What obstacles do you foresee, and how might you deal with them?"
> "What gives you some confidence that you can do this?"

Here is a clinical example of a conversation with a smoker:

CLIENT: How do you think I should quit smoking? I've tried before and it didn't last.

INTERVIEWER: I do have some ideas that have worked for other people, but what really matters is what will work for you. Nobody knows *you* better than you do, so I wonder, given what you know about yourself, what you think it would take for you to succeed. How could you do it?

CLIENT: I don't know. When I've tried before I got really grouchy and hard to live with. I'm not nice to be around.

INTERVIEWER: You really get irritable when you're withdrawing from nicotine.

CLIENT: Yeah. I know there's nicotine gum and all to ease you down, but I think what I need to do is just quit cold turkey, all at once and get it over with.

INTERVIEWER: That's what fits you best. How could you do that?

CLIENT: I think I'd need to be away from people for a couple of weeks *(laughs)*, maybe off by myself in the wilderness somewhere.

INTERVIEWER: For other people's protection.

CLIENT: For *my* protection, if I still want to be married and have some friends when it's over!

INTERVIEWER: You've been that hard to live with when you quit cigarettes.

CLIENT: Well I've only gone 2 or 3 days, but yeah, it's been pretty bad.

INTERVIEWER: So one thing you're not sure about is how long it would take you to get through the really rough withdrawal part, and maybe how you'd spend your time during those days.

CLIENT: I know I'd have to keep busy and be doing something with my hands. I like building cabinets and furniture. I'd probably get a whole house-full done before I was through it!

INTERVIEWER: That's something you know about yourself—that it would really help to stay busy through the hardest days. And you don't want a nicotine patch or gum to ease you down.

CLIENT: No, I just want to get it over with. No messing around.

INTERVIEWER: Once you decide to do something, you just want to get it done.

CLIENT: With something unpleasant like this, yeah. Now, if I'm working on a nice piece of furniture, I don't mind taking my time. I enjoy it.

INTERVIEWER: That could really occupy you and pass the time.

CLIENT: In fact it could be nice just to take some time off from work and build furniture.

INTERVIEWER: You can imagine actually doing that as a way to quit smoking, and enjoying it.

CLIENT: Yeah. I'd have to send my wife away to her mother's for a couple of weeks, and not answer the telephone, but I think that could work.

INTERVIEWER: At least until you get through the really grouchy days. How confident are you that that would work for you?

CLIENT: I think it would. I just need to stick with it and not be around other people, especially other smokers for a week or two.

INTERVIEWER: Is there anything I can do to help you get through this—be your emergency telephone crisis line?

CLIENT: (*Laughs.*) No, I just need to set a date and get it over with.

What you are listening for and working to strengthen is ability language, confidence talk—*could, can, able to, possible*—as well as the person's own ideas for how best to do it. Open questions using this language are a good way to explore the client's ideas: "How could you go about it in order to succeed?"

Confidence Ruler

The ruler introduced in Chapter 13 can be used in a similar manner to elicit confidence talk: "How confident are you that you could do this if you decided to? On a scale from 0 to 10, where 0 is not at all confident and 10 is extremely confident, where would you say you are?" The same follow-up questions discussed in Chapter 13 are then used to elicit the client's perspectives of confidence:

"Why are you at a ____ and not 0?" (or a lower number)
"What would it take for you to go from ____ to [a higher number]?"
"How might I help you go from a ____ to [a higher number]?"

The answers to these questions will be confidence talk. As before, remember not to reverse the questions by asking, "Why are you at ____ and not 10?"

Giving Information and Advice

Sometimes people genuinely don't have ideas about how to proceed and ask you for information or advice. As illustrated in the example above, our initial response to such a request is often to turn it back and solicit the client's own ideas first. Beyond that, though, it is certainly reasonable to offer useful information or advice, and the fact that the client has asked you for it provides permission. As discussed in Chapter 11, when it comes to advice we recommend offering not one possibility but a menu of options from which to choose.

Identifying and Affirming Strengths

Another way of building confidence is to identify more general strengths and resources that the person has that could be helpful in the change process. Affirmation of strengths can in itself bolster self-esteem and confidence. Affirming a person's strengths is a way of bolstering hope and confidence when someone is short on it. As discussed in prior chapters, you can ask people directly about their own positive attributes, exploring these with reflective listening. Because many people are self-conscious about self-affirmation we have also used a more structured procedure called "characteristics of successful changers." The list of adjectives shown in Box 16.2 is simply a compilation of 100 positive attributes that people may manifest. Everyone can find adjectives on this list that describe them, and that is what we typically ask people to do: "Have a look at this list of strengths that people sometimes have, and circle a few that describe you." We try to have people identify at least five. Then explore these strengths with open questions and reflective listening.

INTERVIEWER: Now I'd like to talk to you about how these strengths might help you in your cardiovascular rehabilitation program so that you don't have another heart attack. I see that one thing you have circled is "Forward-looking." Tell me a little about that.

BOX 16.2. Some Characteristics of Successful Changers

Accepting	Committed	Flexible	Persevering	Stubborn
Active	Competent	Focused	Persistent	Thankful
Adaptable	Concerned	Forgiving	Positive	Thorough
Adventuresome	Confident	Forward-looking	Powerful	Thoughtful
Affectionate	Considerate	Free	Prayerful	Tough
Affirmative	Courageous	Happy	Quick	Trusting
Alert	Creative	Healthy	Reasonable	Trustworthy
Alive	Decisive	Hopeful	Receptive	Truthful
Ambitious	Dedicated	Imaginative	Relaxed	Understanding
Anchored	Determined	Ingenious	Reliable	Unique
Assertive	Die-hard	Intelligent	Resourceful	Unstoppable
Assured	Diligent	Knowledgeable	Responsible	Vigorous
Attentive	Doer	Loving	Sensible	Visionary
Bold	Eager	Mature	Skillful	Whole
Brave	Earnest	Open	Solid	Willing
Bright	Effective	Optimistic	Spiritual	Winning
Capable	Energetic	Orderly	Stable	Wise
Careful	Experienced	Organized	Steady	Worthy
Cheerful	Faithful	Patient	Straight	Zealous
Clever	Fearless	Perceptive	Strong	Zestful

Note. From Miller (2004). This page may be reproduced and adapted without further permission.

CLIENT: Well, I like to look on the positive side of things, I guess. I've always been good at seeing the possibilities rather than just how things are.

INTERVIEWER: I see. You're optimistic in a way.

CLIENT: In a way. It's more that I don't dwell on the past with "would have, should have, could have," but just look ahead. I can't do anything about the past, but the future hasn't happened yet. I can do something about it.

INTERVIEWER: That's a real strength for you. You don't get stuck in thinking how bad things are, and instead you ask what you can do to make things better.

CLIENT: Yes, that's right.

INTERVIEWER: So in getting strong and healthy again, it would be important for you to focus on what you want to live for, what lies ahead for you. Is that right?

CLIENT: Exactly. I'm not done living yet. There is a lot I want to do.

Notice that what the patient says here contains a lot of change talk in addition to affirming a particular strength for change. When the client identifies a personal strength, ask for elaboration. In what ways is this characteristic of the person? Ask for examples and follow with reflective listening.

It can also be useful to explore here what sources of social support the client has for pursuing change. Are there others on whom he or she could call for support? In what ways? Who else could help with change?

Reviewing Past Successes

Another source of hope is to explore changes that people have made successfully in the past: "What changes have you made in your life that were difficult for you? Or what things have you managed to do that you weren't really sure at first you would be able to do?" Hearing about one or more of these you explore, "How did you do that?" and again listen empathically, reflecting in particular the skills and strengths implied by the story. Explore past positive changes in some depth. What did the person do that worked? Was there specific preparation for change? You are looking in particular for personal skills or strengths that might be generalized and applied in the current situation. Instead of only asking, "Tell me how you did it," it can be useful to have the person go through in some detail what change occurred and how it came about. Why did the person decide to make this change? What did she do to initiate and maintain change? What obstacles were there, and how did he surmount them? To what does the client attribute her success? What may this mean about his resources, skills, and strengths? Remember that you want the client rather than yourself to be making the arguments for confidence.

Brainstorming

A classic approach for problem solving is brainstorming, which involves freely generating as many ideas as possible for how a change might be accomplished. The list is generated without critique—all ideas are acceptable no matter how silly or unrealistic they might seem. The purpose is to stimulate creative, divergent thinking about how change might be achieved. It's OK to suggest ideas here, but mostly you should rely on the client's creativity to generate possibilities. Write them down.

Once a list has been generated, ask the client which ideas on the list seem most promising or acceptable and why. Don't forget that through all of these methods for evoking hope there runs the common theme of eliciting and strengthening the client's confidence talk. Within the context of MI, brainstorming is not only a method for generating ideas but also another format for eliciting confidence talk.

Reframing

Sometimes a person bogs down in attributions of failure, and a process of reframing or reattribution can be helpful. A common theme is "I've tried several times, and each time I failed," and the general strategy is to reframe "failure" in a way that encourages rather than blocks further change attempts.

The concept of a "try" can be helpful here. It is a short step to recast "failures" as "tries." One need not resort to platitudes ("If at first you don't succeed, try, try again") to discuss what the client has done in the past as successive tries toward a goal. Some knowledge of change research can be helpful here. For example, dependent smokers usually do not succeed in quitting on their first try. On average, it requires between three and four serious tries before a smoker permanently escapes the grip of tobacco dependence, and since that's an average it may require six or seven rounds. With each try, the person is one step closer to success. Whereas a "failure" sounds like a shameful thing, a "try" is laudable. If one has tried several times without success, it may only mean that one has not yet tried the right approach. Even the same approach may work if tried again. Trying is a routine and necessary step toward successful change.

Other reframes can facilitate confidence. Explanations of "failure" as being due to internal, stable factors (like inability: "I can't do it") can be reattributed to external and unstable factors like effort or luck: "The time wasn't right." "I haven't done it yet." "I wasn't quite ready." "I was unlucky that time." "I didn't try hard enough, or long enough." Take a lesson from gamblers, who are notoriously persistent: Maybe next time is my time.

Hypothetical Thinking

If the person is struggling with practicalities, it may be helpful to leap into "hypo-space," to think in the hypothetical. Subjunctive syntax is useful here:

> "Suppose that you did succeed, and were looking back on it now. What most likely is it that worked? How did it happen?"

"Suppose that this one big obstacle weren't there. If that obstacle were removed, then how might you go about making this change?"

"Clearly you are feeling very discouraged, even demoralized about this. So use your imagination: if you were to try again, what might be the best way to try?"

Sometimes the distance of thinking hypothetically can free up a client's creativity. One method we have used for clients who are comfortable with self-reflective writing is a "letter from the future," often as a take-home task to allow some time for reflection:

"What I'd like you to do is imagine that it's 5 years from now and you have succeeded in making this change that you want. Write a letter to yourself from the future. Can you imagine that? Offer some words of encouragement from this future, wiser self and write about how you managed to accomplish this change."

Such creative hypothetical thinking can even work within treatment sessions. On occasion, when feeling stuck during a counseling session we have asked a client to serve as our "consultant":

"Peter, I'd like to try something a little different if you're willing. In a minute I will ask you to move to that chair over there and to take the role of my consultant. When you do, we will talk about your situation together as if you were my consultant, to help me think about what to do. When we do this, talk about yourself not as 'I' or 'me,' but as a third person: 'he.' Do you understand?"

After having the client change chairs, we might say something like this:

"I'm feeling a little stuck at the moment in working with Peter, and I'd like your advice. I really want to help him, and I can't quite see what would be a good next step. What do you think is going on with Peter, and what might I try?"

After this conversation we thank the "consultant," have the client return to his chair, and typically try what he suggested. Not every client can handle this kind of distancing, but sometimes clients come up with surprising insights and ideas. As throughout MI, the working assumption is that the client has wisdom, insight, and creativity to be tapped.

> The working assumption is that the client has wisdom, insight, and creativity to be tapped.

Responding to Confidence Talk

A common purpose that runs through all the methods just outlined is for the client to speak about ways in which change can occur, about confidence: why and how he or she could succeed with change. Consistent with an overall MI perspective, it is useful for the client to make these arguments. When such confidence talk occurs it is important to respond in a manner that supports and strengthens it. The same four complementary responses (OARS) outlined in Chapter 14 apply here, for this is just a special case of responding to change talk.

- *Open question* asking for *elaboration* or *examples*
- *Affirm* the client's strengths and ability
- *Reflect* the client's self-confidence statements
- *Summarize* the client's reasons for optimism about change

Reflective listening remains a central skill here. Listen for themes, experiences, ideas, and perceptions that imply confidence and bespeak the person's ability to make the desired change. Reflect these preferentially, both immediately as they occur and in subsequent reflective summaries. Appropriately affirm the client's expressions of confidence.

As confidence talk emerges, it can also be useful for you to raise possible problems and challenges that could be encountered, asking the client for solutions:

"What might you do if . . . ?"
"How could you respond if . . . ?"
"What do you think would happen if . . . ?"

This in turn elicits further change talk. In fact, it is exactly the opposite of you proposing solutions and having the client point out their limitations. Your role here is not to refute the client's change talk but to stimulate further thought and specificity.

Radical Change with Multiple Problems

There are times when the needed change is not circumscribed but involves a number of interrelated problems that are unlikely to respond to a simple solution. For example, consider the situation of a polydrug-dependent commercial sex worker in a city where prostitution is illegal. Like many such women, she may place high importance on escaping from her conundrum but see no possible way of doing so. Complex though it may be, this is a confidence issue. Change might require escaping from dangerous and resourceful associates; finding temporary food and shelter, geographic relocation, and polydrug detoxification and treatment; resolving legal problems; developing new job skills; and finding employment, child care, and housing. To talk about change in any one of these problems (such as drug dependence) without addressing the others is clearly unrealistic, and low confidence is understandable. Gradually changing one thing at a time is unlikely to work because the problems are interlocking and complementary.

In such situations, the only avenue in which a person can have confidence may be one involving radical change that simultaneously addresses multiple problems. Without underestimating complexity, it is possible to discuss how such radical change might occur. Rather than trying to modify a particular behavior, this requires thinking about the big picture of change.

CLINICAL EXAMPLE

The following clinical dialogue illustrates a MI approach to enhancing confidence using the radical change scenario just described. The dialogue begins after a period of discussion about the importance of change, which the client summarizes so concisely that there is no need for the interviewer to do so. The challenge now, before a concrete change plan can be addressed, is very low confidence.[1]

CLIENT: I just can't do this work much longer. It's too dangerous, and I'm going to end up dead. I have my daughter to think of, too. I don't want her to have the same kind of life I've had. I'm a wreck as a mother—shooting up in the bathroom so she doesn't see me, out half the night. Now the social worker is threatening to take her away from me again, and I don't blame him. I can't go on like this.

On the importance ruler, she rates herself at a 9.

INTERVIEWER: It's a desperate situation you're in, and you really want out.

CLIENT: I came close to getting out the other night, but not the way I want to—in a box.

INTERVIEWER: You said you were nearly killed.

---

[1] With sufficient foundation in place, we add a running commentary now to the clinical example. The entire Julia case example is available at *www.guilford.com/p/miller2* with commentary throughout.

CLIENT: I've come close before, but that one really scared me—the guy I told you about.

INTERVIEWER: So what's the next step? How could you get out?

CLIENT: That's just it. What can I do? . . .

An invitation to provide solutions . . .

INTERVIEWER: You feel stuck, with no way out

. . . which the interviewer simply reflects.

CLIENT: No shit! I have no money. I'm on probation. CC watches me like a hawk, and beats me up and cuts off my drugs if he even thinks I'm holding out on him. We live in a cheap motel room. What am I supposed to do?

One can imagine here the likely result of making suggestions or prescribing solutions ("Well, how about . . . ?").

INTERVIEWER: That's exactly the question you're faced with. You want out, but how in the world can you overcome so many incredible obstacles?

Again the interviewer reflects instead of jumping in with answers.

CLIENT: I just don't see a way. Otherwise I'd be out of here.

Confidence ruler = 1 or 2.

INTERVIEWER: I certainly don't have the answers for you, but I have a lot of confidence that you do, and that working together we can find a way out.

Lending hope.

CLIENT: What do you mean?

INTERVIEWER: Well, for one thing, you're amazingly resourceful. I can't believe how strong you are, to have gone through all you've been through and even be alive, let alone sitting here and talking to me about how you want your life to be in the future. I don't think I could have survived what you've been through.

Utterly genuine affirmation and reframe.

CLIENT: You do what you have to.

INTERVIEWER: How have you come this far and still have the amount of love and compassion that I see in you—not only for your daughter, but for the women you work with and for other people as well? How do you do it?

Affirmation and open question.

CLIENT: Just one day at a time, like they say. I don't know. I just go way inside, like when I'm doing some john. I don't let myself get hurt. I take care of myself.

INTERVIEWER: Like you take care of your daughter.

Linking reflection.

CLIENT: I hope I take better care of her than I do of myself. But yeah, I take care of myself. Nobody else does.

INTERVIEWER: So you have this amazing inner strength, a solid core inside you where you can't be hurt.

CLIENT: Or don't let myself be hurt.

INTERVIEWER: Oh, right! It's not that you can't feel anything, because you do. You have a way of preserving that loving woman inside you, keeping her safe. So one thing you are is strong. How else might you describe yourself? What other qualities do you have that make you a survivor?

Affirmation.
Evocative question.
Asking for personal strengths.

CLIENT: I think I'm pretty smart. I mean, you wouldn't know it to look at me, but I can see what's going on around me, and I don't miss much.

Confidence talk begins.

INTERVIEWER: You're a strong and loving woman, and pretty smart. What else?

A collecting summary.

CLIENT: I don't know.

INTERVIEWER: What might someone else say about you, someone who knows you well? What good qualities might they see in you, that could help you make the changes you want?

CLIENT: Persistent. I'm downright bullheaded when I want something.

INTERVIEWER: Nothing stops you when you make up your mind, like a bull.

CLIENT: I do keep going when I want something.

INTERVIEWER: Strong and loving, smart, persistent. Sounds like you have a lot of what it takes to handle tough changes. How about this? Give me an example of a time when you really wanted something and you went after it.

Reviewing past successes.

CLIENT: You won't like it.

INTERVIEWER: Try me.

CLIENT: I was out of shit last week, and I really wanted it something bad. CC thought I was cheating him, keeping money and not telling him, and so he cut me off. I asked around and nobody had any to give me. It was the afternoon and nothing was happening on the street. So I took my daughter and went over to the freeway entrance. I had to wait until CC went for dinner. I made up this sign that said, "Hungry. Will work for food." In an hour I had enough to get what I needed, and some food for us, too. CC never found out about it.

INTERVIEWER: It's all the things you said. You had to time it all carefully, but you're so aware of what's happening around you that you could do it. You think quickly, and came up with a solution. You stuck with it, and made it happen. How did you make the sign?

Collecting summary of strengths.

CLIENT: Cardboard I found in a dumpster, and I borrowed a marker at the motel desk.

INTERVIEWER: They seem like little things, but I'm impressed at how quickly you solved this one. I'm sad, of course, that all this creativity was spent on getting drugs, but it's just one example of how you can make things happen when you put your mind to it.

CLIENT: Now that's another thing. What do I do about being hooked? The withdrawals are bad.

INTERVIEWER: You've been through them before, then.

CLIENT: Sure. In jail, on the street, even in a detox once, but I don't want to go through it again.

INTERVIEWER: Tell me about the detox. When was that?

CLIENT: Last year. I got real sick and they took me to the emergency room, and from there they took me to detox. I stayed about 5 days, but I got high right afterward.

INTERVIEWER: What was the detox like for you?

CLIENT: It was OK. They were nice to me and they gave me drugs so that I didn't feel uncomfortable. As soon as I hit the street, though, I wanted a fix.

INTERVIEWER: So it was possible, at least, for you to get through the withdrawal process comfortably. The problem came when you went back out. Now let me ask you this. Imagine that you're off the street—like magic. You're through withdrawals and away from the street, out of CC's reach, somewhere else completely. Don't worry for the moment about how you got there—we'll come back to that—but you're free, just you and your daughter. What would you do? What kind of life would you choose?

Using the hypothetical.

Looking forward.

CLIENT: I'd need to find a real job. Maybe I'd go back to school and then get a good job. I'd like to get out of the city—live in a little place out in the country somewhere.

Change talk.

INTERVIEWER: A complete change of scenery.

CLIENT: That's what it would take.

INTERVIEWER: And you can imagine it, a new life somewhere with your daughter.

CLIENT: I can imagine it, yes. But how could I get there?

An invitation to give solutions.

INTERVIEWER: It's such a big change with so many obstacles that you don't think you could do it.

Coming alongside.

CLIENT: I don't know. I might be able to. I just haven't thought about it for a long time.

Confidence ruler = 3 or 4?

INTERVIEWER: Maybe, just maybe, with all your strength and smarts and creativity and stubborn persistence, you could find a way to pull it off. It's what you want, is it?

CLIENT: Yeah, it would be great, getting off the street.

INTERVIEWER: Is this just a pipe dream here, or do you think you might actually be able to do it?

CLIENT: It seems kind of unrealistic, for me at least.

INTERVIEWER: For you. But it might be possible for . . .

CLIENT: I guess I was thinking of my daughter. Or maybe some other women I know, but then I think I'd have as good a chance as they would.

INTERVIEWER: You can imagine yourself doing it, just like others might. Let me just ask you to do one more thing, then, before we get any more specific. Let's think about what it would take for you to get from the street to that place you imagined. And let's be creative. Let's think of any way at all that it might happen, as many different ways as possible. They can be completely unrealistic or unlikely, no matter. What we want is a lot of ideas. OK?

Introducing the idea of brainstorming.

CLIENT: Sure, why not.

INTERVIEWER: So how might it happen?

CLIENT: I could meet a sugar daddy, like that girl in the *Pretty Woman* movie.

INTERVIEWER: OK, good. That's one. What else?

CLIENT: There could be a miracle. (*Laughs.*)

INTERVIEWER: Right. One miracle coming up. What else?

CLIENT: I could talk my mom into bailing me out again. If she thought I was really serious this time, she might do it.

INTERVIEWER: So your mom could help get you out of here with money.

CLIENT: She's worried about her granddaughter, I know. We might even be able to live with her for a while, but I don't know if she'll ever trust me again.

Confidence talk is gradually emerging over the course of this 10-minute segment, and there are the beginnings of a possible change plan. Rather than jumping straight to a how-to-do-it discussion with this high-importance/low-confidence woman, the interviewer spends some time in eliciting confidence in her broader adaptive abilities. The interviewer also resists the invitations to step in and provide solutions. This paves the way for later development of and commitment to a specific change plan (Chapter 20).

FINDING HOPE

Human beings are amazingly resourceful. The mind-set behind this approach is one that profoundly trusts and respects the person's own solutions. It is very tempting for helpers to offer solutions and try to *install* hope and confidence. As discussed in Chapter 10 and later in Part V, there is a role for offering your own expertise, but we have found it wise always to look first within the client for sources of strength and solutions. You don't have to come up with the answers alone, nor is that likely to work well when the challenge is personal change. Finding hope is not a matter of creating it from nothing but rather of calling forth that which is already there. Hoping is a truly collaborative interpersonal process, and one in which it is a profound privilege to participate.

> Finding hope is a matter of calling forth that which is already there.

KEY POINTS

✓ People are reluctant to commit to making a change unless they have some confidence that it is possible.

✓ Clients with high importance and low confidence need a different kind of help from those with low importance and high confidence.

✓ The clinical style of MI can be used to strengthen hope and confidence.

CHAPTER 17

Counseling with Neutrality

What I dream of is an art of balance.
—HENRI MATISSE

If you come to a fork in the road, take it.
—YOGI BERRA

MI was originally developed for a particular purpose: to strengthen people's motivation for and commitment to make a particular change. MI in that sense is about influencing choice, although ultimately the choice of whether to make a personal change always remains with the client.

There are, however, situations in which it is appropriate *not* to nudge a client's choice in one particular direction. This could be because you have no opinion yet about what direction would be best for the person or because you think you should not influence the choice one way or the other even if you do have an opinion. In this case you need to keep your balance so as not to consciously or inadvertently favor one side of the client's ambivalence.

Consider this range of possible clinical scenarios in which you are working with a client who is considering change options:

A couple who want help deciding whether to try to adopt children.
An adult considering donating a kidney for a relative who needs a transplant.
A woman pondering whether to have an abortion.
An adolescent considering whether to use condoms when having sex.
A man who has been injecting "speedballs" (heroin and methamphetamine).

A woman deciding whether to leave her husband who has been physically abusive.

A homeless man who is comfortable with life on the street.

A woman considering whether to enroll in a study you are conducting.

A man who uses self-asphyxiation by hanging to heighten sexual orgasm.

A woman mandated to treatment after a third conviction for drunk driving.

A soldier who in boredom and despair periodically plays "Russian roulette."

A caller to a crisis hotline, pondering suicide by jumping from a building.

A sex offender contemplating new victims.

If you are like most clinicians, your sense of urgency to influence the client's direction of choice varies across these scenarios. There may be some where you feel a professional and ethical obligation to do whatever you can to encourage the client to choose and change in a particular direction. There may be others where you believe it would be ethically wrong for you to try to influence the client to take a particular path, and chances are that some fall into a gray zone for you.

In this chapter we present an MI-informed way of counseling when your intention is to avoid influencing the direction of choice a client makes. In a way this is a more difficult task than moving in one direction. What we have learned about the psycholinguistics of change is quite relevant here, and counseling with neutrality involves being continually conscious of this dynamic throughout the process of exploring options.

EQUIPOISE

The intention to leave a choice wholly up to the client is not a new idea. In the practice of medicine this has been called *equipoise*. The clinician either does not have an opinion about which choice would be best (e.g., among different options to treat a particular cancer), or at least believes that the choice should be up to the patient. A physician may provide information about what the available science indicates so that the patient can make an *informed* choice, but does not want to directly or indirectly nudge the person toward a particular option (Charles & Whelan, 1997; Elwyn, Edwards, Kinnersley, & Grol, 2000).

So what exactly is equipoise? First, it is not a personal or professional trait. Some clinicians do manifest great *equanimity*: they are typically patient, emotionally stable and composed, fair minded, levelheaded and balanced, and this is generally characteristic of them across people, time, and situations. Equipoise, however, pertains to a specific client and situation. Like change talk, equipoise is only definable in relation to a particular decision or change goal. One does not have equipoise about a person, but rather about a particular choice or change the person is contemplating.

Second, equipoise is different from your own opinion or aspiration. It is possible to have a personal/professional opinion or guess about which option would be better for the client, yet choose to practice equipoise because you believe you should not influence the client's decision. Consider, for example, a client who is ambivalent about whether to remain in a 10-year marriage or to seek a divorce. You may have a professional hunch or even personal moral conviction about which would be the better choice but still believe it is proper for this decision to be left completely to the client. In that case you would practice equipoise even though you have a personal opinion or aspiration for the client.

What we are saying, then, is that equipoise is a mental intention or choice that is reflected in practice with regard to a specific client and situation at a particular time. Equipoise is a chosen practice, not a feeling or personality trait. It is a conscious, intentional decision *not* to use one's professional presence and skills to influence a client toward making a specific choice or change.

> Equipoise is a conscious, intentional decision *not* to use one's professional presence and skills to influence a client toward making a specific choice or change.

Can We Influence Choice?

This understanding of equipoise assumes, of course, that it is possible for a clinician to influence which choice an ambivalent person will make. You cannot actually make other people's choices for them or take away their ability to choose. Even if clients "let" you decide for them, that is a choice made by the client. It is clear, however, that interpersonal influences can and do shape the choices people make and that most of us underestimate the extent to which our behavior is influenced by external factors (Bargh & Chartrand, 1999; Bargh & Ferguson, 2000). A wide variety of specifiable factors can influence attitudes, choices, and values and are regularly used in advertising, marketing, and politics (Cialdini, 2007). Much has been written about the extent to which clinicians knowingly or unknowingly influence clients' value choices to resemble their own, calling into question psychotherapies that are purported to be value neutral (Bergin, 1980; Truax, 1966).

This can be unsettling knowledge for professionals and public alike. Western cultures place a high premium on self-determination, which is a cornerstone consideration of medical ethics (see Chapter 10). The assumption of free will underlies much of law and public policy as well: that people are (or at least ought to be) autonomous, freely and willfully deciding their own actions and life course based on their individually held values (Baer, Kaufman, & Baumeister, 2008). Yet Rokeach (1973) demonstrated that values themselves could be shifted with even a relatively simple experimental intervention, a shift that influenced a wide variety of behaviors and choices over subsequent months and years. Thus a clinician's decision of whether to try to influence a client's choice is a serious and consequential one precisely because it is possible to do so.

Choosing Neutrality

A preliminary step in relation to any change goal about which a client is ambivalent is therefore a decision: whether you will maintain neutrality or encourage movement toward a particular resolution. These alternative paths call for different clinical approaches. Much in the foregoing chapters has focused on how to accelerate movement toward a particular change goal by strengthening one side of the client's ambivalence. The same principles of influence, however, can inform how to proceed in practicing equipoise when you choose to maintain professional neutrality. That is the primary focus of this chapter.

It is reasonable and advisable to inform your client when this is what you intend to do. One reason for this is the discomfort that can emerge when a professional explores with equipoise an ambivalence that is emotionally charged. Ambivalence can be an acutely unpleasant, aversive place to remain when the pondered choice is a psychologically significant one with potential long-term consequences. Increasing people's simultaneous awareness of both sides of an internal conflict can be quite distressing for them. Often a client would find movement in either direction more comfortable than pondering the existential dilemma of intense ambivalence. The essential elements of informing, we think, are these:

1. That you want to help the person explore the dilemma that has him or her stuck.
2. That you intend to remain neutral yourself with regard to what the person should do until they decide.
3. That exploring a dilemma like this can be uncomfortable or upsetting, which is one reason people get stuck in ambivalence.
4. That you want to help them work through the dilemma and discomfort, make their own decision, and move on as they choose.

Here's how it might sound.

> "I can see that you've really been struggling with this dilemma and feeling stuck. That's very common in a situation like this. Thinking about either alternative is uncomfortable, and so it's tempting to try not to think about it; but that's uncomfortable, too, because nothing is resolved or changed. What I suggest we do is to explore both sides of this dilemma rather thoroughly. I want you to know that I intend to remain completely neutral about what you should do and not advise you one way or the other, but just help you take a good close look at what your choices are. You may find this process uncomfortable—people often do—but I think that's what you need to do to get unstuck. I will work with you and support you until you decide what you want to do, and then help you move in the direction you've chosen. Do you have any questions about this process I have described? Shall we proceed?"

Avoiding Inadvertent Guiding

A counselor can fall into the taking-sides trap inadvertently, even if not consciously intending to defend or promote one particular side. Consider these two examples of counseling focused on choice in the midst of ambivalence—the decision of whether to have children.

CLIENT: I guess the most pressing issue for me is a family. I'm over 30, and if I'm ever going to have children, it's time.

INTERVIEWER: Your biological clock is ticking.

CLIENT: Yes. I really have to decide about this.

INTERVIEWER: And what have you been thinking?

CLIENT: I guess I always thought I'd have kids at some point. It's just that both of us had to get school out of the way and then we started working, and suddenly I'm 34.

INTERVIEWER: Of course, women are having babies at later ages now.

CLIENT: But isn't it risky?

INTERVIEWER: The risks do go up, yes, but they are still relatively low and there is good prenatal testing available.

CLIENT: If I got pregnant and then found out that there was something wrong, I don't know what I'd do.

INTERVIEWER: There are a number of options.

CLIENT: I know that, but I mean—I guess I'm just not sure if I really want to take the chance.

INTERVIEWER: Why not?

CLIENT: For one thing, it's such a long commitment. You give 20 years of your life—more, really, because being a parent never ends.

INTERVIEWER: Of course there are certain rewards, too. It's a very special kind of relationship that you can never have with another human being in any other way.

CLIENT: I'm not sure, though, that I really want that kind of relationship with just one or two children. I'm a teacher, and in a way I can do a lot more good for children if I'm not tied up for 20 years in raising my own. And it's so *expensive* to raise children these days!

INTERVIEWER: And yet, there is that sense that you might be missing something.

CLIENT: I'd be missing something either way, really. If I have my own children, I miss out on all the opportunities that would have happened in the time I gave to them.

INTERVIEWER: What about just one child. How about that?

CLIENT: I don't think it's fair to make someone an only child. They need to have a brother or sister. It's a special relationship.

INTERVIEWER: Kind of like being a parent.

CLIENT: Well, yes and no. You usually don't spend the better part of your life raising a sibling.

INTERVIEWER: I guess what I'm saying here—what I'm worried about is that if you let your biological clock run out, you might regret it deeply later on.

CLIENT: But I think that's better than the opposite. I know parents who regret having had their kids. They usually don't say so, but deep down they wonder what their lives would have been like if they hadn't had children. I think kids can't help but sense that.

INTERVIEWER: I'm sure that does happen sometimes, but most parents find it very rewarding. It's true that being a mother demands a lot from you, and yet it also gives you something very special . . .

Now consider the same client and scenario, but this time the counselor happens for whatever reason to lean the other way at the outset.

CLIENT: I guess the most pressing issue for me is a family. I'm over 30, and if I'm ever going to have children, it's time.

INTERVIEWER: Your biological clock is ticking.

CLIENT: Yes. I really have to decide about this.

INTERVIEWER: And so you're wondering now whether you want to have a family.

CLIENT: I guess I always thought I'd have kids at some point. It's just that both of us had to get school out of the way, and then we started working, and suddenly I'm 34.

INTERVIEWER: So maybe it's getting a bit late to begin a family.

CLIENT: Oh, I don't know. Lots of people are having babies now who are older than we are. It's fairly common, really.

INTERVIEWER: I'm not saying that it's uncommon. I guess I was just hearing some reluctance in your voice.

CLIENT: Well, of course I'm somewhat reluctant. It's a major life change, but I've always felt like I would have children at some point, and now is the time.

INTERVIEWER: Why? What appeals to you about having a family?

CLIENT: It's hard to say, really—it's mostly a feeling I have. I guess it's good to have children around when you get older—someone to look after you.

INTERVIEWER: Of course that doesn't always happen.

CLIENT: I know. It's also an experience I don't want to miss out on. There's more to life than work. I just feel it would be nice to be a mother.

INTERVIEWER: What other advantages do you see?

CLIENT: Not *advantages* really.

INTERVIEWER: It's not like you have children for what you can get out of them.

CLIENT: Right! There's something about being part of a new life, a part of the future.

INTERVIEWER: Sounds pretty romantic.

CLIENT: Well, I think it is! I know that it's not all roses and it costs a fortune and all, and you open yourself up to pain. It takes a lot of time to raise children. You have to give a lot.

INTERVIEWER: It costs you a lot—not only in money but in time, too.

CLIENT: And yet I feel like it's worth it . . .

The client might leave the first of these sessions feeling more committed to not have a family. In the second example the same person's change talk, elicited by the counselor's inadvertently taking one side, might steer the person in the other direction toward choosing to have children.

EXPLORING AMBIVALENCE

The basic process in counseling with neutrality is to explore thoroughly both the pros and the cons of the available alternatives, and to do so in a balanced way (Janis & Mann, 1977). A common procedure is to evoke systematically the advantages and disadvantages of each option being considered. In a binary choice situation, such as whether to stay in or leave a relationship, a 2×2 decision matrix might look like the one shown in Box 17.1. The diagonal boxes (e.g., advantages of staying and disadvantages of leaving) are complementary and may contain similar entries. Some clients, in fact, find it confusing to distinguish between these, in which case a simple pros and cons list may be better. The point is to give equal attention to each of the boxes by evoking the client's full list in each, exploring each element by asking for elaboration and reflecting (see Chapter 14).

> The basic process in counseling with neutrality is to explore thoroughly both the pros and the cons, and to do so in a balanced way.

BOX 17.1. An Example Decisional Balance

Advantages of staying	Advantages of leaving
Disadvantages of staying	Disadvantages of leaving

Offering Emotional Support

The basic supportive strategy to use when discomfort arises is to acknowledge and reflect it, explaining that it's normal to feel distressed in this situation until one decides what to do.

CLIENT: Oh, I just don't know what to do. I *hate* this!

INTERVIEWER: I know this process is really difficult for you. The temptation is to just turn away and stop thinking about it.

CLIENT: But I know that won't help either.

INTERVIEWER: Yes, that's so. What you're feeling is perfectly normal, and I'm sorry this is so uncomfortable for you. It's been distressing for quite a while.

CLIENT: Yes! It seems like year. I just don't know what to do.

INTERVIEWER: I do understand how confusing this feels, and I want to help you get through it. It's hard but you can do this, and we'll take as long as you need with it.

CLIENT: Oh, I don't want it to take a long time. I want this to be over.

INTERVIEWER: You'd really like to make up your mind and get on with your life.

CLIENT: Yes, I guess so. I can't keep on like it's been. What do you think I should do?

Other people, by the way, are fairly comfortable with ambivalence and become more uncomfortable *after* making a decision and moving toward it, a phenomenon known as "post-decisional regret." This is also a normal personality style, and it becomes apparent which (if either) is true for this particular person as you move through the process (Quenk, 2009).

Can't You Just Tell Me What to Do?

In the midst of the distress of ambivalence, clients may ask what you advise: "What would you do if you were me?" It is a plea to escape the acute discomfort. As described in Chapter 11 we often do provide advice when asked for it if we do have an opinion or relevant information. When in this equipoise situation, however, we have consciously chosen for good reasons to avoid tipping the balance one way or the other. In our hearts we may want to relieve the client's acute distress but we are committed to equipoise. Again, a good response is to acknowledge and reflect the feeling and remind the client of your chosen neutrality.

"You would really like for me to make this decision for you, and in a way I wish I could. I am not you, though, and this is a choice that is definitely not mine to make, or even to point you in one direction or the other. The decision is yours. The way out of this dilemma is to make the tough choice and begin moving in that direction. What are you thinking and feeling at this point? Do you seem to be leaning in one direction?"

The latter question is a parallel to the "key question" described in Chapter 19. It can be preceded by a recapitulation summary of the pros *and* cons expressed by the client.

Persistent Ambivalence

What is a good outcome when you counsel with equipoise? It may be for the person to reach a decision and move on without your consciously or inadvertently favoring one direction over another. Consider an organ donation decision, for example: Will this person donate a kidney for a relative who needs a transplant? Until the decision is made, both the potential donor and the recipient are left in limbo and there may also be medical urgency to find a donor. Yet the health professional believes it would be inappropriate to encourage the person to decide in one particular direction; the choice should be left to the potential donor. In this situation one might facilitate reaching a decision but carefully refrain from favoring one choice over the other.

Having reached a decision, however, does not necessarily resolve inner conflict about it. There may be residual ambivalence or regret regarding the decision that was made. In the case of organ donation, such residual ambivalence is associated with adverse surgical and health outcomes (Simmons, Marine, & Simmons, 1987; Switzer, Simmons, & Dew, 1996), so there is good reason to help people make peace with the decision they have made before acting on it, which may at times involve reconsidering the choice.[1]

It is also quite possible for the outcome of counseling with equipoise to be that the person does not reach a decision. This could be an expected outcome when doing a classic decisional balance grid, because giving equal attention and weight to pros and cons is an operational definition of ambivalence. This is not necessarily an undesirable outcome. The person may simply not be ready to reach a decision and act on it. More information, discussion, or time may be needed.

Sometimes a particular form of affirmation can be helpful in this situation—that the person's worth remains intact regardless of the decision that

---

[1] Thanks to Allan Zuckoff for this insight.

is reached. Spiritual counselors sometimes assure people at this point that, "Whichever path you choose, God will still love you and be with you." A counselor might similarly express confidence in the person's strengths: "Whichever way you go, you'll get through this and can continue to lead a healthy and loving life." Such affirmation can be freeing, helping the person to step back from the immediate situation and view it in a larger life perspective. Another way of conveying this is to say, "Whichever you choose, I will work with you and support you." Of course, that should be true if you say it. Some counselors or programs have a value commitment to one particular choice. Historically, some addiction treatment programs have been willing to work only with clients who choose lifelong abstinence as a goal, and some pregnancy crisis centers are committed to preventing abortions. In such situations the counselor by definition is not counseling with neutrality.

IS THIS MOTIVATIONAL INTERVIEWING?

So if you intentionally choose neutrality as your professional stance and you carefully avoid guiding the client in one particular direction, is that MI? In a way it doesn't matter whether it's MI if it's the right thing to do. Certainly our recommendations here about how to counsel with neutrality arose from what we have learned through MI research regarding guiding and the psycholinguistics of conversations about change. From the earliest description (Miller, 1983) MI has been about strategically evoking the client's own arguments for change, usually with a conscious goal of steering toward a particular outcome. The intended outcome when counseling with neutrality is to help the person make a difficult decision without influencing the direction of choice. The direction is toward making a decision.

> When counseling with neutrality, the direction is toward making a decision.

Sometimes a decisional balance evaluation helps the client realize that in fact the pros far outweigh the cons, or vice versa. This may facilitate the decision process. If pros and cons are really equally balanced, at least the exercise reveals this conundrum and the person may decide to make the choice despite ambivalence. In any event, we believe that it helps to be mindful of these dynamics of interpersonal influence when you wish to counsel with neutrality. In classic "nondirective" client-centered counseling there was little guidance for what to reflect, ask about, or summarize from all the material offered by someone. The decisional balance approach provides a systematic framework for keeping your balance when maintaining neutrality.

KEY POINTS

✓ Neutrality or "equipoise" is not a counselor characteristic but rather a conscious decision to avoid influencing the direction in which ambivalence is resolved.

✓ Understanding the linguistic dynamics of change is helpful in knowing how to counsel with neutrality.

✓ Decisional balance is an appropriate strategy to use when one chooses to counsel with neutrality rather than encouraging change in a particular direction.

CHAPTER 18

Developing Discrepancy

The function of a mirror is to reflect an image
as it is, without adding flattery or faults. From a
mirror we want an image, not a sermon. We may
not like the image we see; still, we would rather
decide for ourselves our next cosmetic move. . . .
Clarity of image, whether in a looking glass or
in an emotional mirror, provides opportunity for
self-initiated grooming and change.
—HAIM GINOTT

We found we had to make haste slowly.
—BILL W.

The idea of developing discrepancy has been part of MI since the very beginning. It was originally framed as cognitive dissonance (Festinger, 1957; Miller, 1983), but a simpler way to conceptualize this important motivational factor is as a discrepancy between present and desired states, the distance between a personal goal and the status quo. Goal–status discrepancy is one of the most fundamental drivers of motivation for change (Ford, 1992).

Discrepancy can be either positive or negative in valence. It can be experienced as discontent with the status quo (Baumeister, 1994) or as an opportunity for betterment (or both). Creating perceived discrepancy through the allure of positive gain or avoiding unpleasant outcomes is a common strategy in marketing and advertising.

Some clients come to a consultation already aware of a large discrepancy, even distressed and ashamed about it. Most smokers are well aware of the hazards and disadvantages of smoking. Most obese people are reminded many times a day of discrepancy: whenever they look in a mirror, cannot fit into a chair, or get short of breath with even minor exertion.

243

So why doesn't such discrepancy produce change? We suggest three inter-related reasons.

First, the discrepancy may seem so large as to be daunting. The "Gold-ilocks principle" applies here: the discrepancy should not be too large or too small, but "just right." If the discrepancy is too small, it may not appear important enough to prompt action. If it is too large, the needed change may seem beyond reach. Scandinavians have a word for this for which there is no direct equivalent term in English: *lagom* in Swedish. It means just so, the right balance, just enough. In order to be motivating, a discrepancy should be *lagom*.

Relatedly, a person may perceive a substantial discrepancy but feel unable to do anything about it. This lack of self-efficacy may be because the discrepancy seems too large, or just because the needed skill is beyond one's ken: "I have no idea how to do it." In order for a discrepancy to be motivating, people need reasonable confidence that they can do something to remove or reduce it.

Furthermore, a discrepancy can evoke such unpleasant experiences that the person simply avoids thinking about it as a matter of self-defense. It is just too painful to look in the mirror. This is exacerbated, of course, if the discrepancy seems too large and beyond one's ability to remedy. It is a peculiar idea that people will change "if you can just make them feel bad enough." If misery cured misbehavior there would be far less of it.

SELF-REGULATION: THE THERMOSTAT OF CHANGE

A thermostat constantly monitors the temperature in the space for which it is responsible and responds accordingly. If the room temperature is within the zone of tolerance nothing needs to be done. Should the temperature go above or below the acceptable range, however, then a change is initiated. Some thermostats are set to tolerate only a small deviation from the ideal before reacting; others have a much wider range of tolerance before change is triggered.

Human beings are similar in some ways. The body adjusts by sweat-ing or shivering when core temperature falls outside a fairly narrow limit. Self-regulation theory uses the same analogy for how people decide when behavior change is needed (Brown, 1998; Kanfer, 1970b). There is a zone of tolerance, a range of behavior or circumstances that feels within nor-mal limits. People are constantly monitoring the world around them and, perhaps to a lesser extent, within themselves and comparing the incoming information with these internal tolerance standards. Moving along a road, for example, one drives straight ahead without thinking much about it, on "automatic pilot" as it were. If an object appears in peripheral vision and seems to be on a collision course, however, attention and muscles kick into gear. Perhaps one brakes or steers to avoid it. The senses have detected something out of the ordinary, something that requires attention and change.

Does self-regulation theory also apply to volitional behavior, to conscious choices that people make? In many ways it does fit (Baumeister et al., 1994; Miller & Brown, 1991). People monitor the status quo and compare it with their sense of how things ought to be. The detection of a discrepancy beyond the zone of tolerance is an instigation to change and triggers a search for options. If an acceptable path is found, the person may try it and monitor the results to see whether the discrepancy has been reduced. In the case of the driver on a collision course, this all happens within a matter of seconds. When it comes to a significant lifestyle change the process may be spread over many months or even years. Often it is not a conscious, rational decisional process, but such adjustments are constant in human life.

Discrepancy within Limits

In Chapter 10 we considered ethical aspects of influencing clients' volition, specifically because of the apparent ability of MI to alter, within limits, one's willingness and readiness to act in a particular way. What are those limits? For example, can a client be caused through MI to behave in a manner directly contradictory to his intrinsic core values? We believe the answer to this question is "No," in part because of our understanding of how MI works. The idea of developing internal discrepancy necessarily raises the question, "Discrepancy with what?" It is discrepancy with the person's own goals and values. Unless a current "problem" behavior is in conflict with something that the person values more highly, there is no basis for MI to work. The focus is on intrinsic motivation for change. It is irrelevant whether the client's behavior is discrepant with someone else's values, unless (1) it is someone highly regarded and valued by the client, in which case intrinsic value discrepancy is again operating; or (2) it is someone with coercive power, discussed in the next paragraph. MI will not induce behavior change unless the person perceives that such change serves an intrinsic value and is thereby in his or her own best interest.

This protective condition of consistency with intrinsic values is not present for coercive methods. People can sometimes be coerced to behave in ways that violate values they hold dear. This is one intention behind torture and brainwashing, and it is also why institutional review boards exist to protect research participants from coercive conditions, such as enticingly high payment to be exposed to risk. Within the realm of counseling a method known as "constructive coercion" used the contingent power of an employer to motivate employees into treatment they might otherwise refuse (Smart, 1974; Trice & Beyer, 1984). An "intervention" as originally propounded by the Johnson Institute (Johnson, 1986) involved a planned and rehearsed group confrontation by family members (and sometimes others such as friends or employers) of a person perceived to have a problem. In addition to expressing compassionate concern, members of the group might also announce negative consequences that would ensue if the person did not comply with the group's aspiration, which was often for the person to enter a treatment program. Such interventions are typically undertaken without the person's approval, with the ethical principle of benevolence being given greater importance than autonomy, at least temporarily.

It is our assertion that MI, by virtue of its reliance on discrepancy with intrinsic values, cannot work in violation of a person's autonomy. It may cause a person to want to do something, but for the reason that the anticipated change is ultimately consistent with important personal goals and values. In this way, it differs from coercive strategies that are explicitly designed to override what a person wants.

FACILITATING DISCREPANCY

Before we turn to how one might instill discrepancy when it seems to be lacking, we consider first the equally important topic of how to make it possible for someone to entertain a discrepancy, to ponder it without triggering a need for self-defense that will shut down the process. In essence, you are creating an atmosphere of safety that helps people to look in the mirror, see an often uncomfortable truth, and let it change them.

Ironically, it is when people experience acceptance of themselves as they are that change becomes possible. Causing people to feel bad and unacceptable usually entrenches the status quo. When you provide acceptance (as described in Chapter 2) you make it possible for people to consider a larger discrepancy, to entertain it without shying away. Remember that acceptance is not the same as approval or agreement. The four elements of acceptance described in Chapter 2 are accurate empathy (accurately understanding the person's own experience), autonomy (honoring the person's choice and self-determination), absolute worth as a human being, and affirmation.

> It is when people experience acceptance of themselves as they are that change becomes possible.

Affirmation itself can have a strong impact in helping people be open to discrepancy and change (Linehan, 1997; Linehan et al., 2002). Perhaps even more powerful than affirmations coming from you are self-affirmations that you can evoke from the client (see Chapter 16). Affirming someone's strengths and good qualities, even ones unrelated to the task at hand, tends to decrease defensiveness and help people attend to potentially threatening information (Critcher et al., 2010; Klein & Harris, 2010; Sherman et al.,

2000; Steele, 1988). Sometimes it is also possible to reframe discrepancy from shame to opportunity, from pessimism to possibility.

There are, to be sure, realities that are best accepted rather than trying to change them. Trying to "not feel" emotions can have an ironic effect of strengthening them (Hayes, Strosahl, & Wilson, 1999). There is wisdom to the prayer penned by Reinhold Niebuhr during World War II asking for "grace to accept with serenity the things that cannot be changed, courage to change the things that should be changed, and the wisdom to distinguish the one from the other." An atmosphere of acceptance and affirmation helps to make this possible. MI thus involves a dialectical tension between acceptance and discrepancy.

Instilling Discrepancy

Most of our discussion thus far in this book has regarded working with people who are ambivalent about making a change: part of their "inner committee" favors making the change and part does not. MI in that case is about evoking and strengthening the client's own existing arguments for change, the pro-change side of the person's ambivalence, before moving on to planning and implementation.

But what about clients who do *not* seem to be ambivalent? Even within a safe empathic atmosphere they seem to have no change talk for you to evoke. In the transtheoretical model of change these people are said to be in the precontemplation stage. They are not even considering change, perhaps haven't even thought about it. They are not truly ambivalent, at least not yet.

The fact that they are having a conversation at all with you about change likely means that someone else besides the client perceives a need for change. It might be an employer, the courts, or concerned family members who have directed the person to treatment. It might be you or another clinician who perceives that a client who is seeking help for other reasons also needs to make a particular change. Consider these examples:

- A parent mandated to treatment for child abuse, who sees nothing wrong with the disciplinary practices that led to referral.
- A patient being treated at a trauma center for injuries sustained in an alcohol-related crash, who blames the other driver and has no apparent personal concerns about drinking.
- A teenager brought to treatment by concerned parents who discovered marijuana and drug paraphernalia during a room check. The teen is incensed about being checked up on and regards cannabis as harmless.
- An overweight patient with Type 2 diabetes who cheerfully admits

that "my blood sugar hasn't been under 200 for years" and shows no inclination to make health behavior changes.

- A college student who failed the first midterm examination in an introductory course and seems unconcerned and unwilling to study differently.
- A pregnant woman who expresses no intention to quit smoking or drinking.

It is actually common for such seemingly "unmotivated" people to begin expressing change talk in MI. Even when you meet someone who genuinely seems to be in precontemplation, a good starting point is to assume that discrepancy is already there and search for it. But what if you do find no apparent perceived need or desire for change, and no matter how skillfully you practice MI there just doesn't seem to be any change talk forthcoming? What then?

The process here is one of instilling discrepancy. We like the verb "instilling" because it means to infuse slowly, gradually, drop by drop. Some have instead advocated flooding people with discrepancy (Johnson, 1986), and that could always be a fallback strategy if all else fails, but we find a gentler, encouraging approach is more effective and less likely to backfire (Meyers, Miller, Smith, & Tonigan, 2002; Miller et al., 1999). There is no in-your-face showdown; quite the opposite. Instilling discrepancy is a process of sitting together and considering reasons why the person *might* consider change.

Exchanging Information

A temptation when encountering precontemplation is to lecture, educate, and try to persuade. An apparent lack of client motivation brings out the righting reflex. Argumentation is, of course, no more likely to be helpful in precontemplation than in contemplation. Providing information (with permission) can be useful, but it is probably not the best place to start.

One approach that we find useful in this situation is to ask clients what they already know about the topic of concern. We came upon this strategy in working with pregnant drinkers (Handmaker, Miller, & Manicke, 1999). Rather than launching into a lecture on potential harms to the mother and unborn child we started out by asking, "What do you know about alcohol and pregnancy?" We discovered several important things in the process. First of all, the women already knew about 90% of what we were planning to tell them. We could add a bit or correct a misunderstanding here or there, but mostly the knowledge was already there. The same is true, we find, with people who smoke or who drink too much. Asked what they know, they can reel off a litany of the untoward effects of what they are doing. Addiction isn't usually a knowledge deficit. People living with a chronic illness also typically have at least a general idea of the consequences of not taking care of themselves.

Furthermore, we found that clients generally appreciated being asked what they know. It is a respectful, collaborative thing to do, and people tend to respond much better to being asked than to being told. The context and the spirit behind your words are quite important here. If you communicate even subtly that you are asking for this information so that you can use it against them, clients clam up quickly. Be careful, then, not to give in to the righting reflex here by thinking or asking, "Well then why haven't you . . .?" That will shut them down like an alligator's jaws, and if you get any answer at all it is likely to be sustain talk.

Perhaps our most important realization in this asking approach, however, was that the client's answers contained a lot of change talk. There is something safer about the hypothetical—to talk not about your own drinking but about what you know, what you have noticed.

A next step in the elicit–provide–elicit sequence of information exchange (Chapter 11) is to provide some information with permission: "Would it be all right if I told you a little about what new research is finding on this?" "Could I fill in a piece or two that I notice you didn't mention? Do you mind?" Remember also that a third form of permission (besides being asked or asking) is to acknowledge the person's freedom to disregard what you offer. "This may or may not concern you . . . "; "I don't know if this applies to you or not . . . "; "I'm not sure if this will make sense for you . . . "

It is also possible to choose information that is most likely to be important to the particular individual(s) with whom you are speaking (e.g., Miller, Toscova, Miller, & Sanchez, 2000). This is far preferable to a "canned speech" going over the same information. For example, what consequences might this person be most concerned about based on age, gender, peer group, and stage of life?

As always in MI, the vital foundation for providing information is the underlying spirit of partnership, acceptance, and compassion. "Getting up on your soapbox" tends to leave people with a soapy taste in the mouth. Emphasizing personal choice helps here ("It's really up to you . . . "; "You're the only one who can decide this . . . ") and it is done without even a hint of irony or sarcasm, because it is the truth.

> Emphasizing personal choice is done without even a hint of irony or sarcasm, because it is the truth.

A tip from *The One Minute Manager* (Blanchard & Johnson, 1982) is also apropos here: If you're going to give corrective information, keep it short. If you must convey a few pieces of information, offer them in digestible bites (see Chapter 11), which raises the third part of the elicit–provide–elicit cycle: to elicit again, this time exploring the client's reaction to what you have said: "What do you think?" "Does that make any sense to you?" "Could I explain that better?"

Providing Feedback

Motivational enhancement therapy (MET), which is a combination of MI with assessment feedback, may be particularly useful with people who are less ready to change. The MET "checkup" format was developed with this in mind: to give the clinician something to talk about when clients volunteer relatively little change talk. The original drinker's checkup (see Chapter 27) included a set of measures that are sensitive to the *early* effects of overdrinking (Miller et al., 1988; Miller, Zweben, et al., 1992). This allowed the therapist to provide personal feedback relative to norms on effects of drinking that might not be readily apparent to the drinker. The nonconfrontational MI style of providing this feedback literally doubled clients' change talk and halved resistance (Miller et al., 1993). Following the information exchange guidelines mentioned above, the therapist offered one piece of assessment feedback at a time, then asked for the client's reaction. The result was often change talk in people who were initially not at all sure that they had any problem with drinking.

Some clients—those who are already more ambivalent—readily offer change talk when asked for it. When spontaneous change talk is not forthcoming it may be useful to ask the person to walk you through a typical day in his or her life. This offers opportunities for asking in more detail about behavior patterns and mood changes, for example, and areas of concern often emerge quite naturally from such discussion. A careful assessment and feedback process can provide some objective information to discuss. Again, the feedback is not used against the client as evidence of what he or she "must" do. Leaving the conclusions to the client is often more powerful. Such feedback has even been effective when offered in written form without an in-person discussion (Agostinelli et al., 1995; Juarez et al., 2006; van Keulen et al., 2011).

Although some assessment instruments are designed to detect high levels of severity, it is useful in a checkup to have instruments that are also sensitive to early-occurring consequences and lower levels of severity. Including normative information (i.e., where this person's scores actually stand in relation to others') can be particularly appropriate for triggering perceived discrepancy and instigation for change (Brown, 1998; Reid, Cialdini, & Aiken, 2010).

Remember that ambivalence is an intended *outcome* in this situation. It is one step closer to change and gives you something to work with using the strategies described in the preceding chapters.

Exploring Others' Concerns

When clients are talking to you because of someone else's concerns about their behavior and welfare, another avenue is to explore how the client understands what those people's concerns are and why they have them. This is best done with a kind of curiosity or even confusion: "Why do you suppose your wife is concerned? What do you think she is seeing?" Ideally here, the client takes on the other's perspective and puzzles with you as to the sources of concern. Along the way some change talk can emerge.

INTERVIEWER: Why do you imagine your wife is worried about your drug use? What do you think concerns her?

CLIENT: She's someone who always comes down on the safe side of every issue. But my drug use is my choice, and it's none of her business.

INTERVIEWER: She's not as much of a risk taker as you are.

CLIENT: That's definitely true. She doesn't like anything that's even remotely risky, and I guess she thinks that my drug use is risky.

INTERVIEWER: Why do you suppose she thinks that?

CLIENT: Well, for one thing it's illegal. She's worried I'll get caught and get in trouble or lose my job or something.

INTERVIEWER: But that's really none of her business.

CLIENT: No, now there I can see where she has some grounds for concern, losing my job and all. That would affect her.

INTERVIEWER: So if it could affect her negatively, it's reasonable for her to worry.

CLIENT: Yes, I guess so.

INTERVIEWER: But if it's just affecting you negatively, that's not her concern.

CLIENT: Well, she'd worry about that, too.

INTERVIEWER: Because . . .

CLIENT: Because she cares about me. She's our family smoke alarm.

INTERVIEWER: Of the two of you, she's the one who watches out for things that might hurt you, even before it's serious. She's cautious.

CLIENT: And I'm not. I'm a go-for-it kind of guy.

INTERVIEWER: You're opposite in that way.

CLIENT: Yeah, and I guess opposites attract, you know.

INTERVIEWER: It's one of the things you appreciate about her.

CLIENT: But I don't think she appreciates my risk taking.

INTERVIEWER: Like using illegal drugs.

CLIENT: Yeah.

INTERVIEWER: What else do you suppose concerns her? What has she told you?

CLIENT: She complains about how much money I spend.

INTERVIEWER: She doesn't like how much you spend on drugs, but from your perspective it's reasonable.

CLIENT: Oh, I admit that I go overboard sometimes and it gets a little hard to pay the bills.

INTERVIEWER: Sometimes. Not all that often.

CLIENT: Well, more often that I'd like. Certainly more often than she would like.

INTERVIEWER: Give me an example. When was the last time that happened?

The interviewer here is primarily using reflective listening. Sometimes reflecting the client's sustain talk elicits the opposite perspective, particularly in the context of discussing the concerns of a loved one.

Exploring Goals and Values

We have previously discussed how exploring clients' goals and values can build rapport (Chapter 7) and evoke change talk (Chapter 13). When change talk is not forthcoming, a good starting point for engaging is to understand what your client *does* want. Take your time in exploring the person's own goals and hopes for the future. This process is engaging in itself, and what you are listening for, although not actually acting on immediately, are points where current behavior may conflict with important goals or values and where a change may facilitate reaching those goals.

In situations like those described above people are often experiencing unwanted sequelae of their choices, even if they regard the consequences to be unrelated to their behavior, arbitrary, unfair, or just bad luck. A top priority for court-referred drug users, for example, may be "I want to get my probation officer off my back." Intrusions into personal liberties evoke reactance, and thus offer an opportunity to negotiate behavior change as a route to restored freedom. The methods presented in Chapter 7 can be helpful both in engaging and in considering implications of the status quo for expressed values. Once the client has identified a set of his or her most important values, the exploration process can create momentum:

"Why did you choose this as one of your most important values?"
"In what ways has this been a central value for you?"
"Why is this important to you?"

"How do you reflect this value in your daily life?"

"How might you be even more true to this value in your life?"

This values exploration process can be complete in itself as a tool for engaging or focusing, and it can provide a context for evoking change motivation. With an identified change target such as smoking cessation, a counselor might ask after completing the values exploration:

> "How does smoking fit in with each of your most important values? Do you think it helps you achieve them, conflicts with them, or maybe is irrelevant? Have a look at these values that you have identified and tell me what you think."

In one smoking cessation study a values-based MI intervention was most effective for those who did *not* initially perceive any discrepancy between smoking and their values (Sanders, 2011). In other words, it helped to develop a latent discrepancy that was there in potential, but that the person had not consciously confronted.

You usually don't need to point out inconsistencies between the client's behavior and values; usually these become apparent to the client. Resist the righting reflex: "Don't you see how your behavior is defeating these life goals?" Let your client connect the dots.

Honoring Autonomy

With your best efforts there will still be clients who choose to continue the status quo. Much as one might wish to do so, the autonomous power of choice cannot be taken from the client. Part of the spirit of acceptance is acknowledging that ultimately it is the person's decision what, if anything, to change. This is one thing that can make it difficult to use MI if, like a parent, you have a personal investment in the person's choices.

If after a consultation process there is still little evidence of motivation for change, leave the door open. "I recognize that you aren't at all interested in stopping smoking now, and that is your choice. If anytime in the future you are thinking more about it, the door is open and I will be glad to talk to you." Perhaps at least you have planted some seeds of ambivalence.

> Part of the spirit of acceptance is acknowledging that ultimately it is the person's decision what, if anything, to change.

KEY POINTS

✓ Change tends to occur when a person perceives a significant discrepancy between important goals or values and the status quo.

✓ In order to be motivating, a discrepancy needs to be large enough to encourage change but not so large as to be demoralizing.

✓ A variety of MI strategies can be used to instill discrepancy within the bounds of the person's own values.

PART V

PLANNING
The Bridge to Change

As noted in Chapter 16, if you merely increase a person's sense of urgency for change but not their belief that it is possible, you haven't done them any favor. Distress without hope is no gift. The reason for developing discrepancy and evoking people's own motivations for change is to help them move on to actual change. If you fail to negotiate this planning process, the person may reduce the distress in some other way and the window of opportunity will close again. You might even inure the person against future considerations of change.

People are more likely to follow through with a change when they have a specific plan and express to another person their intention to carry it out (Gollwitzer, 1999; Gollwitzer & Schaal, 1998). That is the essence of the planning process in MI: to move from discussing importance to developing a specific change plan that the person is willing to implement. The four chapters of this section discuss the transition process from evoking to planning (Chapter 19), how to negotiate a change plan in an MI-consistent way (Chapter 20), strengthening client commitment to a plan (Chapter 21), and supporting the process of change (Chapter 22).

CHAPTER 19

From Evoking to Planning

Our plans miscarry because they have no aim.
When a man does not know what harbor he is
making for, no wind is the right wind.
—Lucius Annaeus Seneca

Action speaks louder than words, but not nearly
as often.
—Mark Twain

When is it time to move from evoking to planning? How do you know when the client is ready to begin discussing not just the *why* of change, but also the *how*? It's a judgment call, but basically your client will tell you. In this chapter we describe some emerging signs to watch for that signal readiness for planning, and how to "test the water" to see whether the person is actually willing to move ahead with you in discussing how change might occur.

Evoking sufficient motivation for change (which we previously referred to as Phase 1 of MI) can feel like an uphill slog. Sometimes it moves quickly, but engaging, focusing, and evoking can be a slow step-by-step process like snowshoeing up the side of a mountain. The progress may be steady, but it feels effortful, there are likely to be a few backslides, and you have to pay attention to where you're going.

Planning, on the other hand, can feel like fun in comparison. It's more like a downhill ski (remember the hill diagram in Chapter 12). There is still danger of running into trees, taking the wrong trail, or even heading off a cliff, so you still have to pay attention, but the process feels different from the uphill climb. It is important to remember that this is still MI, still a collaborative process in which you evoke clients' own ideas, and remember that ultimately the choice is theirs to make and carry out.

A trap to avoid here is thinking, "Well, now we finally have that motivation stuff out of the way! Now I can take the lead and direct." There are at least two problems with this. One is that motivational issues are by no means over at this point. Ambivalence is likely to reappear, particularly if the change plan is one that the client does not own. The other is that planning still involves evoking, asking for, and listening to clients' own experience in what will work for them. Planning is a process of negotiation and collaboration drawing on the client's expertise as well as your own, because ultimately it is the client who (you hope) will carry out the change plan.

With sufficient readiness, developing a change plan improves outcome (Lee et al., 2010). However, if you try to develop a change plan before the client is sufficiently ready you may undo whatever progress you have made through engaging, focusing, and evoking. In Chapter 13 (Box 13.1) we showed a graph of commitment language strength over the course of MI sessions with the two-thirds of clients who subsequently stopped using illicit drugs. (That is the same solid line shown in the chart in Box 19.1.) Now we talk about the remaining one-third of clients, who were not as successful, but nevertheless reduced their drug use by half on average. Box 19.1 also shows (in the dashed line) what was happening with change talk (specifically, strength of commitment language) for these clients who did not stop using drugs (Amrhein et al., 2003). Why does their line look so different? It's not that they never showed motivation for change. Rather, their commitment to change was fluctuating substantially during the session.

Here is what we think happened. The therapists in this study were following a manual to ensure consistency in delivering this one MET session as clients were beginning treatment for drug dependence. They began with a brief period of MI (segments 1–2 in Box 19.1). Next, the therapist provided structured assessment feedback (segments 3–5) as prescribed in MET (Miller, Zweben, DiClemente, & Rychtarik, 1992). When this task was finished the therapist returned to open-ended MI (segments 6–9). Finally, all therapists were required to develop a specific change plan with the client at the end of the session (segments 9–10). For two-thirds of the clients (the solid line) this sequence worked well. But follow the dashed line for clients who had less successful outcomes. They begin at the same (low) level of commitment as the successful clients. During the feedback process, however, change talk is strengthening in the successful group but not in the less successful group. Once that is over, they respond to MI and their commitment strength rises to the same level as the other group. Then comes the change plan. These clients were apparently not ready to commit to a specific plan, but the therapist manual said that it was necessary to do one anyhow—in essence *whether or not the client was ready*—and their commitment level abruptly crashes back to zero.

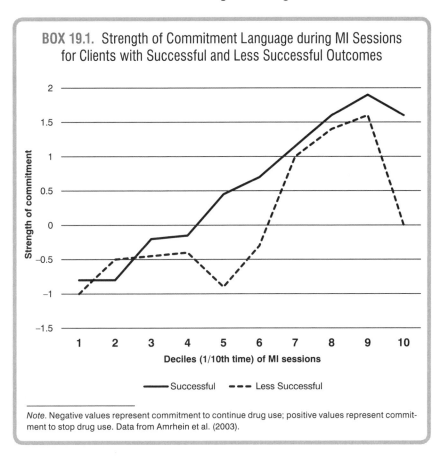

BOX 19.1. Strength of Commitment Language during MI Sessions for Clients with Successful and Less Successful Outcomes

Note. Negative values represent commitment to continue drug use; positive values represent commitment to stop drug use. Data from Amrhein et al. (2003).

Any perceptive MI practitioner who began giving feedback or discussing a change plan and saw the client starting to backpedal and become defensive would stop doing that and switch back to the evoking (or even engaging) process. The problem, we think, was that we did not allow the therapists in this study to use such clinical judgment, but instead required them to proceed to planning. Had the therapist been able to pause at point 9 rather than proceeding, we think that change would have been more likely to happen. Paying more attention to a manual than to the client is not good MI. In one meta-analysis we found that clinical trials in which MI was delivered without a manual (but presumably with good training) had twice the effect size as those in which a manual was used to standardize

> Paying more attention to a manual than to the client is not good MI.

practice (Hettema et al., 2005). Even outline "roadmaps" may distract counselors from empathic focus on the client (Wahab, Menon, & Szalacha, 2008).

So how do you know when it's time to proceed with planning? We offer two guidelines here. First we describe a set of signs that we have observed in practice that signal possible readiness for the planning process. These are clues for the clinician that the client's motivational state may be sufficient to start discussing how change might happen. Then we offer a procedure (recapitulation and key question) to "test the water," to determine whether you should proceed. At this point the client's response is your key in knowing whether to proceed with planning or return to evoking. The client is always right about this.

SIGNS OF READINESS

There is certainly an intuitive aspect of knowing when to proceed. What we describe here are the signs we are aware of attending to as we consider whether to try a transition from evoking to planning.

Increased Change Talk

One sign of possible readiness is an increase in the frequency and strength of preparatory change talk. The more people describe their desire, ability, reasons, and need for change, the more they are opening to consider how it might occur. You don't need to hear change talk in all of these categories, and it's not necessary (although it helps) for people to say specifically that they want to or need to change. You only need *enough* change talk, and therein is the clinical judgment call. Have you heard enough change talk that the person may be leaning in the direction of change? In the language of the transtheoretical stages of change, does it sound like they are transitioning from contemplation to the preparation stage?

The more preparatory change talk you hear, the more likely it is that you will begin to hear mobilizing change talk as well, and this is a particularly good indicator. The key is not to miss low-strength signals. High-strength commitment or activation language is easy enough to recognize:

"I'm ready to do it!"
"Yes, I'm willing to give it a try."
"I'm going to do this, I promise."
"I'll do whatever it takes."

But listen, too, for lower-strength commitment and activation:

"I might do it."

"I'll think about it."

"I'll probably get around to it."

"I hope to."

"I guess I could try."

The righting reflex might cause one to discount or confront responses like this: "What do you mean you *might* do it? How can you sit there and say you'll just *think about it*? Aren't you serious?" The expected result of this, of course, would be sustain talk and discord. When you hear even a little mobilizing change talk, rejoice and be curious about it, but don't get too eager. If you seize on tentative change talk and push for a firm commitment, the person is likely to back away. Don't get ahead of your client's level of readiness.

In any event, change talk is one sign of readiness. Mobilizing change talk in particular is a signal of mental preparation: commitment, activation, and taking steps.

BOX 19.2. Personal Reflection: Selling Executive Jets

On a cross-country flight in the 1990s I found myself sitting next to a gregarious fellow who turned out to be a salesman. More specifically, his job was to select and train sales representatives to sell private jet aircraft to executives. I proceeded to interview him all across the Midwestern states. How do you sell airplanes to people who don't think they need them? What separates successful sales people from those who won't make it in the business? What do you look for when hiring sales representatives? What he told me sounded strangely familiar: "You find out what the executive cares about and what problems or frustrations they face in their daily life." The gradual process is to link how the product to be sold—in this case, jets—would help the customer to better reach their goals. No hard high-pressure selling here: "You would lose the customer immediately." And one thing that a successful sales person needs is a good sense of timing. "You have to be able to see when the customer has privately decided to buy the plane. If you keep on selling after that point, you're likely to lose the sale, but if you push to close before you get to that point you also lose the sale." I kept thinking of what I tell people who are learning MI: Don't let your eagerness for change get ahead of the client's. Some of the tips he gave me about how to know when someone has "decided to buy" clicked with my own clinical intuition and are reflected in this chapter. In any event, it reminded me that interpersonal influence processes are not at all the exclusive province of therapists.

—WRM

Taking Steps

Sometimes as people start leaning toward change they take a small step or two in that direction. These can seem like very halting tentative steps, but they are steps nevertheless. Any step in the right direction is reason for optimism, curiosity, and affirmation. The righting reflex here might be to say, "Is that *all* you did?!"

CLIENT: I went 2 days this week without drinking.

> MI-CONSISTENT: Really! Good for you. How did you do that?
>
> MI-INCONSISTENT: So you drank on 5 days this week.

CLIENT: I did get a newspaper this week and look at the job listings.

> MI-CONSISTENT: What did you see that interested you?
>
> MI-INCONSISTENT: All you did is read the newspaper?

Our inclination is to celebrate and affirm all steps in the right direction. It is viewing the glass as partly full rather than mostly empty.

Diminished Sustain Talk

Along with an increase in change talk there is a decrease in sustain talk— the arguments against change and for the status quo. In a way it is the ratio of these two that signals readiness. Equal change talk and sustain talk is ambivalence. As change talk begins to overbalance sustain talk there is movement toward change. This can feel like "the fight going out of the fish," with less effort needed on your part to respond to sustain talk or discord. The person gradually stops defending the status quo. If this alone happens while change talk remains steady, the ratio is shifting.

Resolve

This one is a clinical intuition harder to measure, but as people work through and start to resolve ambivalence there can be a kind of quietude that settles over them. It may seem like resolution or resignation, pensiveness or passivity, but before people directly voice mobilizing change talk we often sense this quiet kind of resolve. Maybe there is just less discussion about the problem. Sometimes there are sighs or tears. It is as if the realization is settling in, the mind is shifting.

Envisioning

Envisioning statements indicate that the person is thinking about what it would be like to make the change. In imagining a possible future, clients may verbalize positive or negative aspects or both. Positive envisioning statements may just sound like preparatory change talk: "Imagine what I could do with all the money that I would save if I quit!" sounds like a reason for change, and it is, but there is also something more here. The person is *imagining* it. "I wonder if my family would take me back" is not just a possibility but a wondering. The mind is imagining possible positive outcomes. And don't overlook envisioning if the imagined outcomes sound negative:

"How would I make a living?"
"I wouldn't have any friends if I quit drinking."
"What if I try and they turn me down?"

What is happening here is that the person is envisioning having made the change and considering problems that could arise. These are obstacles to be discussed, but the important point here is that the person is imagining the change even if it sounds like sustain talk.

Questions about Change

Finally, it is common for the client to ask questions in the process of considering a possible change. The person may or may not be envisioning it, and in fact may have difficulty imagining it at all, but the questions bespeak a search for options.

"What happens here in this treatment program?"
"How could we make our marriage better?"
"What do people do to quit smoking?"
"How likely am I to be able to get my blood sugar down without medication?"

The timing and art of providing information and advice were discussed in Chapter 11, and it's not necessary (or even a good idea) for you to come up with all the answers. The point here is that when a client asks questions about change, it signals increasing openness to the possibility.

TESTING THE WATER

When you sense that a client may be ready to talk about a change plan, you face an important decision point. Is it actually time to open up the planning process? One way to find out is just to ask the client directly (Magill, Apodaca, Barnett, & Monti, 2010):

"Would it make sense to consider how you might go about
_____?"

"Are you willing to think about how you might _____ or is
that getting ahead of things?"

Another procedure that we suggest for testing the water is a recapitulation
and a key question.

Recapitulation

A recapitulation is basically a transitional collecting summary of all the
change talk that the client has provided thus far. It is the big bouquet, a
bunching together of all the "flowers" of change talk that you have collected (Chapter 14). It might be introduced with some words that announce
a transitional summary, followed by a gentle recitation of the person's own
change talk. There is no need for editorial commentary here. You are summarizing the motivations for change that the person has already given you.
This may be the first time that the person has ever looked at the whole
bouquet together, and it can be a powerful experience.

This means, of course, that you need not only to recognize but also
to *remember* change talk when you hear it. Some people are very good at
doing this within the same conversation at least, and after a session make
notes to recall the change talk that occurred. Other people choose to take
notes during a session as a memory aid. We recommend not taking notes
during MI so that you can devote your full attention to the client, but if you
must, here are a few general tips.

- Mention briefly and in a matter-of-fact way that you are planning
  to take notes: "I like to jot things down from time to time if that's
  all right with you, to help me remember what you say." This simple statement does several positive things: it normalizes your note-
  taking as routine, it respectfully asks permission, and it communicates that "What you say is important enough to me that I want to
  remember it."
- Keep your notes brief—just enough words to help you remember
  later. Note-taking should not break your eye contact for more than
  a few seconds.
- Never let your note-taking distract you from the present moment.
  Listening, experiencing, and responding to what is happening is
  more important than having detailed notes.

How much of the client's sustain talk should be included in a recapitulation? It's a clinical judgment call, but our general advice is: not too much.
Certainly we do not recommend recapitulating all of the client's arguments

against change. If there has been a particular point of sustain talk that the client has emphasized, you might include this like a few leaves in a floral bouquet (bearing in mind that too many leaves can obscure and distract from the flowers). The primary content of a recapitulation should be the client's own change talk.

Key Question

Having pulled together the big bouquet, ask a short and simple question, the kind that we call a key question. A key question is about doing, about the far side of the motivational hill in Chapter 12 (Box 12.2). There are countless ways to ask essentially, "So what's next?" A typical key question that we often use is, "So what do you think you'll do?" Some other examples:

> "So where does all this leave you?"
> "So what are you thinking about [area of concern] at this point?"
> "I wonder what you might decide to do."

Notice that key questions are not asking for commitment. That comes later. Asking a commitment question puts pressure on the client at what can be a critical juncture, which can evoke defensiveness and a setback in motivational momentum. Don't ask "What are you *going* to do?" That's more pressuring than "What do you think you might do?" Closed questions are usually not a good idea as key questions: "So are you going to do anything about this or not?"

The underlying rhythm of a recapitulation and key question is, "Here are all the motivations for change that you have told me. It's in your hands what, if anything, you choose to do. What do you think?" You pull together all of the person's *own* desire, ability, reasons, and need, revving the engine of change, and then get out of the way by asking a key question.

Pregnant Pause

We have not said much about silence thus far, and silence can be an important tool in MI. Many people feel a need to speak, to fill in the silent space when it has been quiet for 5 to 10 seconds in a conversation. Clinicians should not respond to this pressure and feel a need to start talking if the client has been silent for a while. Allowing some silence to pass gives clients time to process and increases the likelihood that they will voice a product of their reflection. People also differ in how long they need to process before speaking. In Jungian tradition, extroverts process *by* talking, whereas introverts prefer to process

> An unhurried mind is an asset in MI.

before speaking (Quenk, 2009). Trust the process and allow time for things to "sink in" and for the client to reflect on them. Don't feel rushed when you do MI, even if your available time is short. An unhurried mind is an asset in MI. Some clinicians tell us, "I don't have *time* to do this!" We often reply that when client behavior change is needed and you don't have a lot of time, you can't afford *not* to do this (Rubak, Sandbaek, Lauritzen, & Christensen, 2005).

We think of silence, of a pregnant pause here because it is particularly useful to wait a bit at this transitional moment after a recapitulation and key question. Some clients will answer right away. Others will reflect for a while. That reflection time at this moment is rich.

RECAPITULATING JULIA

Once again we continue the case example of Julia. We last heard from her in Chapter 13 when illustrating the evoking process. What might the clinician include in a recapitulation of the process thus far to test the water for how ready she is to get on with specific planning for change? The immediate goal toward which the clinician is now focusing is for Julia to do something to alleviate her depression.

INTERVIEWER: Well, thanks for all you've told me, Julia. You've been feeling a lot of turmoil in your life and I appreciate how honest and open you have been with me. *Affirmation.*

Let me just pull together what you've told me, and then we'll see what the next step *Orientation to* is. *transition.* You would really like to start feeling better, in general and about yourself, and *Change talk (desire).* to feel interested in things again. When you got to feeling bad enough that you cut *Change talk (reason).* yourself, that kind of startled you and got *Change talk* your attention, and it helped you decide *(activation).* that it was time to do something about it. You've been feeling really bad, like you *Change talk (reason).* have been dragging a great weight around with you, and you're rather tired of feeling like your friends avoid you. Friends are important to you. In the longer run you *Change talk (reason)* also want to have an open, warm, and *and further focusing.* loving relationship with a man. You're a pretty resourceful person. You moved here *Affirmation.* from Ireland all on your own and set up a new life for yourself. You're also a stubborn and persistent person. Once you make up your mind to do something it's likely to happen. You would like to understand what's been going wrong in your relationships because somewhere down the line you would like to be married, and you also mentioned finding a better job as a longer-term goal. You've been through a lot of emotional pain, and you're eager for a calmer and happier life. So what would you like to do?

Change talk (ability).

Change talk (desire).
Change talk (reason).

Change talk (reason).

Key question.

JULIA: I'm not sure what to do, but I know I can't keep going like I have been. Something has to change.

Change talk (need).

INTERVIEWER: It sounds like you're ready to do whatever it takes to feel better and get on with a new life.

Reflection and testing the water.

JULIA: I am. I don't want to keep living the way I have been.

Change talk (desire).

INTERVIEWER: Well, shall we talk about some possibilities then?

JULIA: Yes, please.

In this case, Julia clearly signals a readiness to proceed to planning. That doesn't always happen, of course. One might offer a recapitulation and key question for a smoker, only to have the person say: "I don't know. I'm not really sure I want to quit. Smoking is a big part of my life." That is a signal that the person is not ready to talk about planning yet, and there is more evoking work to do. It is even possible that the focus of consultation might change. "I think what I really need to talk about is . . . " Recapitulation and key question is a testing of the water, of your hypothesis that the person may be ready to discuss *how* to change. Whatever signal the client gives you, follow it.

KEY POINTS

✓ The time to move from evoking to planning is a clinical judgment call guided by signals of readiness from the client.

✓ Recapitulation and a key question is one procedure for discerning whether planning is timely.

✓ It is unwise to proceed with change planning before clients are ready.

CHAPTER 20

Developing a Change Plan

Faith is taking the first step even when you don't see the whole staircase.
—MARTIN LUTHER KING JR.

Easier to change the course of a river than a person's natural habit.
—CHINESE SAYING

Habit is habit, and not to be flung out the window by any man, but coaxed downstairs a step at a time.
—MARK TWAIN

Technologies and frameworks for developing change plans abound in service settings worldwide. Guidelines, workbooks, maps, self-monitoring diaries, and computer-driven change plans have harnessed the wisdom of behavioral science to bridge what is sometimes called the intention–action gap. It's one thing for clients to really want to change, but how do you help them succeed?

The contribution of MI here is a modest yet potentially important one. Helping someone to form a change plan is not necessarily a simple practical transaction, a matter of advising someone to do this or do that. If it were that simple, clients would probably do it for themselves. The quotation from novelist Terry Pratchett that opened Chapter 14 was no doubt written with wry humor, but it contains more than a grain or two of truth. Often people don't really want advice, but they want you to be there while they talk to themselves. The planning process in MI is to be with someone while they form a change plan that will work. Of course, you don't just sit there passively. Engagement is important, and you keep a keen eye focused on the horizon, modestly offering your own

> The planning process in MI is to be with someone while he or she forms a change plan that will work.

268

expertise as needed to help develop a plan that makes sense to the client. Readiness to adjust and to tolerate uncertainty will serve you well. In short, MI has a contribution at the heart of planning, compatible with using whatever practical tools you may use.

We note in passing that there is a difference between a change plan and a treatment plan. The latter is required in many service settings, but "treatment" at most forms only one part of a person's plan for change, and often a minor part. Most human change happens without any formal treatment. A change plan is broader, addressing how a person will proceed and how the change will fit into his or her life. What contribution (if any) will happen via treatment is just one part of the picture.

This chapter illustrates how the language of change and your skillful response to it can support the emergence of a change plan that champions clarity of action and is something the client is more likely to do. How you speak to someone about a change plan is probably just as important as what you talk about.

CHANGE TALK IN THE PLANNING PROCESS

The planning process is not a different form of MI. There is the same attention to change talk, the same collaborative spirit, plenty of OARS, and a clear direction toward change. In other words, the planning process builds on the same skills that are used in engaging, focusing, and evoking.

Does change talk differ at this point? Certainly the interviewer listens carefully for change talk that is about specific action, moving toward implementation intentions. Mobilizing change talk (CATs) is particularly about action, but DARN also occurs (see Chapter 12). For example, here are change talk statements about taking a particular action; in this case, a college student setting aside a specific daily block of time for study.

"That's what I want to do: study from 6:00 to 8:00 each day." [Desire]
"I think I can do that; it seems reasonable." [Ability]
"I like it because at 8:00 I'm done and can do other things." [Reason]
"That's what I need to do to keep up with my classes." [Need]
"That's what I'm going to do: save 6:00 to 8:00 for study 6 days a week." [Commitment, and also an implementation intention]
"I'm ready to give it a try." [Activation]
"I tried it out yesterday and it worked well for me." [Taking steps]

Note that change talk statements could be about a goal ("I want to get my grades up"), a general plan ("I need to study more"), or a specific action as illustrated above ("I intend to save 6:00 to 8:00 every day except Saturday just for studying"). It's not a different type of change talk; the key is that as a plan progresses from general to specific the change talk you're particularly attending to is about a particular change plan.

One more issue to which to attune your ear in planning is language about efficacy. Does the person think this plan will work? Bandura (1982, 1997) distinguished between general efficacy ("Would it work for people in general?") and self-efficacy ("Am I able to do it, and would it work for me?"). For example, it is possible for people to believe strongly that stopping smoking improves health and prolongs life (high general efficacy), and also be convinced that they are unable to do it (low self-efficacy).

THE DYNAMICS OF PLANNING

While there are rich research data on what happens in the evoking process, the role of MI in change planning is less well understood. However, the interpersonal dynamics of the planning process are those of MI more generally. Watch out for the righting reflex: "Now let me tell you what to do." Stay attuned to how the person is responding (such as any signs of disengagement or doubt) and don't get ahead of your client's readiness to develop and commit to a change plan. If you become the change advocate the result may be reluctance, sustain talk, and discord. The task is to elicit a change plan (and related change talk) from the client. This doesn't mean that you can't help, but ultimately it is the client who must own and implement the plan.

Don't get ahead of your client's readiness.

Clarity of planning depends on clarity of the goal. Sometimes the focusing process yields a goal that is clear and discrete, like quitting smoking or finding a job. Other identified goals are more diffuse, like "eating better" or "helping my son learn to be more responsible." It helps to have a more specific goal because this can clarify steps toward it, which also makes it easier to see progress.

Three Planning Scenarios

With an agreed goal, a journey begins from a conversation about whether and why to the arrival at a specific plan for how and when. Any single guideline about this journey is bound to run afoul of the obvious diversity among clients, and even within one person on different occasions.

In the rest of this chapter we discuss three scenarios for the planning process and provide examples. They mirror the continuum of scenarios that we described for the focusing process in Chapter 8. This is no coincidence. While focusing is about the intended destination of a change journey, the planning process is about the route of travel to arrive there. To oversimplify a bit:

Engaging is about "Shall we travel together?"
Focusing asks "Where to"
Evoking is about "Whether" and "Why" and
Planning is about "How" and "When"

Clearly, in any conversation about travel these threads will intertwine and evolve over time. As we discuss below, the planning process relies on evoking as well as engagement and a clear focus.

The three planning scenarios differ in complexity of the plan, though the process has similarities in each. The simplest scenario is when one clear plan already exists as you arrive at the planning process. This can happen when there is only one way to pursue the goal, or when clients have already made up their minds about how they want to proceed, and the struggle was just about whether to do it.

Scenario 2 is when there are several clear options and the task is to choose among them. For example, if a man or woman wants reliable contraception, there are finite possibilities to consider. The process leads toward choosing the path that seems best.

In Scenario 3 there is a clear goal (otherwise, it's not time for planning yet), but it is not at all apparent how to get there. It's not just a matter of choosing from a set menu of options. This scenario requires developing a plan from scratch when the way forward is unclear.

SCENARIO 1: WHEN THERE IS A CLEAR PLAN

Once people have decided on a change destination, the path sometimes is clear. They know how to do it. There is not much need for considering paths because they know the way. It's always possible that they will still get lost along the way, but it seems clear what they choose to do and how to do it.

> "I know what I need to do, because I've quit smoking before. What I need to do is to get off by myself, away from anybody else because I'm impossible to live with for about a week. There is this cabin I like to go to up in the mountains, and I could go up there for a week with no cigarettes. There's no store anywhere near there—this is really out in the woods. If I know there are no cigarettes around, the craving isn't as bad. I'm going to take along things I've been wanting to read, or just spend time out walking. I think that will work. After a week I'm

through the worst of it. The last time I got through a whole week it lasted for 3 years, but I was pretty hard on people that first week and I didn't do myself any favors either."

The plan seems clear. There is solid change talk about the plan, but notice that it is all preparatory (DARN) so far—no mobilizing language (CATs) yet.

Summarizing the Plan

A first step in helping to consolidate a specific plan like this is to offer a clear summary of it, to make sure you and the client both understand and agree about it.

> "What you plan to do, then, is to go to that cabin and stay there for a whole week, taking everything you'll need, but no tobacco."

Calling the CATs: Eliciting Mobilizing Change Talk

A summary like that just seems to beg for a question to go with it. What might that question be? Here are some possibilities:

Evoking activation talk
"How ready are you to do that?"
"Are you willing to give that a try?"

Asking for commitment
"Are you going to do it?"
"Is that what you intend to do?"

Getting more specific
"What reading would you take?"
"How would you get ready?"

Setting a date
"When could you do that?"
"When do you think you'll go?"

Preparing
"What would be a first step?"
"What would you need to take along?"

These are questions for which the answer is likely to be mobilizing change talk: commitment, activation, or taking steps. Also notice that some of these are closed questions, to which the intended answer is yes or no. ("Are you willing . . . ?"; "Is that what you're going to do?")

Troubleshooting

Another possible help at this point is to troubleshoot the plan. What might go wrong? What are possible obstacles or unanticipated difficulties that could arise? If you raise these points and ask the client how he or she could respond to them, the answer is likely to be more mobilizing change talk. Avoid providing the solutions yourself. From an MI perspective, if the client is raising the problems and you're providing the answers, you're in the wrong chair.

> If the client is raising the problems and you're providing the answers, you're in the wrong chair.

Case Example

For a practical example of the planning process in Scenario 1 we return to the student who planned to study from 6:00 to 8:00 P.M. each day to improve grades. Here is how the conversation might unfold.

INTERVIEWER: So let me see if I understand your plan. You definitely want to improve your grades, and to do that you know that you need to spend more time studying. What you're thinking of doing is to set aside 2 hours every day except Saturday, from 6:00 to 8:00 P.M., and do nothing but study during that time. Is that right?

CLIENT: Yes. I think that will help.

INTERVIEWER: It should help. You might need to do more, but this would be a very good start.

CLIENT: Definitely. If I did that, it would make a difference in my grades.

INTERVIEWER: OK. What could you do to stick with your plan better?

CLIENT: I'd need to work it out with my roommate not to bother me or play music during that time. Or maybe I'd have to go to the library or a coffee shop.

INTERVIEWER: Someplace where you can concentrate and not be distracted.

CLIENT: Right. It would be tempting to get distracted and not study.

INTERVIEWER: You know that about yourself, that you need to be in a place where you can focus. What else?

CLIENT: I get hungry, and it would be better if I had something to eat before I start.

INTERVIEWER: I see. That might also help you concentrate on studying. You're really thinking about how to do this. When do you think you'll start?

CLIENT: Well, this is Monday, I have a date tomorrow and a meeting on Wednesday evening, so I guess I could start Thursday.

INTERVIEWER: Do you think you will?

CLIENT: Yeah, I don't see why not. Thursday.

INTERVIEWER: If it's all right, I'd like to ask you a few more things about your plan. Would that be OK?

CLIENT: Sure.

INTERVIEWER: You seem to know a lot of people, and I can imagine that whether you're in your room or the library or a coffee shop there's a good chance that you'll see somebody you know, or they'll see you.

CLIENT: I'm not too likely to see my friends in the library. (*Smiling.*)

INTERVIEWER: All right, so that might be a safer place, but imagine if it happened. It's 6:15 and a friend spots you, comes over and says, "Hey, how are you doing?" How could you stick with your plan if that happened?

CLIENT: Easy. I'd just say that I'm glad to see them, but I'm studying until 8:00 and maybe we could talk after that.

INTERVIEWER: "Oh come on! You don't have to study right now!"

CLIENT: Oh, like she might say that. OK, I'd say, "Yeah I really need to, but I'd love to see you later on."

INTERVIEWER: OK. Most friends would probably honor that. And what about when there's something else happening between 6:00 and 8:00 that you'd really like to do, and it's not Saturday?

CLIENT: Yeah, I thought about that. I don't think I'd stick with this 100% of the time.

INTERVIEWER: You're not perfect.

CLIENT: Right. I mean sometimes I'm going to want to do something else in that time. I guess I could study later, then, or double up another day.

INTERVIEWER: To get in the same number of hours. Do you think you'd really do that?

CLIENT: Yeah, I usually would. I'm serious about getting my grades up.

There are the basic elements in Scenario 1: summarizing the plan, eliciting mobilizing change talk, and troubleshooting. When people verbalize their intention to take a specific action, it's more likely to happen. These same elements also carry over into Scenarios 2 and 3, along with some additional wrinkles.

Getting More Specific

Even with a clearly stated goal it can be helpful to get a bit more specific about steps toward it. This can help in the planning process and also in knowing when progress is happening. The method of goal attainment scaling (Kiresuk, Smith, & Cardillo, 1994) can be useful in honing a goal within any of the three scenarios described in this chapter. It was originally developed to provide a standard way of evaluating treatment outcome in mental health settings across multiple problem areas.

At the heart of this method is finding a way to specify degrees of change for the goal. The intent it to provide a way to ascertain from a simple conversation how the person is doing in pursuing a goal. A variation that we find useful involves developing a scale from −3 to +3. The zero point on the scale describes the status quo at the outset (for example, when entering treatment). The best imaginable outcome is +3, with +1 and +2 being approximations. Similarly −3 is the worst imaginable outcome, with intermediate levels of deterioration at −1 and −2. Using the study time example above, a scale based on the number of hours spent studying in one week might look like this:

+3	16 or more hours
+2	10–15 hours
+1	5–9 hours
0	4 hours (current level)
−1	3 hours
−2	2 hours
−3	1 hour or less

Ideally, with such a scale any interviewer (as well as the client) could easily determine progress toward (or away from) the goal in any given week. This same method can be used for several change goals with the same person, as illustrated in Box 20.1.

SCENARIO 2:
WHEN THERE ARE SEVERAL CLEAR OPTIONS

In the second planning scenario, there are several clear alternatives for action toward a goal, and the task is to prioritize and choose among them. We like the term *path mapping* here as a parallel to agenda mapping,

BOX 20.1. An Example of Goal Attainment Scaling

	Goal 1: Exercise more (cardiovascular)	Goal 2: More quality time with my children	Goal 3: Decrease my alcohol use
+3	200 minutes or more	8 hours or more	0–7 standard drinks
+2	131–199 minutes	6–7 hours	8–14 standard drinks
+1	61–130 minutes	4–5 hours	15–20 standard drinks
0	50–60 minutes this week	About 3 hours this week	21–28 standard drinks/ week
–1	31–49 minutes	2 hours	29–35 standard drinks
–2	11–30 minutes	1 hour	36–49 standard drinks
–3	10 minutes or less	Less than 1 hour	>50 standard drinks

because the process is one of choosing from among possible routes the best path toward the destination. Some component tasks here are:

1. Confirm the goal, and as appropriate, subgoals along the way.
2. Itemize the options that are available or have been discussed.
3. Elicit the client's hunches/preferences as to the best way forward.
4. Summarize the plan and strengthen commitment.
5. Troubleshoot—raise any concerns you have.

Confirm the Goal

The goal may seem quite clear at this point, but it doesn't hurt to confirm the destination before setting out on a journey. What is the change that the client chooses to pursue? There may be a larger long-term goal and more proximal subgoals. A good guide finds out first where the person wants to go; then they consider different possible routes to get there. If there are several proximal goals, which of them should be pursued first?

Itemize the Options

With a clear goal in mind, the next task is to enumerate the alternative paths that are available for getting there. Options may already have emerged from earlier processes in the conversation. Your own professional expertise can also be of service here. For the change that this person wants to make, what are the sound, evidence-based ways to achieve it? With the client's permission (see Chapter 11) you can offer a menu of options. This is not meant to supplant the person's own ideas and preferences—not at all. Your expertise is a resource in the planning process, and the client also brings important resources. The key task is to develop a list of the options that are available without spending too much time critiquing them. The evaluation process comes next.

Elicit the Client's Hunches

Among the alternative routes available, what are the client's own preferences and hunches as to the preferred path? A good guide offers: "Here are the different routes that we could take. Which one appeals more to you?" What are the good things and the not-so-good things about each option? Like a good guide you would advise (again with permission) against paths that you believe to be dangerous or that would not lead to the destination.

It is also useful to think of whatever path is chosen as Plan A. There can be unanticipated obstacles along the way, and there are alternative routes if Plan A proves problematic. "What would be the best route to try first?" is a helpful mind-set to share in this process. This leaves the door open to consider alternative paths if the chosen way is not working.

Summarize the Plan

This is much like Scenario 1. Once a plan has emerged, offer a summary of it to make sure you're both clear about it, then evoke mobilizing change talk. We say more about strengthening commitment in Chapter 21.

Troubleshoot

With Plan A in mind, a further task is to consider what obstacles might be encountered along the way. Again a good guide does this: "If we take that route, here are some things you should be prepared for." What tools does the person need to take along? What might go awry, and how could the person respond if this happens?

Remember not to switch into a prescriptive directing style here. The evoking process continues throughout planning. A modal approach would be to ask clients how they might respond if certain obstacles are encountered. When the person asks for or seems to need your ideas you can provide them; when you do, beware the pitfall of offering one at a time (thus inviting the person to respond with what is wrong with your idea). Ultimately it needs to be the client's plan. Asking how the person might respond to obstacles is also likely to evoke further change talk.

Case Example

Scenario 2 is one often encountered by diabetes practitioners. In order to promote health and quality of life, people with diabetes need to maintain reasonably tight control over their glucose levels, and there are a finite number of effective strategies for managing blood sugar. Here is how a planning process might proceed building on prior engaging, focusing, and evoking.

INTERVIEWER: I can see you're aware of the problems that can result from high blood sugar, and it sounds like you're eager to get your glucose levels under better control. Is that right?

Confirming the goal.

CLIENT: Sure. I want to stay as healthy as I can.

A long-term goal of better health.

INTERVIEWER: OK, good for you. You're willing to make some changes in order to stay healthy.

Specifically checking willingness to make behavior changes.

CLIENT: Yes.

INTERVIEWER: Well, let me ask you first, then, what you have thought about that you might change to manage your glucose levels.

Eliciting the client's own ideas.

CLIENT: I haven't really thought about it that much. This is pretty new for me. I'm only 46.

INTERVIEWER: You certainly didn't expect to be diagnosed with diabetes at your age.

Reflection.

CLIENT: No, I didn't! I know I probably need to change how I eat.

Change talk.

INTERVIEWER: What kinds of change?

Asking for elaboration.

CLIENT: Well, I drink a lot of sodas, cola mostly. I sip them all day, and I know they have a lot of sugar.

INTERVIEWER: Yes, they do—quite a lot. So that's one way you could cut down your sugar intake right away.

"One way," inviting more.

CLIENT: I don't really like how the sugar-free colas taste, but I guess I could get used to them.

Sustain talk.
Change talk.

INTERVIEWER: What else?

CLIENT: Sweets? I mean, I guess it's a matter of not eating sugar, isn't it?

Gives permission for information exchange.

INTERVIEWER: And cutting down on carbohydrates more generally. What do you know about those?

CLIENT: Like bread, potato chips, pasta?

INTERVIEWER: Exactly. The body turns those into sugar quite quickly. Now, changing how you eat is one good strategy. What else do you know that helps?

CLIENT: Getting enough sleep, maybe? Why don't you tell me since you're the expert.

INTERVIEWER: I can certainly tell you some things that people with diabetes do to manage their sugar, but you're the one who decides if those could work for you. Shall I give you a short list?

Emphasizing personal control.

Asking permission.

CLIENT: Sure.

INTERVIEWER: Changing your eating patterns, especially carbohydrates, is one good step. Exercise is also important, and we could talk about that; it helps reduce insulin resistance. It's a good idea to check your blood sugar regularly to see what drives it up and down, and you can do that at home with a simple device. In addition to sleeping well, it can help to decrease stresses in your life. And there are medications we can discuss that help. Those are five possibilities: eating, exercise, monitoring, managing stress, and medication. Which of those sounds like something that you could do?

A menu of options.

CLIENT: What about medication—that sounds easy. Are there side effects?

INTERVIEWER: There are some good oral medications that help reduce insulin resistance, and usually there are few side effects. So that's one thing that sounds reasonable to you.

CLIENT: I guess so. Is that enough?

Activation (willingness).

INTERVIEWER: Honestly, the medications work much better when you also help them with some lifestyle changes. Are there other areas I mentioned where you think you might be able to make some changes?

CLIENT: What I eat, I guess. I don't exercise much;   *Change talk.*
    I really have never liked running or going to   *Sustain talk.*
    a gym. But maybe I could do more there, too.   *Change talk.*

INTERVIEWER: You might be able to bump your   *Summary.*
    activity level up some, and you're willing
    to make some changes in how you eat in
    addition to trying medication. That could
    make quite a difference!

CLIENT: What should I do first?

INTERVIEWER: That's a good question, and it's   *Emphasizing*
    really up to you. Managing your glucose is   *personal control.*
    a long-term process, and most people make
    changes gradually over time. We could
    certainly start you on a medication, and
    between changing your diet and increasing
    your exercise, which seems like a better place   *Looking for Plan A.*
    to start?

CLIENT: I probably need to change what I eat first,
    like cutting out those colas.

INTERVIEWER: Shall we begin there, then? I can   *Summarizing Plan*
    give you a prescription to fill, and we can talk   *A.*
    now about how you might change your eating
    patterns. Is that a good place to start?

CLIENT: OK.

This is one example of Scenario 2. There was a clear goal and a finite list of ways to pursue it. The interviewer confirmed the goal, enumerated the menu of options (with permission), and helped the client map a path toward it.

SCENARIO 3:
DEVELOPING A PLAN FROM SCRATCH

Sometimes one has neither a clear single plan nor an obvious set of options from which to choose. Asked a key question like, "So what's the next step for you?" a client may answer, "I don't know," and you may not be much clearer yourself at the beginning of the planning process. The task here is one of collaboratively developing a change plan. If you do have an aspiration the righting reflex can kick in mightily in this situation: "Well then, let me tell you what to do." A minority of clients may want and respond to such direction (you can find out by asking), but usually motivation to follow through is higher when the client has more ownership of the plan.

The starting point here is the same as for Scenario 2: Confirm the goal(s). Make sure you understand the client's chosen destination. If this is not clear, there is a need for additional focusing (Chapter 9) and possibly evoking as well to confirm motivation for the goal itself.

Because there is not a predetermined menu of alternatives for pursuing the goal (as there was with the Type 2 diabetes example in Scenario 2), a next step is to generate possible options, steps, or plans. Both your client and you are resources for generating alternatives. Instead of itemizing ready possibilities, the task is to generate them, guided in part by your formulation (Chapter 9) and by the client's own hunches about the cause(s) of the problem (Khalsa, McCarthy, Sharpless, Barrett, & Barberr, 2011). If you make a suggestion (with permission), try to offer several options rather than just one, and keep the process collaborative.

Compared to Scenario 2, the process here may be more like traditional brainstorming, where the task is to generate a variety of ideas while temporarily suspending evaluation of them. Sometimes this can be fun—to think creatively about *any* approach that might work, even if it seems silly at first. As you generate ideas keep a list of them, at least in memory if not in writing.

Now with a list of options available, the process converges again with that described for Scenario 2 earlier. What are the client's hunches or preferences among the possibilities considered? What are your own best guesses? From these you negotiate a Plan A, a first approach to try. As appropriate, break it down into doable steps, and troubleshoot as needed.

As an example of this more complex scenario we return to the case of Julia last visited with a recapitulation summary in Chapter 19. The development of a change plan takes into account the client's own preferences and hunches about the cause(s) of the problem (Khalsa et al., 2011). Here is an example of a guided change planning process in which the interviewer and Julia combine their expertise to arrive at a beginning plan.

INTERVIEWER: First of all, Julia, I would like to know what ideas you have for how you might start feeling better. No one knows you better than you do, and I'm sure you have tried some things in the past to lift your mood a bit. Tell me about those.

CLIENT: Sometimes I have gone to a funny, romantic movie and it makes me smile, but it also reminds me of what I don't have in a relationship.

INTERVIEWER: Um-hmm. A pleasant movie is one thing that can lift your spirits sometimes. What else?

CLIENT: Getting out of my apartment. If I just sit there watching television with the curtains drawn, that's not good for me.

INTERVIEWER: You know that about yourself—getting out helps. And what do you do when you go out of your apartment?

CLIENT: I might just take a walk or arrange to see my friends. But like I said, it seems like they don't want to be around me so much anymore because I bring them down with me. What do you think I should do? Do you have some suggestions for me?

INTERVIEWER: Yes, I do. I already have a few thoughts of things you might try. I don't know very much about you yet, but you do, and I think together we can find what works for you. [The counselor supports hope, emphasizing partnership and Julia's expertise regarding herself.]

CLIENT: So what do you think I should do?

INTERVIEWER: Well, let's consider some options. You already know some things that have helped lift your mood in the past, like getting out of your apartment to take a walk, see friends, or go to a pleasant movie. I'm very interested in your own hunches about what you need and what will help you, so let's talk about some possibilities, and then discuss together where to start, what might be best to try first.

CLIENT: OK.

INTERVIEWER: One thing that seems clear to me is that you're struggling with depression right now. Tell me this, Julia. What do you already know about how depression can be treated? [Beginning an elicit–provide–elicit sequence of information exchange.]

CLIENT: Not much. I've seen ads for pills.

INTERVIEWER: You've mentioned that several times, and it's one good option. What other possibilities do you know about?

CLIENT: I don't know—talking about it, maybe? What causes depression?

INTERVIEWER: The good news is that there are several different approaches that work well. If you want, I can describe them to you briefly and you can tell me your hunches about which of them seem to fit you best.

CLIENT: OK.

INTERVIEWER: It seems there are several different things that can contribute to depression, a variety of ways that people sink into it. One of them has to do with thought patterns. Some people are super critical of themselves; they are often running themselves down or thinking about things in a negative way that keeps them upset. One approach helps people to examine and change their thought patterns. Does that make sense? [Providing a bit of information, and now eliciting her reaction]

CLIENT: Uh-huh. I do that.

INTERVIEWER: You run yourself down. All right. Well, let me continue, because there are other possibilities as well. Some people just get into a situation or a lifestyle where they have very little happening that is positive. There's not much that is enjoyable or pleasurable in their lives. They spend a lot of their time doing things they don't enjoy or hearing negative feedback from other people. How does that fit?

CLIENT: I don't know, it doesn't sound quite like me. I do enjoy going for a walk or seeing my friends, and when I have a good relationship with a man it's a real high for me. My work isn't all that great, but it's OK.

INTERVIEWER: So that one doesn't seem to fit your situation as well.

CLIENT: Right. I mean, you're the expert, so you would know better.

INTERVIEWER: Actually I think we will know best together, and I trust your judgment on this. Ready for another one?

CLIENT: Sure.

INTERVIEWER: Sometimes people feel like they can't express their own needs or feelings very well. They let people walk all over them, or spend their time trying to meet other people's needs rather than their own. Inside they feel frustrated or angry, but they don't often express it openly.

CLIENT: Oh, I express it all right. I don't think that's my problem.

INTERVIEWER: Let me just check one more thing, though. Some people go back and forth between stuffing their own feelings and frustrations, and then blowing up. It's like the pressure builds up until there's an explosion. What about that?

CLIENT: Like I told you, I've had some explosions in my relationships, but I don't think it was because I wasn't expressing my needs. I'm pretty good at asking for what I want, and sometimes that's what gets me into trouble.

INTERVIEWER: OK—one more idea. Sometimes depression just seems to come out of nowhere. Life is going along all right, and then gradually the person starts having trouble sleeping, breaks out crying, feels fatigued, and feels sad and worthless for no apparent reason. If you try to think up a reason to explain it you can probably find one, but the depression just seems to have a life of its own.

CLIENT: Maybe there's some of that with me. Is that when people take medication?

INTERVIEWER: That's one reason, yes, but there can be other reasons to try medication as well.

CLIENT: It seems like I have more than enough reasons for feeling down and upset. But I do wonder if medication would help me.

INTERVIEWER: That's very helpful, thanks. There are different treatments to try depending on which of these seems to be contributing to depression, and your strongest hunch seemed to be about how you run yourself down in your mind—things you tell yourself that get you feeling worse about yourself. A treatment that helps with this is called cognitive therapy.

CLIENT: I definitely do that.

INTERVIEWER: And then you also have wondered whether an antidepressant medication might help. Those are the two that you mentioned as seeming most promising.

CLIENT: Which do you think I should do?

INTERVIEWER: It's not a matter of having to choose between them, because it's possible to do both. The research on this indicates that both cognitive therapy and medication are about equally effective, and we could start with either.

CLIENT: That's a relief. I don't want to take medication if I don't have to—the side effects and all. If I can do it myself, I'd prefer that.

INTERVIEWER: One plan, then, could be to start with cognitive therapy and see how that goes for you. We can always keep other options open depending on your experience.

KEY POINTS

✓ Developing a change plan usually involves moving from general intention to a specific implementation plan.

✓ Three planning scenarios are (1) the change plan is already clear; (2) there are options among which to choose in path mapping; (3) the way forward is unclear and a change plan needs to be developed from scratch.

✓ The planning process retains the core spirit and skills of MI and builds on the prior processes of engaging, focusing, and evoking.

CHAPTER 21

Strengthening Commitment

> Until one is committed, there is hesitancy, the chance to draw
> back, always ineffectiveness, concerning all acts of initiative and
> creation. There is one elementary truth, the ignorance of which
> kills countless ideas and splendid plans: that the moment one
> definitely commits oneself, then Providence moves too. All sorts
> of things occur to help one that would never otherwise have
> occurred. A whole stream of events issues from the decision.
> —JOHANN WOLFGANG VON GOETHE

> Unless commitment is made, there are only promises and hopes,
> but no plans.
> —PETER DRUCKER

Most change happens gradually. It is a process that emerges over time. Sometimes there is a discrete, even dramatic moment in which the decision to change suddenly crystallizes (Baumeister, 1994), as for the smoker at the library who was described in Chapter 7 (Box 7.3) or the transformative "white light" experience of Bill W., cofounder of Alcoholics Anonymous (Kurtz, 1991; Miller & C'de Baca, 2001). More commonly, a person's commitment to a particular action fluctuates and grows over time. MI is a way of facilitating the natural growth of commitment.

When a change plan has been developed is the planning process complete? Not necessarily. There is a further step from plan to action (Ajzen, 1985, 1991). An important question is whether the person is actually satisfied with the plan and intends to carry it out. That is the focus of this chapter.

LISTEN FOR MOBILIZING LANGUAGE

In Chapter 12 we introduced the concept of mobilizing change talk, language that indicates momentum toward change. It is language on the far side of the ambivalence hill, using the metaphor from Chapter 12. Mobilizing change talk includes activation language that, while falling short of actual commitment, nevertheless signals increasing openness to and readiness for change:

> "I am willing [ready, prepared] to . . . "
> "I will consider [think about] doing it."
> "I might . . . "
> "I probably will . . . "

None of these would be a satisfactory commitment to seal marital vows or a business contract, but they are getting close to intention. These types of speech are different from the preparatory change talk of desire ("I want to"), ability ("I could"), reasons ("I would feel better"), and need ("I have to"). Mobilizing change talk has to do with *doing*. The word *do* usually fits naturally into the sentence: "I am willing to [do]"; "I will consider [doing]"; "I might [do]."

> Mobilizing change talk has to do with *doing*.

Another previously discussed form of mobilizing change talk is taking steps. These describe something the person did that represents a step toward change. The taking of even small steps toward a goal is another predictor of subsequent change.

Committing speech, in contrast, signals an intention to carry out the plan. The language varies somewhat in strength, but in essence says, "Yes, I'll do this."

- A bit weaker: "I plan to"; "I intend to."
- Solid: "I will"; "I am going to."
- Stronger: "I promise"; "I guarantee"; "I swear."

There are surely other kinds of statements from the far side of the hill that represent mobilization toward change but do not fit neatly into one of these categories. The key is to tune your ear to recognize both preparatory and mobilizing change talk. These are the signals that people normally use when negotiating with each other about change.

As a change plan emerges listen carefully for mobilizing language. To what extent is the person intending to carry it out? What is the person willing or ready to do? What steps has the person already taken toward this goal?

IMPLEMENTATION INTENTIONS

Research in cognitive psychology has explored language that signals increased likelihood that an action will occur. One such form of speech is termed an *implementation intention* (Gollwitzer, 1999; Gollwitzer &

Schaal, 1998; Rise, Thompson, & Verplanken, 2003), which includes two components: (1) a specific plan of action, and (2) an interpersonal statement of intent to do it.

Both components are important. A general intention (e.g., to be a better person) is less predictive of behavior than is a specific intention (e.g., to tell the truth, the whole truth, and nothing but the truth today). Like a contract, the specificity usually includes a description of the particular action to be taken and a time frame to carry it out (e.g., to buy bread on the way home from work today). The description of specific action is accompanied by a committing verb that signifies the person's intention to do it, witnessed by at least one other person. ("Yes, dear, I will buy bread on the way home from work today"). Together these two elements form an implementation intention.

An MI style for developing a specific change plan was described in Chapter 20. Consistent with the principle of specificity, it may be easier for a client to agree to take a particular step in the direction of change than to commit to the ultimate change goal itself.

Taking a step	*Ultimate goal*
"I will fill the prescription today and start taking this medication."	"I will keep my HbA1c [blood glucose] level under 7.0."
"I intend to lose 5 pounds this month."	"I will lose 50 pounds."
"I plan to not drink today."	"I will never drink again."

The examples of ultimate goals given here are quite specific. It would not be difficult to observe whether they have actually been accomplished, but they do represent large changes, and implementation intentions are easier for smaller, more achievable goals. If a change plan is general or ambitious it can be helpful to break it down into smaller pieces. What would be a reasonable next step? When and how will that step be taken?

> If a change plan is general or ambitious, break it down into smaller pieces.

EVOKING INTENTION

Change planning feels complete when the person can say "yes" to the plan, and that "yes" can involve a range of activating and committing language. It is often easier to ask for activation language than bald commitment. "What steps are you *willing* to take this week?" "What part of this plan do you think you are *ready* to do?" This hones down the bigger plan to a specific doable step.

The same procedure of recapitulation and key question that was introduced in Chapter 19 can be useful in consolidating commitment. The recapitulation here could include the person's broader goal as well as the specific step(s) that had been discussed and whatever mobilizing change talk the person has expressed. It may also incorporate some of the person's own preparatory change talk as a reminder of the "why" as well as the "how" of change. Following this summary, the key question could, for once, be a closed yes/no question that focuses on commitment ("Is that what you're going to do?") or activation ("Is that what you're willing to do?"). You could also ask it as an open question ("How ready are you to do this?") and ask how you or others might help.

Once more we return to the case of Julia to illustrate this process of consolidating commitment, picking up with a recapitulation of the plan developed in Chapter 20.

INTERVIEWER: All right, Julia. Let me see if I understand what you want to do. The first time we talked you were feeling a bit out of control, scared about the explosion with Ray and cutting yourself. As we talked, much of what you're experiencing fits together as depression, and addressing that seems like a first priority. I know that you have other important goals as well, like understanding what has been happening with your relationships. First, though, it makes sense to do something about your depression—to have more energy, sleep better, feel better about yourself. Is that about right?

CLIENT: Yes.

INTERVIEWER: And as we discussed different ways to alleviate depression, you particularly picked up on your thought patterns as a contributing factor. I mentioned cognitive therapy as one approach that has been shown to work well, keeping other options open depending on your experience. So far so good?

CLIENT: How long does that take?

INTERVIEWER: It varies, but normally we would meet weekly for about 2 months, probably twice a week in the beginning to get started.

CLIENT: And how long before I get better?

INTERVIEWER: Again it varies, but certainly you should feel quite a bit better within a month or two. If not, we will explore other options.

CLIENT: Like pills.

INTERVIEWER: Like medication if that seems the next good option. I will work with you until we find what works for you. So that's our plan as I understand it. Are you willing to do that—come once or twice a week, work together for about 2 months, and see how it goes?

CLIENT: Yes, that sounds good.

INTERVIEWER: So that's what we'll do then?

CLIENT: OK.

INTERVIEWER: Then let's get started on Thursday. Is 4:00 possible for you?

CLIENT: Yes, that's fine.

COVERT COMMITMENT

This all sounds very linear and orderly: develop a clear plan and ask for commitment, like drawing up and signing a contract. What we have said about implementation intentions here might imply that *unless* you get the person to give you commitment language, change is not going to happen. We definitely do not believe that you *must* hear the language of commitment for MI to be effective. You will hear whatever the client is ready to say, and pushing for more commitment than the person is ready to give is likely to be counterproductive. The common failure of New Year's resolutions reflects the insubstantial nature of commitment language without having done the preparatory motivational work.

> It is not necessary to hear the language of commitment for MI to be effective.

Whether or not it is evident in overt speech there is a deliberation going on inside. You continue to explore the forest of change, moving from tree to tree in a reasonably straight line. Beneath the surface, seeds are germinating. Preparatory change talk itself can predict change whether commitment is actually voiced (e.g., Baer, Beadnell, et al., 2008; Gaume, Gmel, Faouzi, & Daeppen, 2009; Moyers et al., 2007, 2009). We have learned to trust the process of MI and the natural process of change. A physician in one of our advanced workshops told us:

> "When I used to sit with patients who needed to make a lifestyle change, it just looked overwhelming to me. It was as though I was staring at an enormous retaining wall of rock. I knew there was water behind it, but told myself, 'I don't have time to take down this whole thing rock by rock!' and so I didn't try. Then in learning about MI I realized that I don't have to worry about removing all those rocks. All I need to do is remove a few of them and not add any more on top, then get out of the way and let the water do the rest."[1]

---

[1] Thanks to Cleve Sharp for this metaphor.

It is not simply speaking the words themselves that causes change. Otherwise you could give people a script to read aloud and the change would happen. Rather, preparatory and mobilizing change talk represent an underlying process, the normal process by which change happens. The underlying shifts are reflected both in change talk and in change itself. Commitment happens when a person feels ready, willing, and able to change. Accept whatever level of activation and commitment the person is willing to voice and affirm all steps in the right direction. The water will do the rest.

FURTHER WAYS TO STRENGTHEN COMMITMENT

The processes that we have discussed thus far can go a long way to strengthen commitment to change:

- Engaging in a supportive, collaborative working relationship.
- Focusing on clear goal(s) for change.
- Evoking the person's own motivations for change.
- Developing a specific change plan.
- Determining what step(s) the person is ready, willing, and able to take.

There may be other ways to strengthen commitment to change as well. A first resource in finding these is, of course, your client: "What might help you strengthen your commitment to this plan?" Evoke and explore the client's own ideas.

One common method is voicing commitment to significant others in one's life: "If I tell my friends that I'm quitting, that would be a serious commitment." To this the client could add a specific request for how others can help and be supportive. Social support from even one significant other can substantially facilitate change (Barber & Crisp, 1995; Longabaugh, Wirtz, Zweben, & Stout, 1998).

Self-monitoring is another self-control tool for remembering a goal and tracking one's progress toward it. This can take many forms—a diary, notecards, counting systems, even stepping on the bathroom scale each morning—and the essence is to remain aware of one's own ongoing behavior, decisions, or thoughts. In Julia's case, the therapist might prepare for cognitive therapy by asking her to record specific kinds of thoughts that occur. The record keeping represents a step toward change, and self-monitoring can itself facilitate change (Kanfer, 1970a; Safren et al., 2001). People who are trying to reduce their alcohol use, for example, can be encouraged to keep detailed records of every drink that contains alcohol, writing it down *before* drinking it (Miller & Muñoz, 2005). Clients report that taking out the card to record a drink reminds them of their goal and can deter them from taking it. Average alcohol consumption has been found to decrease by about one-third on the first week of self-monitoring (Miller & Taylor, 1980; Miller, Taylor, & West, 1980).

If self-monitoring reinforces commitment, what about supportive monitoring by others? In weight-reduction programs a simple weekly weigh-in provides some public accountability that can be helpful. Effective pharmacotherapies are available to help in self-management of mood disorders, psychoses, and substance use disorders, but poor medication adherence is a substantial obstacle. Procedures are available for both practitioners (Borrelli, Riekert, Weinstein, & Rathier, 2007; Daley, Salloum, Suckoff, Kirisci, & Thase, 1998; Gray et al., 2006; McDonald, Garg, & Haynes, 2002; Pettinati et al., 2005) and significant others (Azrin, Sisson, Meyers, & Godley, 1982; Meyers & Smith, 1995) to monitor and support medication adherence and to facilitate behavior change more generally (Bellg, 2003; Harland et al., 1999; Knols, Aaronson, Uebelhart, Fransen, & Aufdemkampe, 2005; Mallams, Godley, Hall, & Meyers, 1982; Meyers & Wolfe, 2004).

EXPLORING RELUCTANCE

A further aid to commitment can be exploring any reluctance and concerns the person has about change and the change plan. In a way this seems contradictory to an MI approach in that it involves intentionally evoking and exploring sustain talk, but with a solid foundation of engagement and of motivation established during the evoking process this can unearth some potential pitfalls that may lie in the path of change. Some examples of open questions of this kind are:

> "I wonder what concerns you may have about making this change?"
> "What might get in the way of your succeeding with this plan?"
> "Let me ask what lingering doubts you may have about moving ahead."

Follow with reflection and be careful not to fall back into the righting reflex by providing uninvited advice or solutions. Rather, evoke solutions from your client:

> "And I wonder how you might keep that from derailing your plan."
> "It would take a creative person to find a way through that. What ideas do you have?"
> "Knowing yourself as well as you do, how could you handle that?"

In this way you can problem-solve collaboratively with your client regarding possible obstacles to change. You can also raise specific obstacles or concerns that occur to you:

> "Now suppose that you're on day 4 of not smoking. You're through some of the worst of the withdrawal, and you're at an outdoor café with a friend who takes out a pack, taps one out and offers it to you. Suddenly you feel a tremendous desire for a cigarette. How might you get through that without smoking?"

> "Sometimes patients have told me that they just forget to take their medication, or don't have it with them if they have meals away from home. What would work for you to be sure you take it with breakfast and dinner every day?"

The client's answer is likely to be further change talk, and you're also anticipating strategies for coping with difficult aspects of change. The key is that you're not providing the ideas yourself (although you could if invited—see Chapter 11), but they are coming from the person who knows the client best and who ultimately has to use them.

KEY POINTS

✓ Developing a plan is not a final but a beginning step.

✓ Implementation intentions involve both a specific plan and the intention or commitment to carry it out.

✓ The clinical style of MI can help to strengthen commitment to a change plan.

✓ Public commitment, social support, and self-monitoring can also reinforce the best of intentions.

CHAPTER 22

Supporting Change

If you do not change direction, you may end up
where you are heading.
—LAO TZU

Change will not come if we wait for some other
person or some other time. We are the ones we've
been waiting for. We are the change that we seek.
—BARACK OBAMA

From one perspective MI is complete when there is a change plan in place
to which the client is committed. Viewed in this way, MI is something that
might be done at the beginning of a treatment process to prime the pump
for change. We have ourselves voiced this view at times: that one puts down
MI when it is time to move on to implementing a change (e.g., Miller &
Moyers, 2006).

Yet clinicians who have learned MI often do not experience their work
in this way, that MI is somehow disconnected from the rest of practice.
There may be at least two reasons for this. The first is that the spirit and
methods that characterize MI can be more generally applied in clinical
practice. Indeed, Carl Rogers (1959, 1980b) taught that a client-centered
way of being with people is not only necessary but also sufficient to promote change. Thus at least aspects of MI can permeate one's clinical work.
A second reason is that change is often not a
linear process. Motivation to initiate and
persist in change fluctuates over time regardless of the person's stage of readiness. From
the client's perspective, a decision is just the
beginning of change.

> The spirit and methods
> that characterize MI can be
> more generally applied in
> clinical practice.

This chapter focuses on how the four processes of MI discussed in the foregoing parts of this book can be useful after an initial change plan has been elicited and the person has decided to proceed. We considered adding a fifth process of implementing, but because it is ultimately the client who carries out any change it seemed sufficient to subsume the clinician's interpersonal role here within the fourth process of MI (i.e., planning).

Before proceeding we emphasize that some people need little or no additional help once they have decided to make a change. This was one of the unanticipated findings of our early research (see Chapter 27); that MI by itself often triggered change without any further treatment. In retrospect this should not have been surprising; the unexpectedness arose from our overestimation of people's need and desire for help in changing once they have decided to do so. Some clients, however, do want continuing support and assistance through the process of change. The style and spirit of MI can remain useful while many other clinical skills and tools are being used to facilitate people's progress through the implementation of change.

SUPPORTING PERSISTENCE

Some changes happen quickly, but many require sustained attention and effort over time. Overweight people yearn for rapid weight loss, but stable change may consist of a pound or two per week over many months, followed by permanent lifestyle changes to promote maintenance. Overcoming depression or relationship problems can take time. Effective treatment of some conditions can require persistence in difficult, uncomfortable, or painful procedures (Slagle & Gray, 2007). Medication adherence may necessitate enduring some unpleasant side-effects for a period of time. While it may seem clear what a client needs to do, it is often less clear how best to support the persistence that is required (Arkowitz et al., 2008; Westra, 2012).

Then there is the problem of a setback; a client is making good progress when suddenly something happens. It might be a family crisis, an unexpected visitor, an accident, or a loss. Sometimes it is simply a recurrence of old behavior patterns: the New Year's resolution problem. When people set up an absolute black-or-white perfection goal for themselves (e.g., "I will not eat sweets"), the first rule violation can trigger a breakdown in self-control (Baumeister et al., 1994; Cummings, Gordon, & Marlatt, 1980). Once the rule has been broken it seems there is nothing to lose. The very term *relapse* is a pejorative label implying that there are only two possible states: perfection or relapse (Miller, 1996). It can help to catch these setbacks early, normalize them, and keep them from derailing the person's entire plan. This kind of support can be useful in the maintenance of change (Marlatt & Donovan, 2005).

Some changes also entail larger shifts in lifestyle or sense of self. Being a nonsmoker is different from thinking of oneself as a smoker on temporary leave. To support changes in their children, parents may need not only to do some things differently but also to reconsider what they think about and expect of them. A significant lifestyle change can have unanticipated consequences and pose new problems. Decision points also arise about whether it is better to continue pursuing change or to accept what is. Members of Alcoholics Anonymous seek "the serenity to accept the things I cannot change, courage to change the things I can, and wisdom to know the difference." Ongoing support can be helpful when encountering such oft-unexpected aspects of implementing change.

The Spirit and Style of Motivational Interviewing

At the broadest level, the same relational spirit underlying MI can support persistence in a difficult change process. The client-centered skills of accurate empathy, unconditional warmth, and genuineness have been positively, albeit modestly, linked to client change, with substantial variability across studies (Bohart et al., 2002; Norcross, 2002). Rather than falling into a directing style when difficulties arise, a counselor can continue to evoke the client's own wisdom and solutions. Affirmation and self-affirmation can bolster clients' confidence and persistence. Imperfection can be reframed as partial progress, affirming headway that has been made. The way of being

---

BOX 22.1. Personal Reflection: On the Sense of Self

I used to do it quite a lot. What the particular behavior is seems less important here than what the change was like. I noticed that I had some quiet times when I wondered about change, one of which was with a professional. What helped was a realization that I was "filling a hole in my soul" with the behavior. Once I accepted that this was what I was like, it seemed easier to do it less. I was beginning to accept myself more; it felt like there was less fighting in me. Maybe this was a natural maturing process? It was incredibly helpful to have a little space with a professional who let me wonder aloud what change might be like, and who enjoyed with me the easy feeling when I made some progress. It wasn't, and isn't just about the behavior, but also about my sense of who I am!

—SR

with people that Rogers (1980b) described can support clients throughout the process of implementing change.

An MI style also supports client ownership of the change process. Whose plan is being implemented? What will it take to implement? Given clients' expertise on themselves, what would they see as a reasonable next step? In a sense, all change is self-change, to which clinicians are sometimes privileged witnesses and facilitators.

> All change is self-change, to which clinicians are sometimes privileged witnesses and facilitators.

BOX 22.2. Personal Reflection: Learning Behavior Therapy

The clinical training program at the University of Oregon strongly emphasized cognitive-behavioral approaches to psychological treatment, although we were also guided in learning the client-centered style of Carl Rogers. Each clinical faculty member had an active lab group to implement behavioral therapy and research in a particular problem area. This gave us far more than lecture and reading knowledge of therapies. We had the opportunity to try out our new skills in supervised community clinics, observe each others' work, and discuss with peers and mentors every week our practical experiences and challenges.

One of the labs in which I participated focused on behavioral family therapy. I understood the basics of how parents should track their children's behavior and reinforce the right stuff (Miller & Danaher, 1976). Yet when I tried to help families do this, I ran into many obstacles. Homework was a problem not only for children but also for the parents. They would come back with incomplete or no records. Reading assignments weren't done. And even when a child's behavior was improving, the parents might still view them pessimistically. Although I was doing what the textbooks said to do, it just wasn't working for me.

Then we had the privilege of going over to the Oregon Research Institute to observe Gerald Patterson, the grandfather of behavioral family therapy, in action. He did use the procedures that he had described (Patterson, 1974, 1975), but he was also doing much more. He was a warm, engaging, compassionate man who listened empathically to his clients' concerns and problems. He spoke in simple language that people could understand, and families loved him. They did what he suggested in part because of who he was as a person. Too often these important relational aspects of practice are not addressed in therapist manuals. "Oh, so *that's* how you do it!" I thought. He let us hear the music behind the words. I went back to the clinic, tried practicing in that way, and it worked much better.

—WRM

Flexible Revisiting

In Chapter 3 we emphasized that the four processes of MI are not a one-way linear sequence. It is common to revisit processes in the course of implementing change. Here we consider how one might return to each of the four processes to support persistence in change.

Replanning

Perhaps the most common revisiting during change is to the planning process. Something seems to be wrong with the plan, or at least it needs some adjusting.

A good question is often "What next?" Changes typically consist of successive approximations, a series of small steps in the right direction. People are easily overwhelmed when thinking about a larger change goal, but can more readily entertain one small step. Coming up with the right next step is a collaborative process, combining your own expertise with the client's. Of course, ultimately it is up to the person whether to take a step. That is the person's prerogative and autonomy. Even though major negative consequences may ensue, a client does not "have to" take action. It is always a choice. What's the next step?

Another common question is "What now?" This commonly follows a setback, an unexpected interruption or obstacle to change. Is some adjustment needed in the plan to prevent such setbacks in the future? How will the person get back on track? Such challenges call for some replanning.

Then there is "What else?" If one approach is not working, what could be tried instead? What else might work? Here the old plan may be scrapped rather than adjusted and a new plan formulated for pursuing the same goal(s).

The very same methods described for planning in the preceding chapters also apply to replanning. Don't succumb to the righting reflex or overrely on a directing style. Eliciting a change plan is a collaborative process, and the client's own ideas and resources are key (Chapter 20). When a new plan emerges, offer a reflective summary of the plan and ask for the client's assent to it (Chapter 21). Explore any reluctance that the client expresses verbally or nonverbally, and ask how the client might respond to foreseeable obstacles.

Reminding

Sometimes the obstacle to change is wavering commitment to the goal. Whose goal is it? Even with a sound plan, people sometimes seem less sure about whether to pursue the goal that it was designed to accomplish. We could have called this "re-evoking" because it is a revisiting of the evoking process, or "recommitting" as a renewal of prior commitment. It can be either or both, but we liked the everyday term "reminding" instead. It is a bringing back to mind, to conscious awareness, the power of choice and the reasons behind it. A simple checking-in process of "Is this still what you want (need, choose) to do?" may indicate whether you should revisit evoking. The person may need to hear his or her own arguments for change (DARN) again. This could be a recapitulation summary of change talk that the client previously offered. Avoid a "Let me remind you . . . " tone that blatantly confronts the client with discrepancy. That kind of "reminding" is likely to evoke discord. You might begin, "Let me see if I can remember what reasons you gave me for making this change, and tell me whether these things still seem important to you." You could revisit the importance ruler to assess whether there has been a shift in self-rating, and again evoke why the person is at that number rather than zero.

Sometimes slippage in confidence undermines importance. Some failed attempts may undermine self-efficacy for change. It is simply uncomfortable to keep attending to a discrepancy when one is unsure whether it is possible to do anything about it. Doubts about self-efficacy can lead to rationalization that the goal really wasn't all that important or realistic. The confidence ruler may provide clues in this regard, and tools to address a crisis of confidence may come in handy (Chapter 16).

The purpose of reminding is to review and renew the person's intention to pursue the identified goal(s). Is that still the direction in which the person wants to move? If so, then move again to the planning process to consider how best to proceed, and as appropriate elicit an implementation intention. If not, then refocusing is probably needed.

Refocusing

In extended consultation it is common for the focus to shift. Achieving one goal can open up another. Efforts to change may reveal a more pressing or underlying concern that requires attention. People may decide not to pursue a goal that previously seemed important. Changed circumstances can alter priorities. When the goal itself needs adjustment (not just renewing commitment to it), then refocusing is the task.

If the client does not present a salient alternative focus, there may be a need to clarify priorities. The values exploration approaches discussed in Chapter 7 may help in this regard. Focus is a process of choice, and as discussed in Chapter 9 candidate goals can arise from the client, the context, or the clinician. What will be the focus of consultation? Is it possible to move together toward particular goals? When a focus is clear, move on to evoking and planning.

Is the client avoiding change by finding something to focus on instead? This is, of course, the person's prerogative—to choose not to pursue a particular change for the time being. Our inclination here is just to discuss this openly and directly. Is the person, in fact, deciding that another focus is a higher priority than the previously discussed change? This should not be done in an accusatory fashion ("You're just avoiding what you really need to do because it's hard"), which reverts to the expert model that you know better than the client does. It is the client's irrevocable domain to decide what kind of change (if any) to pursue. If you are concerned that the client may not be aware of a desire to avoid, raise your concern (with permission). The point is to make the person's autonomous choice conscious and explicit, not in a blaming or shaming way, but recognizing and honoring the person's power of choice.

It is also possible that the client is considering whether to continue in this counseling relationship. In that case, the appropriate process may be reengaging. That can also be the case when at least one focus of consultation is not negotiable, as in probation or child protective services.

Reengaging

When a client seems to be disengaged or disengaging, it is time to revisit the methods described in Part II. Regular feedback from clients after each visit can provide early warning signs of disengagement (Lambert, Whipple, Smart, Vermeersch, Nielsen, & Hawkins, 2001; S. D. Miller, Duncan, Brown, Sorrell, & Chalk, 2006; S. D. Miller, Duncan, Sorrell, & Brown, 2005). Without engagement it is difficult to make much progress with the other processes of MI.

Take the initiative when there are signs of disengagement. OARS skills are important here (Chapters 5 and 6). If a client misses an appointment, get in touch to renew contact. A simple phone call, handwritten note, or other message expresses your continuing commitment to a helping relationship. Ask for your client's advice as to how you could be more helpful or supportive in the change process. If reasonable engagement is reestablished, move back to refocusing.

> Take the initiative when there are signs of disengagement.

Another service is to follow up with clients after a period of consultation has ended. Many kinds of change do require persistence over time, and clients are often slow to reengage when problems arise. With addictive behaviors, for example, it is fairly predictable for setbacks to occur within 3 to 6 months after initial consultation, and routine follow-up contacts at that time may avert the reversal of gains (Miller et al., 2011). Similarly, continuing supportive contact can be vital with lifestyle changes to address diabetes, weight loss, heart disease, and other long-term self-management challenges.

INTEGRATING MOTIVATIONAL INTERVIEWING
WITH OTHER APPROACHES

Because MI is a clinical style for conversations about change, it can be integrated with a wide range of specific treatment methods. It has been combined, for example, with cognitive-behavioral therapy (Buckner & Schmidt, 2009; Marijuana Treatment Project Research Group, 2004; Westra, 2012), transtheoretical (Erol & Erdogan, 2008; Moe et al., 2002; Velasquez, von Sternberg, Dodrill, Kan, & Parsons, 2005), and gestalt approaches (Engle & Arkowitz, 2005). MI has been used to enhance retention and adherence with both medical and psychotherapies (Baker & Hambridge, 2002; Heffner et al., 2010; Hettema et al., 2005; Olsen, Smith, Oei, & Douglas, 2012). In this sense MI can be more than a prelude to other treatment. As discussed in this chapter, MI is applicable throughout the stages of change to facilitate engagement, focus, and motivation, and to adjust planning in response to challenges that arise. Ways for integrating MI with other approaches are still in relatively early stages of development, but doing so makes more sense to us than regarding MI as an alternative stand-alone treatment to compete with other approaches.

THE CASE OF JULIA: OUTCOME

We did pursue cognitive therapy as a remedy for Julia's depression. She stayed with the process very well, did her homework assignments, kept journals of her thoughts and resulting feelings, generated antidote self-talk to practice when she was running herself down ("Now wait a minute . . . ") emphasizing her strengths and inherent worth, and began feeling substantially better. Flagging motivation was not really a problem during the treatment process, but still she longed for an explanation that would account for her experience. Even though she recognized that changing her self-talk was helping her to maintain a more positive mood, she wanted to understand why she was having so much difficulty in relationships and she feared continuing to repeat the pattern. Then during our eighth session, on a hunch I (WRM) asked her:

INTERVIEWER: Julia, what was your father like?

JULIA: He was gone a lot. He traveled, but when he was in town he was usually around at night. My sisters and I were always glad to see him, and he liked to tell us stories sometimes. He wasn't very affectionate—physically, I mean. He didn't hug or kiss us much. We always knew that deep down inside he loved us. He just wasn't the kind of man who showed it.

INTERVIEWER: Inside he loved you, but outside he was pretty reserved.

JULIA: Right. It's like he was a little afraid of us maybe, afraid of getting too close.

INTERVIEWER: So sometimes you probably wondered whether he really loved you.

JULIA: No, not really, but it would have been nice for him to show it more. He wasn't even very affectionate with our mum, at least not as far as we could see.

INTERVIEWER: Like it was uncomfortable for him. He kept his distance.

She went silent and I saw it hit her. She began weeping, and I waited. After a while she broke the silence: "Oh my God! I'm trying to make my father love me and show it." It was a classic insight breakthrough, and it satisfied her yearning to understand.

Julia reminded me once again that people have wisdom about themselves. I was skeptical that insight would heal her, but I remained open to her own intuition and in the end it provided closure for her. Her insight also helped me with several subsequent clients who had a similar pattern of repeated relationship difficulties. By virtue of her history she was attracted to precisely the wrong kind of man for her. Her romantic passions were aroused by men who were uncomfortable expressing feelings, with the fantasy that she could somehow "get to" the real, warm teddy-bear person she envisioned to be inside them. But then as the relationship developed and she wasn't getting the warm affection that she longed for, she began pressing harder for it. The natural response of her partner in this demand–withdraw pattern was to withdraw more, further frustrating her desire until finally it ended in a cataclysm of rage. We continued to meet for a few more weeks, and she began experimenting with dating men to whom she didn't feel a chemical attraction, but who were overtly warm and loving. She found these relationships less intense but considerably more rewarding.

KEY POINTS

✓ The core style of MI can be useful throughout the implementation of change as, for example, in supporting persistence.

✓ Integrated MI involves flexible revisiting of the processes of planning, evoking, focusing, and engaging as needed.

✓ MI combines well with a variety of other treatment approaches and may enhance retention and adherence.

PART VI

MOTIVATIONAL INTERVIEWING IN EVERYDAY PRACTICE

Motivational interviewing is simple but not easy. The processes of change that are involved are natural, and in an intuitive sense we all know and recognize them. Perhaps this is one reason why MI has had such broad appeal. Yet the practice of MI involves the integration of some quite complex skills. Reflective listening alone is challenging to master. Someone who is good at it makes it look easy, as natural as breathing, until you try to do it. These are skills that can be honed throughout the course of a career.

MI also is but one of a broad array of competencies used by any clinician in daily practice. A further challenge is to integrate MI with other practices so that one can use them flexibly and weave them together in responding to clients' needs. Then there is the challenge of implementing MI within programs or systems: effective treatments also need effective implementation strategies in order to be expressed and maintained in ongoing systems.

These are some of the issues addressed in Part VI, which we unfold like layers on an onion. We begin in Chapter 23 with the clinician's inner experience when practicing MI. Next we address challenges in developing proficiency with this clinical method (Chapter 24) and applying it in practice (Chapter 25). Then we turn to how MI can be implemented in systems and how organizational structures in turn can facilitate or impede MI-consistent practice (Chapter 26).

CHAPTER 23

Experiencing Motivational Interviewing

In theory there is no difference between
theory and practice. In practice, there is.
—DEAN FIXSEN

A picture is worth a thousand words.
—NAPOLEON BONAPARTE

Having discussed each of the four component processes of MI we turn now
to some issues that arise in the experience of clinicians when practicing MI.
We introduce these as four questions that you may wonder about as you
gain practical experience with this style:

1. "How do I know when I'm doing MI?"
2. "How do the four processes fit together in practice?"
3. "How brief can MI be?"
4. "What about my own inner experience?"

We use these questions as springboards to illustrate some challenges that
arise when putting MI into practice.

AWARENESS: "HOW DO I KNOW WHEN I'M DOING MI?"

MI can be defined, described, and even quantified (see Chapter 28), but
what does it look and feel like in practice? Defined as a style, the parallels
of MI with dancing are striking. How do you know, for example, when

305

someone is dancing in tango style? If it's done really well it is almost unmistakable. The spines are straight, the faces are pointed in unison, and the four feet move as if belonging to one being. If the dance is in another style such as flamenco, it's easy to see that it is not tango. Different styles can be blended, of course, but few dance instructors would recommend trying this before you are skilled at both forms.

Spot the Difference

What differences can you spot between the following two interviews? Both conversations start in the same place, but there are many differences in technique as well as style. Here's the situation: A doctor is concerned about whether a man in his early 80s might be depressed following a mild right hemisphere stroke 2 weeks earlier. A nurse on the ward offers to speak with the patient about his future before he is discharged, keeping in mind the possibility of a referral to the psychiatric liaison service. Ask yourself: Is this nurse doing MI? How do you know?

Nurse A

CLIENT/PATIENT: I feel worried about going home now. I hardly know where to begin.

INTERVIEWER: Oh, that's very understandable for someone with your condition. I'm sure you will get much better, you'll see. It's only been 2 weeks, and you could get back a lot of functioning in the year ahead. Have you been working with the physical therapist here?

CLIENT: Yes I have, but I live alone, you see, and now I can't even walk properly. I don't know how I am going to cope.

INTERVIEWER: Well, we've scheduled a physical therapist to come to your home for a while, and we have also arranged for you to see the social worker so you can talk about how things will go at home. From our point of view here on the ward you're recovering very well, and we think you will keep regaining some of your functioning over the next few months. This is quite likely, and so you'll gradually find it easier to cope than you can imagine right now.

CLIENT: I miss my friends.

INTERVIEWER: We also have outpatient recovery group meetings where you can meet new friends and talk together about coping with a stroke. I know other stroke patients who have gone there and they have found it very helpful. Do you think you might be interested in that?

CLIENT: I don't know. I used to go golfing a few times a week and then for a drink at the clubhouse afterward, but now I can't even walk properly.

INTERVIEWER: Don't worry, you will get to feeling better bit by bit. The drinking probably wasn't good for you anyway. The social worker will work with you, and if you need it we'll also get the occupational therapist to come around to your house and help you cope with all the changes. It's important that you make yourself try a little harder each day to move around and do the normal things like washing and walking and that sort of thing. That will help you feel better, too.

CLIENT: Well thanks, but that's the problem, because I can't imagine myself doing all this. It all feels like too much.

INTERVIEWER: You just take it a day at a time. If you like, we can ask the hospital psychologist to come around and talk to you, because I can see you are feeling pretty down about this all.

CLIENT: Wouldn't you? How could a psychologist help with my situation? I don't understand.

INTERVIEWER: Well, the psychologist can help you to adapt to these changes better and to make the best of your situation. They have a lot of experience in helping people like you. I'm sure you'll do fine.

CLIENT: I just don't know.

INTERVIEWER: Well, wait until you've had some time to work with the physical therapist, the social worker, and the psychologist. You're just getting started, and it takes time to recover from a stroke like you had. You just need to be patient.

CLIENT: I just don't see how it's possible for me to get my life back.

Nurse B

CLIENT/PATIENT: I feel worried about going home now. I hardly know where to begin.

INTERVIEWER: It all seems rather overwhelming for you.

CLIENT: That's right. I live alone, you see.

INTERVIEWER: And you're wondering how life will turn out now that you've had this stroke.

CLIENT: Yes, I like to play a round of golf and have a drink with friends, and now I can't see how it's possible to get that life back again when I can't even walk properly.

INTERVIEWER: It seems like a real uphill struggle.

CLIENT: Yes, exactly. More like a mountain! The doctor told me I might get a bit better but we'll have to wait and see.

INTERVIEWER: There's still a lot of time and room for improvement.

CLIENT: That's what the doctor says. It's only been 2 weeks.

INTERVIEWER: And you've already made good progress. What do you think would help you the most right now?

CLIENT: I don't know, but thank you. I need to figure out how to get my life back and carry on, even if it's for my grandchildren. They were here this morning and that was good.

INTERVIEWER: You really enjoy being with them.

CLIENT: I was in tears after they left and I decided that I have to get better, but then the reality hit me that I can't even get to the toilet on my own!

INTERVIEWER: Your independence is a very precious thing.

CLIENT: Well, I want to go out with my golfing group. It was me who started that foursome 40 years ago.

INTERVIEWER: Wow! You've been together for a long time with those friends.

CLIENT: Yes, and they came to see me yesterday. It was good to see them, you know.

INTERVIEWER: I'll bet they want you back with them one way or another.

CLIENT: I can't see how it's possible and that's what makes me just, well, really upset.

INTERVIEWER: I wonder how you could keep in touch with them while you're recovering.

CLIENT: They'll come around to see me, I know, and maybe we can do some other things together.

INTERVIEWER: Like what?

CLIENT: Well, I'll probably be able to have a drink and play cards with them even if I can't play 18 holes.

INTERVIEWER: So it feels like you have a mountain climb ahead of you. It looks so difficult that you can't quite imagine it yet, since this is all so new. And you also have some good friends to go on this journey with you. Is that about right?

CLIENT: Yes, that's how I feel.

INTERVIEWER: I'll tell you what. How about if I come back tomorrow morning—I'm on duty then—and I'll bring us a cup of tea and we can talk again, see how you're feeling, and think together a bit about getting up that mountain. Would that be all right?

CLIENT: Yes, thank you, that will be good. It helps to talk about this.

Was It Motivational Interviewing?

Clearly both Nurse A and Nurse B were concerned and trying to be helpful, and both conversations took about the same amount of time. It is possible that both nurses thought of what they were doing as MI. But was it? How can you tell? Here are some questions to consider related to the four processes of MI.

1. *What was engagement like?* To what extent did the nurse seem to be interested in understanding the patient's perspective? What was the quality of reflective listening? How engaged do you think the patient felt in the conversation? Was a foundation laid for further conversation? In terms of technique, Nurse A asked two closed questions and offered no reflections. Nurse B offered nine reflections and asked three open questions before closing: a 3-to-1 ratio of reflections to questions. Quality listening didn't take any longer, and it might be argued that it saved time, allowing Nurse B to get closer to the heart of the challenge. Sometimes *not* listening can prolong the process.

2. *Was there a clear focus?* Both conversations did focus on issues related to recovery from stroke. Nurse B homed in on the patient's relationship with his golfing friends, a somewhat more specific topic that is of obvious importance to him.

3. *Was the interviewer evoking change talk?* With Nurse A the patient offers only sustain talk, no change talk. Through reflective listening and open questions Nurse B is already evoking change talk (did you spot it?), with the patient seeming more activated and engaged in the conversation. Specifically, Nurse B asked three open questions, the expected answer to which would be change talk:

"What do you think would help you the most right now?"
"I wonder how you could keep in touch with them while you're recovering."
"Like what?" [Asking for elaboration or an example]

4. *Was there collaborative planning?* Perhaps the biggest difference between these two conversations was the extent and style of planning. Nurse A jumps right in with advice and solutions (never with permission, by the way). The righting reflex is flagrant, and the patient seems unimpressed with the ideas being provided. No advice was asked for, and none was given by Nurse B. Instead, all three of the open questions listed above were such as to elicit the patient's own ideas for what to do.

With these four considerations in mind, the latter conversation was clearly MI whereas the former was not. Nurse A's obvious concern is channelled into a directing style and unilateral problem solving. The well-intentioned reassurance peppered across Nurse A's conversation clearly falls within Thomas Gordon's description of a roadblock to listening, to understanding the client's predicament (Chapter 5). Nurse B's conversation is much closer to a guiding style. As a dance it has a firm sense of direction, with a gentle and fluid approach to movement. Even in this short exchange the elements of the underlying spirit of MI (Chapter 2) are apparent.

How are the two participants in each of these conversations likely to be feeling? It can feel comfortable to take the lead as Nurse A does, confident in one's expertise, and it can also quite soon feel frustrating—a bit like pulling someone across the dance floor, trips and all. One can imagine Nurse B feeling fairly calm, engaged, happy to offer advice when needed, yet trusting of the client's good judgement. And what about the patient? Defensiveness is apparent in the many "buts" in the first conversation. Discord is also beneath the surface: "Wouldn't you feel down? You don't understand." Nurse B gives him room to say how he feels, and he is likely looking forward to continuing the conversation. Rather than offering him vague reassurances and uninvited solutions, Nurse B finds particular points to affirm.

Who is doing the talking about change? In the first conversation it's the nurse who gives voice to change while the client states the case against it (sustain talk). In the second conversation the client expresses the desire, reasons, need, and to some extent ability to change. In essence, these two conversations illustrate two very different styles when encountering ambivalence.

> A conversation about change is MI when you are listening to understand the person's own perspective, have a clear focus on one or more change goals, and actively evoking the person's own motivations for change.

In summary, it's MI when there is a conversation about change in which you are (1) using empathic listening to understand the person's own perspective and to engage in a collaborative relationship, (2) have a clear focus in the form of one or more change goals, and (3) are actively evoking the person's own motivations for change. Planning may or may not ensue but tends to flow naturally from evoking.

NAVIGATION: "HOW DO THE FOUR PROCESSES FIT TOGETHER?"

"Where am I, and where are we going in this conversation?" It is common in MI to experience a temporary loss of clarity about what is happening

---

BOX 23.1. Am I Doing MI?

Here are some questions to ask yourself, reflecting on your inner experience as well as your conversational style.

1. **Engaging.** How well do I understand how this person perceives the situation or dilemma? Could I give voice to what this person is experiencing? How many of my responses are reflective listening statements? How engaged in our conversation does the person seem to be?

2. **Focusing.** Do I have a clear sense of focus? Do I know the direction in which I hope change occurs? What goal(s) do we have for change, and to what extent do we agree about them?

3. **Evoking.** What do I know about this person's own motivations for change? Am I hearing change talk? What am I doing intentionally to evoke and strengthen change talk? What concerns, goals, or values does this person hold that would encourage this change?

4. **Planning.** Am I hearing mobilizing change talk that may signal readiness to discuss when and how change might occur, even a first step? Would it be premature at this point to be discussing a plan? To what extent am I evoking mobilizing change talk from the person rather than providing solutions myself? If I am giving information and advice, is it with permission?

---

and where to go next. Reflective listening is an excellent fallback strategy in moments like this while you seek clarity, and the four processes may be a helpful map for finding your way. What progress have you made together in engaging, focusing, evoking, and planning? Which process seems to be the immediate challenge?

The four processes are sequential and layered upon one another, which makes it possible to move flexibly between them in response to the situation. They are also interwoven so that what occurs in one process can affect the others. Discord during the planning process may foster disengagement. Increased self-efficacy may enhance change talk and readiness to consider planning. High-quality listening during the evoking process can deepen engagement.

Despite these overlaps and interactions among processes it can be useful to step back and ask yourself which process needs emphasis at present. One of the clearest windows into MI is to consider these moments when you have a choice to steer the conversation one way or another. The client says something, and what you say next can and probably will affect the course of the interview. Here is a case example to illustrate how an interviewer might use OARS skills differently depending on which process is being emphasized.

A young man with a quiet and passive manner finds himself unhappy at work to the point of wanting to phone in sick in order to avoid the discomfort. He's not being bullied or harassed, but thinks he is being taken advantage of and always given the worst jobs. His doctor referred him, concerned about apparent depression manifested in low energy, sleep problems, and self-deprecation.

If your emphasis were on engaging you might be exploring the man's experience and demonstrating your grasp of his dilemma.

- *Open question*: "How have you been feeling when you're at work?"
- *Affirmation*: "You're really trying to do a good job at work, even coming here to talk it over."
- *Reflection*: "It seems to you that you're being taken advantage of, even pushed out at work, and that's really uncomfortable."
- *Summary*: "You're not happy with how things are at work and this is creeping into other parts of your life. You aren't sleeping well these days, and you've been to see a doctor about your nerves. At this point you dread even going in to work because you seem to be disrespected there."

If focusing were your emphasis you would be seeking clarity about the direction for your conversation together.

- *Open question*: "What change do you think might make the biggest difference for you?"
- *Affirmation*: "You're really trying to do a good job and sort out what might be the best way for you to make it work."
- *Reflection*: "You'd like to talk about how you could be more assertive at work."
- *Summary*: "You decided to seek help because you've looked to the future and think you can't keep on like this. We've talked about what's happening at work, how you are feeling about it, and how it's affecting you at home, too. I wonder if we might talk about how you could be more assertive at work and what effect that could have."

If you have arrived at a clear focus (in this example, to become more assertive at work) your emphasis could be on evoking, building motivation and commitment to this change.

- *Open question*: "What do you think could be some advantages if you were to express yourself more assertively at work?"

- *Affirmation*: "You know that you can stand up for yourself because you've done it before."
- *Reflection*: "You've thought about looking for another job, but you think the same problems could arise and it might be best to focus on solving this where you are now."
- *Summary*: "You've been so uncomfortable at work that you've considered just leaving this job, which could bring some immediate relief. You also know that finding another job would be hard and you could have the same challenges there. Wherever you work, you want to be more assertive and you'd like to try that in this job."

When there seems to be enough readiness to move ahead, then your emphasis might shift to planning, developing specific ideas about how to move ahead.

- *Open question*: "How might you approach a meeting with your boss?"
- *Affirmation*: "You're going to use that persistence of yours to find some new ways of communicating at work."
- *Reflection*: "So one thing you can imagine doing is to ask for some more responsible tasks to do, and you feel ready to give that a try."
- *Summary*: "You want to ask for a meeting with your boss where you won't just complain, but talk about how you would like things to be better for you at work. You plan to start by writing him a letter to ask for the meeting, and then we'll look at this together next week before you send it out. Is that what you're going to do?"

Deciding which process needs to be emphasized at present can help you know how to proceed.

Of course, the four processes of MI are not the only things going on in clinical consultations. Practitioners bring a wealth of clinical experience and expertise, and regularly encounter in-session choice points about what to do next; for example, choosing between reflecting or offering advice and encouragement. One choice is not necessarily better than another; they just move in different directions. Being aware of these choice points and experiencing the results of choosing one path versus another helps to hone practice skills over time.

TIME PRESSURE: "HOW BRIEF CAN MI BE?"

A common inner experience is a sense of time pressure, of needing "to get on with it." This is particularly common in settings like health care, where visits tend to be short and there is much to do, but even with longer consultations one can feel an urgency to get moving. When you don't have much time or things seem to be moving too slowly there is a particular temptation to resort to a directing style in order to "take charge." This can be exacerbated by system pressures to work quickly and produce results.

> A directing style can be exacerbated by pressures to work quickly and produce results.

How possible is it to practice MI in relatively short spans of time? Conversations about change can and do occur in very brief episodes. One of the briefest we've ever encountered was in a dental clinic where a practitioner asked the patient, whose mouth was wide open with instruments, whether he smoked. "Erghhh" was the reply, to which the dentist responded, "You really should stop, you know." The patient said "Urglll," and the drilling continued. Not exactly MI!

Our interest in brief applications of MI began with a trial in a hospital setting (Heather, Rollnick, Bell, & Richmond, 1996), and ever since, this issue of brevity has arisen frequently as clinicians learn MI. Can MI be done in a few minutes? If "done" means "provided," the answer is surely "Yes." Nurse B's conversation above is a good example. If "done" means "completed enough to result in change," then the answer is "Often." Clinical trials do clearly show that relatively brief MI interventions can trigger significant change (e.g., Bernstein et al., 2005; Nock & Kazdin, 2005; Rubak et al., 2005; Senft, Polen, Freeborn, & Hollis, 1997; Soria, Legido, Escolano, Lopez Yeste, & Montoya, 2006). There are also published trials in which brief MI-based interventions have yielded no effect (e.g., Juarez et al., 2006; Marsden et al., 2006), and longer exposure to MI may be more effective (Longabaugh et al., 2001; Polcin, Galloway, Palmer, & Mains, 2004; Rubak et al., 2005). We know of no evidence, however, that directing-style interventions are more effective than MI when time is brief. If patient behavior change is what's needed and time is short, MI is likely to be more effective than telling people what to do and why (Rubak et al., 2005).

Understanding the critical components of MI that facilitate change may be particularly important with brief interventions (Heather, 2005). When time is short, what is most important to do (and not do) in order to promote change? We consider this issue further in Chapter 28.

Listening under Time Pressure

The style of MI is wrapped around the skillful use of empathic listening. What might seem brief to a psychotherapist (say, about four 50-minute sessions) could be impossibly long to a health care practitioner, who often has less than 15 minutes. We know it is quite possible to practice MI within conversations of 15 minutes or less. A challenge, of course, is that MI is usually not the only thing that needs to be done in a short visit. Nevertheless, if you do have a few minutes for a conversation about positive change, it's possible to do so with an MI style and with an unhurried mind. Skillful reflective listening can give both parties the sense of having had quality time together.

MI is not a treatment protocol that requires a specific amount of time. It's a particular way of talking with people, of asking questions and responding to what they say. It's possible for a single utterance to be more or less "MI-like." Sure, a longer conversation usually affords more opportunity to make progress, but when clinicians have a relatively brief amount of time, MI can still make a contribution to conversations about change. A switch as simple as replacing "Why don't you try . . . ?" with "What do you think will work for you?" could change the outcome of an interaction. We caution, though, against oversimplifying and thereby distorting MI to make it fit in small spaces. This can take the form of stripping away the spirit that lies at the heart of the style and reducing it to formulaic techniques that have the feeling of something that is applied *to* or *on* people. "Just ask them these questions." "Have them list their pros and cons." "Just use the ruler." It is one thing to search for ways of evoking thoughtfulness about change in just a few minutes, a feat of considerable skill, and quite another to imply that the solution is a technological one that resides in the delivery of this or that ploy or procedure, like doing the steps of a dance without any music. When techniques become tools to use on people, one has abandoned the spirit of MI.

> When techniques become tools to use on people, one has abandoned the spirit of MI.

Spot the Difference

This consultation occurs in a busy prenatal clinic where a pregnant woman with HIV-AIDS is facing the need to maintain a healthy diet, adhere to an antiretroviral medication regimen, and practice safe sex. Her first language is not English.[1] In this example we use a very brief segment to illustrate the directing style and then an example of a guiding style.

Counselor A

INTERVIEWER: Good morning. We are talking today because we don't want you to have an HIV-positive baby.

CLIENT: Uh-huh. It's difficult because what about if my husband wants to have sex with me?

---

[1] Thanks to Bob Mash and colleagues for this practical example.

INTERVIEWER: You need to use a condom.

CLIENT: But he doesn't want to use a condom.

INTERVIEWER: The problem is that you can get reinfected. For the sake of your baby you need to discuss this with your husband if you want this baby.

CLIENT: Yes, I want the baby.

INTERVIEWER: Well, if you want a healthy baby you need to discuss this and work it out with your husband to use condoms as responsible parents.

CLIENT: But he gets mad and hits me sometimes.

INTERVIEWER: You have to protect your baby. Are you taking your medications?

CLIENT: Yes, when I can. Sometimes I miss doses.

INTERVIEWER: You really need to take all your medications faithfully. That's very important. If you miss doses the medicines don't work as well.

CLIENT: I do take them most of the time.

INTERVIEWER: I'm afraid most of the time isn't good enough. You need to take them all as we discussed.

CLIENT: I'll try.

INTERVIEWER: And how about your diet? Are you eating good food for you and your baby?

CLIENT: Yes.

INTERVIEWER: Because you are eating for two people now, so watch the beer also. It's not good for the baby. Do you have any questions?

CLIENT: No.

INTERVIEWER: All right, I'll see you again in 3 weeks.

CLIENT: OK.

Counselor B

INTERVIEWER: Good morning. I'm glad you came back to see me today.

CLIENT: I must do this for my baby.

INTERVIEWER: This baby is very important to you and you want it to be healthy.

CLIENT: Yes, I told my husband and he is supportive but there are some issues he is not helping me with. He doesn't want to use the condoms.

INTERVIEWER: The condoms are an issue. We can talk about that, about your medication, your diet, or anything that's important to you.

CLIENT: I want to talk about the medicine.

INTERVIEWER: Yes, fine, we can come back to other things. The medication feels important to you.

CLIENT: I know it's very important. If I miss some doses, is that bad?

INTERVIEWER: Tell me what difficulty you're having.

CLIENT: I don't want my mother to know about this. I hide the medicines from her, but she can see what I am doing all the time.

INTERVIEWER: So sometimes it's a challenge for you to take the medicine on time.

CLIENT: Yes, I want to do this for myself and my baby, and sometimes she looks at me strangely.

INTERVIEWER: How might you be able to take them without her seeing?

CLIENT: When I go to the toilet.

INTERVIEWER: That's good. When else could you take them?

CLIENT: After she's gone to bed.

INTERVIEWER: It sounds like that could work. With just those two options I think you could take them when you need to, and maybe there are even more possibilities. What do you think?

CLIENT: I don't want to miss doses. I'll see how that works.

INTERVIEWER: Good! You're right that it's important to take them regularly, and that sounds like a good plan. Now, could we talk a bit about how it's going with your husband and using condoms?

CLIENT: All right.

MI at its best is both simple and skillful, though not necessarily easy. These two brief conversations are the same in length: 10 exchanges in each. Consider these questions:

- How engaged was the patient in each conversation? How well was the interviewer listening to the woman's own perspective? How is she likely to be feeling at the end of each exchange?
- In each conversation about change how was the focus established, and by whom?
- Is there change talk? If so, what did the counselor do to evoke it and how did the counselor respond when it occurred?
- How willing would the woman be to continue the discussion if the clinician has time to do so?

AN UNCLUTTERED MIND:
THE CLINICIAN'S INNER STATE

The practical issues discussed thus far in this chapter have focused on matters of definition, boundaries across processes, and brevity. This might leave you with the impression that the practice of MI is a tough and cerebral matter of grasping and applying specific clinical strategies. Our experience is that the harder you try to do this, the more difficult it can be. If you are focused on internal chatter about how to use techniques, then you are probably not sufficiently engaged with and attending to your client. Rather than effortful cleverness, what is needed is an emotionally aware, thoughtful, and responsive manner. One shorthand that we use for this is "an uncluttered mind."

Much of this skillfulness rests on restraint in the face of distractions and even provocations, with an awareness of there being strength within the client that is responsive to calm and purposeful guiding. Distractions come aplenty and can affect your emotional state. How you handle them might be critical to your progress.

Also don't balk when a client seems to throw out an obstacle. Just keep going with a calm and uncluttered mind. Such a pivotal moment arrived when a colleague was conducting an interview about losing weight. The conversation could easily have turned in quite a different direction, but it didn't. It went like this[2]:

INTERVIEWER: This weight loss idea is really important to you.

CLIENT: I know I should do something about this. I mean, I want to really lose weight.

INTERVIEWER: How confident are you that you can succeed?

CLIENT: No, forget it, absolutely not at all. [The pivotal moment, when the interviewer might have backed off]

INTERVIEWER: What *would* success look like for you?

CLIENT: I would make healthy eating a sort of habit, like a daily routine rather than a special event.

INTERVIEWER: A routine that makes sense to you.

CLIENT: It can't be too radical, it must be gentle and enjoyable . . .

The conversation continued to consider constructive routes to change, even though the client had apparently shut the door to confidence talk ("Forget it—absolutely not at all"). It illustrates very well how MI consistency

---

[2] Thanks to Nina Gobat for this example.

BOX 23.2. Personal Reflection: The Inner Experience of MI

Over the course of 30 years I have had plenty of opportunity to reflect on the inner world, the phenomenology of practicing MI. This reflective process began for me with my Norwegian colleagues asking me to verbalize what was going on in my mind as I counseled, to say what I was trying to do and not do from moment to moment (see Chapter 27).

I would say first that there is a joy for me when practicing MI. I am excited knowing what potential there is for change in the person across from me and in not knowing exactly where the process will go. It's challenging, but it doesn't really feel like work to me anymore, nor is it ever boring. When practicing MI I feel about as awake and alive as I can be. In part this is because there is so much going on under the surface of MI. Watching me interview, Steve once said to me, "Miller, you're a duck!" I knew he wasn't referring to my roots at the University of Oregon.

"A duck?"

"Yes," he replied, "a duck. On the surface it looks like you are moving along slowly, smoothly, effortlessly, while underneath the water you're paddling like mad."

In a way that's how it feels. It's not an anxious, exhausting process; usually I feel quite relaxed about it, even on videotape, but I am very conscious about what is happening and (once we have focused) where I'm heading, where the sunrise horizon is. There are several things constantly in my consciousness. As a prime directive I mean to stay with the person in the present, paying attention and not letting my awareness drift off into plans or distractions. At the same time I am remembering what has already transpired, logging away what the person has said. I am also sorting what I have heard, storing away in the person's own words the bits (like change talk) that seem particularly important. I may not respond to these bits immediately; it is wise, I think, not to pounce on what seems important. Let it rest a while and allow the process to unfold. I will come back to it later. Thus it can look like I have missed something (and of course I do sometimes). "Why didn't you challenge that right away?" I don't usually feel in a hurry about it; I will come back to it when the time seems right, and probably sooner rather than later.

It seems to me that at its best the inner experience of MI is holding past, present, and future simultaneously. I am clearly hearing and attending to whatever the person is saying in this moment and adjusting my own course accordingly. I hear it in the context of what has already transpired, putting together pieces like the flowers of a bouquet. And I am conscious also of direction, of the compass that tells me where I'm headed and how to get there. No wonder it's such a rich experience!

—WRM

involves a combination of attitude and technique. The former in this case was a curious, compassionate, and accepting attitude; the latter was a purposeful intervention, in this case a question: "What would success look like for you?" based on the conviction that the client had strengths, knowledge, and competence.

Distractions from Outside the Interview

Some distractions arise from outside the interview and apart from the particular person with whom you are conversing. Distressing news, conflicts at home or work, or time pressures can mean that you enter into an interview some distance from an ideal emotional state. We find it can be helpful before an interview to take a moment for centering on the person or task at hand. This might be a quiet meditation (see Box 2.3 in Chapter 2) or simply a review of notes from prior contacts. Some practitioners keep a short "Remember to . . . " list of self-guidance reminders handy to review just before an interview. The content of the list depends on what you most need to remember at this point in your learning and practice of MI. Some examples include:

> Listen and reflect.
> Be sure to affirm what the person is doing well.
> Listen for change talk.
> Call upon the person's own motivation, wisdom, and strengths.
> Resist the righting reflex.

Distractions Inside the Interview

Other threats to an uncluttered mind arise within the interview from what the client says to you. An emotional response in you is not a problem in itself; it's how you recognize and respond to it. Consider these questions, pausing to consider and answer each one.[3] What might a client say in session that would predispose you to feel:

> Angry?
> Concerned?
> Bored?
> Overenthusiastic?
> Alarmed?
> Challenged?

---

[3] Thanks to Jeff Allison for this training exercise.

What could a client say that might:

> Warm your heart?
> Trigger a desire to rescue?
> Remind you why you love your work?

If you were to write down client responses that could evoke these responses in you, some patterns might emerge.

Now consider how you might respond to each of these situations if you simply allowed your emotions free rein. Might you reply with defensiveness or a righting reflex? Would your mind wander off to other situations or concerns of which it reminds you? Do you have any "prerecorded message tapes" that might be triggered? How much of your immediate response you share with clients is an issue of professional judgment discussed in Chapter 11.

In general, though, we counsel restraint when negative emotions are tweaked by a client. The responses to sustain talk and discord that we discussed in Chapter 15 ideally come from a calm, curious, and thoughtful stance that places the client's welfare first and foremost. A reflective listening statement is a good default and tends to be calming for both you and your client. When you focus on understanding the client's own frame of reference you may experience a shift in your own emotional state and feel more curious and reflective. This allows MI to proceed through moment-to-moment responsiveness to what is happening with both the client and yourself.

KEY POINTS

✓ What constitutes MI is a combination of (1) an engaged understanding of the client's internal frame of reference, (2) a clear change focus, and (3) evoking of the client's own motivations for change. If appropriate, it may also include a collaborative planning process.

✓ Even within relatively brief consultations MI can be practiced with integrity and has been found to facilitate client change.

✓ The four processes of MI are layered upon one another, making it possible to move flexibly between them in response to the immediate situation.

✓ The skillful practice of MI is promoted by an uncluttered mind.

CHAPTER 24

Learning Motivational Interviewing

You need knowledge and you need skill. Knowledge you
can even get just from reading a book. Skill you cannot
get from a book—you need to practice again and again.
—PAUL EKMAN

There is no such thing as teaching; there is only learning.
—MONTY ROBERTS

We are sometimes asked how many hours of training are enough to learn
MI. In a way that is like asking how long rope is or how many hours of
lessons are required to learn to play a musical instrument. Enough for what
purpose? What level of skill is needed in a particular context or application? How much learning is required before it makes a difference to your
clients? It's not a matter of completing a certain number of hours of training and then you have it. Learning MI is an ongoing process, and more
than knowledge is involved. When learning to fly an airplane one may
begin with hours of classroom instruction, but ultimately it's a matter of
guided practice in the air. With practice and feedback you can become
more proficient.

THE VALUE OF FEEDBACK

The feedback piece is important here. One of the better replicated findings in psychotherapy research is that therapists with many years of practice have no better client outcomes on average than those who are recently
trained. In contrast, one of the most replicated findings in medicine is the
effect of experience. A surgeon who has done a particular procedure 2,000
times is simply better at it than someone who has done it twice: better

outcomes, fewer complications and adverse effects. What's the difference between psychotherapists and surgeons? The surgeons get constant feedback. They rarely practice alone behind closed doors, and when there are complications or adverse outcomes they find out soon enough.[1]

As in mastering a sport or musical instrument there are also large differences in how quickly people learn MI. We have worked with people who took to MI very quickly; it was like putting a fish into water. They just seemed to have an intuitive grasp of it, and once exposed to the ideas and examples they quickly developed proficiency. We have also met people who had a great deal of difficulty learning MI. Perhaps they thought that they had mastered it, but after many hours of training and coaching there was still little skill. Both of these extremes are exceptions. Most people develop skill with guided practice, and we have not found any relationship between years of graduate education and the ability to learn MI (Miller et al., 2004; cf. Hartzler & Espinosa, 2011; Naar-King, Outlaw, Green-Jones, & Wright, 2009). Even people with advanced degrees are able to learn it!

Feedback is fundamental for any kind of learning, and immediate feedback is even more helpful. It is difficult to learn archery in the dark. It is hard to learn if you receive no accurate information as to whether your guesses or tries were on the mark. With no reliable feedback it is possible to practice for decades without much improvement in skill.

> Feedback is fundamental for any kind of learning; it's hard to learn archery in the dark.

An advantage in learning MI is that once you learn what to listen for, your clients provide you with immediate feedback. Like a surgeon, you can tell during a session how it's going and what outcome is likely. When learning empathic listening (Chapter 5) every reflection yields immediate feedback from the client as to its accuracy. When you hear change talk you're on the right track in MI, and clients also quickly tell you when you're going astray. A key is the knowledge that, of all the things clients say, change talk and sustain talk are particularly important signals for what to do next, just as when you strike a key on the piano you get immediate feedback as to whether it was the right note.

Just as there are self-taught musicians there are people for whom this immediate feedback from clients is enough to help them learn MI. For most people, though, just reading about MI or taking a 2-day workshop is not enough to make a difference in their proficiency (Madson et al., 2009; Miller & Mount, 2001; Miller et al., 2004). This is not unique to MI, but seems to be true in learning new therapeutic skills more generally (Fixsen, Naoom, Blase, Friedman, & Wallace, 2005; Miller, Sorensen, Selzer, &

---

[1] Thanks to Theresa Moyers for this insight.

Brigham, 2006). To develop proficiency with a sport or musical instrument people often engage a coach with a higher level of skill than their own to provide feedback and make specific suggestions for further development. One would not say to a tennis coach, "Don't watch me," or to a piano teacher, "Don't listen to me playing."

Similarly, coaching in MI needs to be based on direct observation, which is usually accomplished via recorded sessions. It is for good reason that most professions call their consultations "practice," and like archery in the dark, practice without reliable feedback (literally "private practice") is unlikely to improve skill. We learned long ago that when supervising therapists in training, the places where we could be most helpful were in regard to what they *didn't* hear during the session. Consequently, it was insufficient for a trainee to come out of a session and describe what had happened. The problem with "private practice" is that it's private! As coaches, we needed to be in the room, if only indirectly through audio or video recordings. Even a modest amount of expert coaching can significantly improve MI proficiency (Miller et al., 2004).

> Coaching in MI needs to be based on direct observation.

A MENU FOR LEARNING

MI is not a single technique but rather an integrated set of interviewing skills. It is possible to think of specific learning tasks that correspond to component core skills of MI (Miller & Moyers, 2006). We think of at least 12 such tasks:

- Understanding the underlying spirit with which MI is practiced: partnership, acceptance, compassion, and evocation (Chapter 2).
- Developing skill and comfort with reflective listening (Chapter 5) and the client-centered OARS skills (Chapter 6).
- Identifying change goals toward which to move (Chapter 9).
- Exchanging information and providing advice within an MI style (Chapter 11).
- Being able to recognize change talk and sustain talk (Chapter 12).
- Evoking change talk (Chapter 13).
- Responding to change talk in a way that strengthens it (Chapter 14).
- Responding to sustain talk and discord in a way that does not amplify it (Chapter 15).
- Developing hope and confidence (Chapter 16).
- Timing (Chapter 19) and negotiating a change plan (Chapter 20).

- Strengthening commitment (Chapter 21).
- Flexibly integrating MI with other clinical skills and practices (Chapter 25).

We have not numbered these tasks because they are not necessarily learned in order. Clinicians may come to MI already with well-developed skills in some of these areas. Some component tasks can be learned apart from the others. For example, one might learn to identify change talk in a classroom or by reading. That is mostly a knowledge task, although it is far easier to recognize change talk on a transcript than within the fast-emerging flow of a clinical consultation.

Some component tasks are fundamental, and it is difficult to develop further skills until these are in place. Reflective listening is a good example. In the beginning, one struggles to remember to reflect and to come up with a good reflective listening statement rather than, say, asking a question. It feels effortful. With practice and the immediate feedback provided by the people with whom you converse, forming reflections becomes easier. Then with more practice and good results with clients, empathic listening begins to feel natural. It becomes the default response rather than asking questions or giving advice. You can always fall back to reflective listening, and at worst, you're unlikely to do harm. Then for some it becomes not only easy but a pleasure, a joy, a privilege. While, thankfully, one need not reach this level of proficiency in listening to begin doing MI, a certain level of comfort or naturalness with reflections is important. Until one can comfortably follow a conversation with reflective listening it is difficult to take the next step to evoking, where one uses the OARS skills in a strategic manner to elicit and strengthen change talk. Similarly, you need to have a change goal and be able to recognize change talk, to know it when you hear it, before you can evoke and respond differentially to it. A reasonable question to ask when learning is, "What would be one good next step for me in developing and being comfortable with the clinical style of MI?"

> You can always fall back to reflective listening; at worst, you're unlikely to do harm.

CODING

A coach's subjective feedback can be valuable, and there are also coding systems to provide more reliable and objective feedback on practice (Madson & Campbell, 2006; Moyers, Martin, Catley, Harris, & Ahluwalia, 2003; Moyers, Martin, Manuel, Hendrickson, & Miller, 2005). These systems have the merit of identifying specific areas in which practice might be improved. A variety of MI coding instruments can be found at *www. motivationalinterviewing.org/library.*

Some coding systems, such as the Motivational Interviewing Treatment Integrity (MITI), focus only on the interviewer's responses, including both global ratings and specific response counts to document intervention fidelity (Hendrickson et al., 2004; Moyers, Martin, et al., 2005). Others code only what the client says, with particular focus on change talk and sustain talk (Glynn & Moyers, 2010). More complex systems like the Motivational Interviewing Skills Code (MISC) quantify both interviewer and client responses and thus permit therapeutic process research (Baer et al., 2004; Daeppen, Bertholet, Gmel, & Gaume, 2007; Moyers et al., 2003; Welch et al., 2003). Coding systems like these require substantial training and quality assurance in order to establish and maintain coders' reliability. Experienced MI coaches often use coding systems like these and provide feedback from them (e.g., *www.mi-campus.com*).

It is possible, however, to use simpler strategies in listening to your own MI sessions, which we strongly encourage you to do. In the midst of a clinical consultation the mind can be busy attending to multiple tasks. Listening to the consultation again afterward can reveal insights and patterns that were not apparent in the initial experience of the session. Besides simply listening to your own sessions, here are some more structured tasks that can help you focus on the process and not just the content of the client's story.

- Count your reflections. Were they simple (basically just repeating what the person said) or complex (making a bit of a guess)? Keep a count of each. When you have trouble deciding whether a reflection was simple or complex, count them in the simple category. One learning goal is to offer more complex than simple reflections.
- Count your questions. Were they open questions (providing plenty of room to respond) or closed questions (short answer, yes/no, rhetorical, etc.)? Keep a count of each. A learning goal is to ask more open than closed questions.
- Count both reflections (R) and questions (Q). What is your ratio of R to Q? Most counselors when learning MI ask far too many questions. A learning goal here is an R:Q ratio of at least 2:1—two reflections for every question.
- Listen for change talk and sustain talk. Keep a count of each and consider the ratio between them. Equal frequency reflects ambivalence and predicts no change, but over the course of an MI session the balance normally shifts toward more change talk. When change talk appears, what were you doing just before it? What in

your practice seems to evoke change talk? Remember that change talk often comes intertwined with sustain talk and you may have to listen closely to find it.

- When change talk occurred, what was the *next* thing that you said? Count your OARS responses: Open question asking for elaboration, Affirmation, Reflection, Summary (Chapter 14).
- Listen for any of your responses that would be inconsistent with an MI style such as giving advice without permission, confronting or arguing with the client, or other "righting reflex" responses. How did the client respond to these?

Don't try to attend to all of these. Pick out one or two that seem important and track those as you listen to your sessions. Try setting a specific change goal for yourself, such as increasing your ratio of reflections to questions, and use these counts to track your progress.

LEARNING COMMUNITIES

Learning together is often more fun than learning alone. Not everyone has access to an expert MI coach, but it may be easier to find colleagues who are also interested in developing their skills in MI. We have been experimenting with such learning communities as a resource to support continued development. There need not be an identified expert in the group, although some do invite an experienced coach to visit with them occasionally. The idea is peer-supported learning, to puzzle together over questions like:

"How could I apply MI in this particular situation?"
"What is a good next step in practicing MI?"
"How else might I have responded at that point in the session?"
"Should I be trying MI in this situation?"
"What interviewer responses seem most likely to evoke change talk?"

We believe that, as with coaching, listening to each other's practice is a crucial resource for learning. So is practicing skills together. Talking *about* MI is not as likely to promote learning as actually practicing skills within a supportive learning community. We recommend that every meeting include some listening to practice recordings and some skill practice. Some clinicians who have developed a learning community of this kind have told us that they look forward to the meetings as one of the most rewarding experiences of their week or month. Here are some practical suggestions for skill practice within learning communities.

1. Focus on a particular interviewing skill or task. If you're trying to increase your use of complex reflections, focus on that. One chapter from this or another book (e.g., Rosengren, 2009) can provide plenty of material for discussion and practice.

2. Try using "real play" instead of role play. That is, have the colleague who is speaking as a "client" talk about something real, such as a change that he or she is actually considering or wanting to make. We find that this tends to promote learning better than enacted role plays. One reason is that even experienced actors do not respond like real people; they are taking on a role and sticking to it. We have used actors in our research, and while this does allow trainees to try out their skills the actors rarely respond as an actual client would. Similarly, when clinicians role-play a case they are often tempted to portray "the client from hell," the most difficult, intractable, unresponsive sort. There are few actual clients as difficult as those portrayed by clinicians during role play! It is easier to learn when someone is responding *in vivo* and not in role.

3. Don't let practice go on too long before you stop for discussion. Usually 10 minutes is enough time to get in some good practice without boring observers.

4. Give observers something to do while watching. If there is more than one observer they could use different coding tasks from the list above so that they can provide feedback from different perspectives.

5. When a practice is done, the first person to comment on it should be the one who was practicing MI. What were they experiencing during the interview? Next, the "client" should comment on the experience of the conversation. If it was a real play this is straightforward. What did the speaker experience during the interview? What seemed particularly helpful? Then observers can say what they saw. If they were using a structured coding task, discuss their objective observations. When commenting on a practice that you observed, focus on the positive. In fact, consider limiting yourself to the good things you saw. What did you observe that you liked? What seemed to be particularly effective? What specific MI skills did you see? It is very easy (and demoralizing) for observers to make many specific critiques and suggestions: "Well, I would have said that this way . . . " Avoid the righting reflex here, too. Mostly these stylistic preferences are unhelpful. There are many right ways to do MI. The two of us have very different styles when practicing MI, but we are fundamentally doing the same thing. What was *good* about what you observed?

6. If someone is to make a recommendation of something to try, let it be just one suggestion. Changing one thing is plenty to try in subsequent practice. A good tennis coach would probably not make five suggestions to implement on the next serve.

Other elements that people have added to MI learning communities are to watch and discuss demonstration videos and to have an ongoing journal club with participants taking turns presenting recently published research that is relevant to practice.

A caution here is that with solely peer-led learning groups it is possible to get off track without realizing it, and some rather strange variants can develop when individuals or groups try to teach themselves MI. At least periodic check-ins with a well-trained observer/coach are advisable. Trainer-members of the Motivational Interviewing Network of Trainers can be found through *www.motivationalinterviewing.org.*

SOME GUIDELINES FOR TRAINING

This section is particularly for policy and decision makers who are arranging for training in MI. As with the practice of MI there are many different styles and preferences for training MI. What is the state of the art for MI training? What guidelines emerge from the rapidly growing research on MI training and practice to inform those who wish to implement MI with a particular staff or system?

Initial Training

One thing that is relatively clear at this point is that self-study or attending a single workshop is unlikely to improve competence. Do you want your staff to know *about* MI or do you want them to actually be able to deliver it effectively? Reading or a single workshop can increase knowledge of MI, but there is little reason to believe that it will instill skill. Worse, we know from firsthand experience that if we imply that participants will become skillful in MI through attending our workshop, they are likely to *believe* mistakenly that they have learned it. In a first evaluation of our own 2-day training workshop, participants showed very little improvement in skills, certainly not enough to make any difference in how their clients responded, but we did manage to significantly decrease their interest in learning more about MI (Miller & Mount, 2001). Why? It was not because they didn't like MI or thought it was ineffective. It was because they believed they had already learned it.

We pause here to say again that there are those rare individuals who come to a workshop and do "get it." These prodigies are somehow able to integrate what they have learned and demonstrate reasonably good, sometimes brilliant practice of MI. We don't know why that happens, but it's fascinating. People do seem to learn MI faster if they are already reasonably skillful in reflective listening (Miller, Moyers, Arciniega, Ernst, & Forcehimes, 2005; compare Miller et al., 2004, with Moyers et al., 2008). So it's not the case that no one learns from workshops; it's just that on average you shouldn't expect practical skill to emerge from sitting in a classroom workshop, even a very good one, any more than you would expect proficient pianists to emerge from a 2-day piano class. An introductory workshop is just the beginning in learning a new clinical skill.

Follow-Up Training

Addictions were once treated primarily in inpatient programs that, by historical accident, tended to be 28 days in length. What became clear was the importance of "aftercare"—continuing outpatient care back home in the community where ultimately the person had to work out his or her own sobriety. Without aftercare, inpatient treatment was a bit like a car repair model: bring them in, fix them up to run right, then put them back on the street. It works reasonably well for cars and for repairing broken bones, but not so well for people when behavior change is needed. Likewise, short-term "inpatient training" alone is not likely to change practice behavior much.

What is needed is continued learning over time, and as discussed earlier, learning requires individual feedback. Our recommendation, then, is not more workshops but ongoing coaching with feedback based on observed practice. This need not be extensive. In one study we found that six individual expert coaching sessions of half an hour each conducted by telephone were sufficient to bring trainees on average up to a level of proficiency that would be satisfactory for delivering MI in a clinical trial, whereas our workshop alone was not (Miller et al., 2004). Introductory workshop training alone is not likely to provide much return on investment. In truth, one cannot say how much coaching will be required to bring a particular clinician up to proficiency. It is a matter of learning to criterion, not a fixed dose of training hours completed (Martino, Canning-Ball, Carroll, & Rounsaville, 2011).

Another sensible goal in implementation is to develop on-site expertise in MI so that there is someone in house who can support continued skill development and train new staff as they are hired. This allows ongoing supervision/coaching with a goal of continuous quality improvement in clinical skill. Short of this is to provide the time and administrative support for an ongoing learning community as described above.

Maintenance of Skills

Many skilled professions require periodic recertification of practitioners to demonstrate that skills are still up to current standards. Medical specialists, airline pilots, firefighters, and lifeguards cannot continue to practice without periodically updating and verifying their skills. Check pilots come along on flights. Paramedics and lifeguards must demonstrate their skills in cardiopulmonary resuscitation.

There is a good reason for this. Skills tend to drift over time. People develop their own variations or simply forget key elements. It is also important to keep up with new developments. New research on MI has been emerging at a rapid pace, and much more is known now than was true when we wrote our second edition just a decade ago. Demonstrating the ability to provide a service does not guarantee that it is actually being delivered in practice or that the same skills will be present a few years down the line. Self-perception and self-report of proficiency are unreliable, which is why recertification programs tend to require observed practice.

This is why we encourage ongoing direct observation of practice as a norm. This is more accepted in some professional settings than others. Medical professionals and airline pilots are accustomed to being observed at work as part of their job. In some other settings, private practice behind closed doors has been the norm with little more than case notes to audit what is happening. The latter situation inhibits new learning for practitioners and continuous quality improvement for the organization.

Client confidentiality is sometimes thought to prohibit direct observation or recording of sessions. The issue here is proper consent. Sessions should not be observed or recorded without client knowledge and consent. We have found, however, that most clients readily agree to audio or video recording of sessions with secure protection of their confidentiality. Written consent should be revocable, include an explanation of the purpose(s) for which recording will be used, specify how confidentiality will be protected, and indicate when and how recordings will be destroyed. Clients are also allowed to request that the recording be turned off for a particular segment of a session, although we find that in practice this seldom happens.

Clinical skill development is not a one-shot time-limited event but a continuing process. Helping staff to continue improving their clinical skills will benefit all concerned. As discussed earlier, coding systems are available to provide more standardized assessment than subjective impressions alone. To be sure, there is much more to skillful practice than can be detected by such structured coding systems, but they do provide at least a foundation for skill development.

Content of Training

What should be included in MI training? Here again we wish to be conservative and stay close to what research has demonstrated to be important. We suggest four broad components that we believe should be represented in any comprehensive training regardless of format (see Box 24.1).

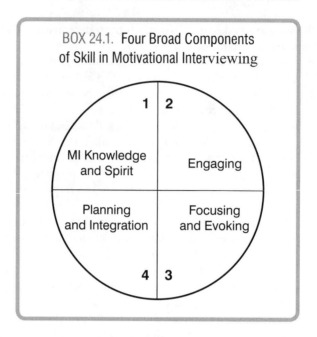

BOX 24.1. Four Broad Components
of Skill in Motivational Interviewing

1	2
MI Knowledge and Spirit	Engaging
Planning and Integration	Focusing and Evoking
4	3

Motivational Interviewing Knowledge and Spirit

Most basic is up-to-date knowledge about MI. Providing that foundation is a primary purpose of this book. An introductory workshop can also provide this, presuming the trainer is keeping up with developments in the field. From the trainee's perspective some of the central questions to be addressed include:

> "What is MI?"
> "How might it help me in my day-to-day work?"
> "What is the evidence for its efficacy?"
> "How does it work?"
> "How different is this from what I am already doing?"
> "Do I want to learn more about how to do this?"

An introduction to MI should include not only knowledge about but a demonstration of the method. This can be done via any of a number of available video demonstrations, but trainers should also be able to demonstrate skillful MI on the spot as it applies to particular issues or populations relevant to participants. This is why we have emphasized that before people become trainers they should be competent in the practice of MI. Instruction should focus not only on technique but also on the underlying spirit of MI practice.

Engaging

A second *sine qua non* of MI training is the development of proficiency in client-centered counseling skills, exemplified in earlier chapters by OARS. These are useful clinical skills in themselves and are fundamental to the practice of MI. We are particularly confident in the importance of accurate empathy as a key skill to facilitate client change. The skill here is to be able to practice OARS comfortably and well without necessarily using them in a goal-directed manner.

Focusing and Evoking

The method becomes uniquely MI with the addition of a clear focus and the goal-directed evoking component. The importance of these two processes has sometimes been missed in MI training. The skills here involve finding a clear focus, recognizing, evoking, and responding to change talk in ways that strengthen it. When training groups of clinicians, greater homogeneity of the trainees' practice contexts or clinical specialty may be particularly helpful in learning these skills.

Planning and Integration

Another component that has been underemphasized is the planning process with the negotiation of a change plan. Necessary skills include timing, developing a change plan, evoking commitment to change, and integrating MI with other clinical skills needed for the implementation of change. A goal here is to apply MI flexibly in concert with other clinical skills in order to facilitate change.

Not everyone needs all four components of training. Thus if training can be individualized it makes sense to assess each person's current proficiency with each of these skills. This would necessarily involve observation of practice samples. If client-centered engaging skills are already solid, it makes sense to emphasize focusing and evoking next. An understanding of MI knowledge would be needed for evoking to make sense. Planning could be learned as a separate skill set, but flexible integration of MI with one's everyday clinical skills is likely to come after developing a reasonable level of skill and comfort with evoking.

At a minimum, the content of MI training should cover these four components. There is much more to MI than these elements, but evidence is clearest that these are important. Understanding the overall style and spirit of MI is important (not just techniques). An empathic client-centered style matters. Change talk and sustain talk can be influenced by MI practice, and their balance predicts client outcome. Saying yes to a specific plan of action significantly increases the likelihood that it will happen.

KEY POINTS

✓ MI is not a technique but an integrated set of interviewing skills.

✓ Feedback and coaching are important in learning MI and need to be based on observed practice.

✓ Skill development in MI is not a one-shot event but an ongoing process.

CHAPTER 25

Applying Motivational Interviewing

> The great thing in the world is not so much where
> we stand, as in what direction we are moving.
> —OLIVER WENDELL HOLMES

> Act as if what you do makes a difference. It does.
> —WILLIAM JAMES

We are often asked, "Can I apply MI in my setting?" The range of contexts in which MI has been applied is broad indeed, and our response is likely to be, "Try it and see (and let us know)." If we know of relevant research on the use of MI in this particular context or population we also pass it along. A comprehensive bibliography of MI applications can be found at *www.motivationalinterviewing.org*.

But most often it is not just a closed question to be answered "yes" or "no." The underlying open question is "How can I adapt MI?" for this problem, population, or setting. Does it make sense in this context? What changes might be needed? What is essential to keep and what can be modified without losing the essence or impact of MI?

That is the subject of this chapter: applications and adaptations of MI. We begin with a set of questions to ask yourself when you are wondering about the applicability of MI, whether those being served are clients, patients, students, trainees, supervisees, or families.

1. Are there (or should there be) conversations about change happening?
2. Will the outcomes for those you serve be influenced by the extent to which they make changes in their lives or behavior?

3. Is helping or encouraging people to make such changes a part of your service (or should it be)?
4. Are the people you serve often reluctant or ambivalent about making changes?
5. Are utilization of and adherence and retention in your services significant concerns?
6. Do staff struggle with or complain about people who are "unmotivated," "resistant," or "difficult"?

"Yes" answers to these questions suggest a potential role for MI in your context. In itself this does not guarantee that MI will be useful or effective in your setting; it is just reason to consider the possibility if there seems to be a good fit between MI and the needs or challenges of your service.

There is also a question of goodness of fit. It is possible to answer "yes" to all of the above questions and have a work setting where MI will not easily take root. Imagine a service in which the dominant perspective includes assumptions like these:

"We are the experts here, and it's up to us to take charge."
"We don't have time to listen to people. We have too much to do."
"We're not going to waste our time with people who are unmotivated."
"Our clients are in denial, dishonest, out of touch with reality, and incapable of changing on their own. There is no point in listening to them."
"The only language these people understand is to get in their face, scare them, and tell them what to do."
"They're not going to change anyhow, even if we do our best."

Such a philosophy of service is so opposite to the underlying assumptions described in Chapter 1 that one would expect little interest or receptiveness to MI on a servicewide basis. Culture change can occur, of course. The person(s) responsible for new hires can have a substantial impact on future climate as turnover happens. Within the current climate, however, MI would probably not be welcomed.

We hasten to add that this does not preclude any role for or benefit from MI. Having even one person who can work with clients in this person-centered way may make a difference, particularly if it occurs early in service delivery. That was our experience in a rather confrontational 21-day residential alcohol treatment program where adding a single MI session soon after admission (in a randomized trial) doubled abstinence rates after discharge relative to treatment as usual (Brown & Miller, 1993). The staff of this program (who were unaware of

> Having even one person who can work with clients in this person-centered way may make a difference.

group assignment) also rated clients who had received MI as more motivated, adherent, and having better prognosis (which turned out to be correct). Even one person can make a difference.

MODES OF DELIVERY

In most outcome studies MI has been delivered as an individual face-to-face consultation. Can MI be delivered effectively in other ways?

Telephone and Televideo

MI is a conversation about change, and it is possible to carry on conversations remotely. Some technologies provide only the audio portion, while others make it possible to see each other as well. Dozens of studies have successfully delivered MI via telephone or other audio link, for example, to promote physical exercise (Ang, Kesavalu, Lydon, Lane, & Bigatti, 2007; Bennett, Lyons, Winters-Stone, Nail, & Scherer, 2007; van Keulen et al., 2011), colorectal cancer screening (Wahab et al., 2008), medication persistence (Berger, Liang, & Hudmon, 2005; Cook, Emiliozzi, Waters, & El Hajj, 2008), dietary change (Campbell et al., 2009; Resnicow et al., 2001; van Keulen et al., 2011), tobacco cessation (Persson & Hjalmarson, 2006; Severson et al., 2009), and blood donation (Sinclair et al., 2010). Visual contact adds some nonverbal cues and may increase client satisfaction (Baca & Manuel, 2007), although it is unclear whether this increases the impact of MI.

Group Counseling

In the interest of efficiency, counseling may be delivered in group rather than individual sessions. Can MI be provided effectively to groups? If individual versus group-delivered interventions yield similar outcomes, there could be a cost-effectiveness advantage for the group format (Sobell, Sobell, & Agrawal, 2009).

The transfer from individual to group delivery of MI is not straightforward. We do strongly recommend that providers hone their skills in individual MI first before attempting to conduct MI groups, because the management of group processes adds a layer of complexity.

If evoking and voicing change talk is an important component in the efficacy of MI, then an immediate challenge with groups is individual airtime. Each member of a group necessarily has less time to speak and receive the counselor's individual attention than would be the case in individual MI. Thus there is less opportunity for individuals to voice their own change talk. Furthermore, group dynamics can alter the probability of change talk.

Clients may reinforce each other's sustain talk, and such collusion for the status quo can cause a group to backfire with less favourable outcomes than no treatment or standard treatment (Brown et al., 2007; Walters, Ogle, & Martin, 2002). A key, then, is to arrange the group to maximize opportunities for each member to generate and explore change talk.

There is reasonable evidence that MI can be delivered effectively in group format (Bailey, Baker, Webster, & Lewin, 2004; LaBrie et al., 2008; Santa Ana, Wulfert, & Nietert, 2007; Schmiege, Broaddus, Levin, & Bryan, 2009), although research is still at a relatively early stage. Our reading of the current literature is that group-delivered MI tends to have less predictable outcomes relative to individual MI, although there is certainly variability in both. Relatively little is known about the "active ingredients," the mediators and moderators of efficacy in group MI (LaChance, Feldstein Ewing, Bryan, & Hutchison, 2009; Webber, Tate, & Quintiliani, 2008). A state-of-the-art summary of knowledge and experience along with practice guidelines for group MI are provided by Wagner and Ingersoll (in press).

Text Formats

Can MI be delivered in text formats via printed material or interactive computer software? Here, too, research is at a rather early stage, but there is some encouraging evidence.

Most evaluated in this regard has been computer-based delivery of the "drinker's check-up," the prototype for motivational enhancement therapy (Squires & Hester, 2004; Walker, Roffman, Picciano, & Stephens, 2007; Walters, Hester, Chiauzzi, & Miller, 2005). At 12-month follow-up sustained reductions in drinking and related problems were reported following a computer-delivered checkup (Hester, Squires, & Delaney, 2005). Positive outcomes with a computer-based program including an MI component have been reported for smoking cessation (Hollis et al., 2005), sexual risk reduction (Kiene & Barta, 2006), and depression and marijuana use (Kay-Lambkin, Baker, Lewin, & Carr, 2009). Computer-based intervention has also been explored for drug use during pregnancy (Ondersma, Chase, Svikis, & Schuster, 2005; Ondersma, Svikis, & Schuster, 2007). A randomized trial of face-to-face versus computer-administered feedback found that the in-person intervention yielded significant behavior change relative to control groups, whereas the computerized version did not (Wagener et al., in press).

It is unlikely that these computer-based interventions exerted their effect by expressing empathy or evoking change talk. Within the checkup format, an active ingredient is likely to be providing individualized feedback, which in itself can trigger change (Agostinelli et al., 1995; Juarez et al., 2006). MI-based computer interventions may yield outcomes intermediate between those for in-person MI and no treatment (Barnet et al.,

2009). Motivational feedback can also be provided through individually tailored letters (Agostinelli et al., 1995; Miller et al., 2004; van Keulen et al., 2011).

It is also possible to design print materials for specific therapeutic purposes (Christensen, Miller, & Muñoz, 1978). The potential therapeutic benefits of evocative journaling have been widely recognized (Pennebaker, 1997; Progoff, 1975), with effects similar to those of talking in therapy (Donnelly & Murray, 1991; Murray & Segal, 1994). Interactive journaling is a specific method that elicits clients' written responses while reading related information (Parr, Haberstroh, & Kottler, 2000; Proctor, Cowin, Hoffmann, & Allison, 2009). Controlled trials with offenders have reported reductions in recidivism with interactive journaling (Loudenburg, 2008; Proctor, Hoffman, & Allison, 2012). Such interactive materials can be designed specifically to evoke client change talk and enhance motivation for change (e.g., Miller & Mee-Lee, 2010; Parks & Woodford, 2005). Such journaling materials can also be presented in online interactive format (Childress, 1999).

Family Consultations

What about including one or more family members in a motivational interview? MI-based interventions have incorporated the option of including a significant other (SO) to support motivation for change (Longabaugh et al., 2005; Miller, Zweben, et al., 1992; Tevyaw, Borsari, Colby, & Monti, 2007; UKATT Research Team, 2001; Zweben, 1991). Doing so can increase social support for the client in pursuing change and may also provide important information not offered by the client alone (Burke, Vassilev, Kantchelov, & Zweben, 2002). A challenge when including a concerned SO is to manage the interaction within the session so that the SO does not elicit sustain talk and defensiveness from the client. Often there has been a history of the SO arguing for change and the client arguing against it, and this is easily rehashed in a joint MI session unless specific steps are taken to prevent it. Practicing MI with both partners can accentuate positive change. You may establish certain ground rules at the outset to shape how the SO and client participate (e.g., no blaming; focus on positive change).

It is also possible to practice MI with relationship enhancement as your goal rather than having one partner as the identified client (Burke et al., 2002). Here, too, you are providing MI for both partners. The MET approach of providing personalized feedback in combination with MI has been adapted to various family checkup interventions (Connell & Dishion, 2008; Cordova, Warren, & Gee, 2001; O'Leary, 2001; Rao, 1999; Roffman et al., 2008; Slavet et al., 2005; Uebelacker et al., 2006; Van Ryzin, Stormshak, & Dishion, 2012).

Combining Motivational Interviewing with Other Treatments

How does MI fit with the rest of what you do? It would make little sense for one's practice to be limited to MI, since it is just one clinical tool for the particular problem of helping people move from ambivalence to enduring change. Other important clinical tasks and skills are included in most any practice, some of which are more centered on directing or following than on guiding.

One way to think about integrating MI within a larger panoply of practice is an alternation model. One makes use of MI when motivation for change is the challenge and then puts it down when it is time for other tasks (Miller & Moyers, 2006). In one study where we preselected therapists for high empathic skill we found that they took quite naturally to the MI components of a combined treatment but seemed to have more difficulty shifting into a more directing style for behavioral components (Miller, Moyers, et al., 2005). In an alternation model one would switch flexibly back and forth between MI and other styles depending on the clinical task at hand. In this way of thinking one stops and starts doing MI. Consultation might begin with MI and then transition into other strategies once clients are ready for action (Longabaugh et al., 2005; Miller, 2004). If motivational obstacles emerge later, MI can be taken back off the shelf.

Yet clinicians who are experienced in MI sometimes find this an unsatisfactory model. "I don't really ever put MI aside," they say. It is not just that they keep MI in reserve in case it is needed again. Their experience is that MI is somehow integrated with and infused in all of their clinical practice. It has become a clinical style with which to practice a wide variety of treatment tasks. More than something specific that one does, MI has become for them a way of doing, of practicing.

Within our current understanding of MI as comprising four clinical processes, the latter integration model makes more sense. Engaging, focusing, and planning (understood broadly as including implementing) are processes found in many different forms of practice. The process of evoking, which is more unique to MI, is appropriate when strengthening motivation for change, and as with each of the processes there are times when it is needed and others when it is not. The practice of MI as we have described it here involves flexible movement among these four processes. This is not, then, an alternation into and out of MI, but rather a nimble interweaving of processes that is responsive to the client's immediate state.

Another aspect of this integrative model of practice is the underlying spirit of MI (Chapter 1) that can be sustained behind a wide range of specific practices. This *Menschenbild* and understanding of one's own facilitative role in the dynamics of change is not something easily turned on and off. The mind-set and heart-set of partnership, acceptance, compassion, and evocation can be a firm foundation for good practice. This is, we think, another reason why clinicians do not experience themselves as "putting down" or "turning off" MI when moving with clients through the change process.

An MI style appears to be compatible with a wide range of other clinical practices. When MI is combined with another active treatment, the efficacy of both can be enhanced (Hettema et al., 2005; Westra, 2012). By far the most common admixture thus far has been of MI with cognitive-behavioral procedures (e.g., Ali, Hagshenas, Reza, Ira, & Maryam, 2011; Arkowitz & Westra, 2004; DiLillo, Siegfried, & West, 2003; Kertes, Westra, Angus, & Marcus, 2011; Longabaugh et al., 2005; Merlo et al., 2010; Parsons, Golub, Rosof, & Holder, 2007; Runyon, Deblinger, & Schroeder, 2009; Smith, Heckemeyer, Kratt, & Mason, 1997). Hybrid combinations of this kind pose special challenges in assuring treatment fidelity (Haddock et al., 2012). It is equally feasible to combine MI with educational (Gance-Cleveland, 2007; Leak, Davis, Houchin, & Mabrey, 2009; Sherman et al., 2009), pharmacological (Anton et al., 2005; Heffner et al., 2010), public health (Thevos, Kaona, Siajunza, & Quick, 2000), case management (Robles et al., 2004), or other interventions. Clinically, such integration may make more sense than head-to-head horse-race comparisons of MI with other approaches, although MI is a reasonable comparison condition in clinical trials to determine whether other treatments improve over a more minimal active treatment (e.g., Davidson, Gulliver, Longabaugh, Wirtz, & Swift, 2007).

> An MI style appears to be compatible with a wide range of other clinical practices.

DIFFERING ROLES AND CONTEXTS

MI has most often been used in treatment contexts where a health professional (e.g., social worker, psychologist, pharmacist, physical therapist) talks with people about change. Recently, applications of MI have been broadening to include other service contexts. We consider briefly several of these newer adaptations.

Coaching

Coaching is the process of helping someone to acquire skill and is a common component of various professions. "Life coaches" offer consultation on a wide range of topics:

> The coaching process addresses specific personal projects, business successes, general conditions and transitions in the client's personal life, relationships or profession by examining what is going on right now, discovering what your obstacles or challenges might be, and choosing a course of action to make your life be what you want it to be. (Retrieved August 12, 2011 from *www.lifecoaching.com*)

In this regard, coaching can have much in common with MI. The processes of engaging, focusing, and planning are apparent in such descriptions, and the MI process of evoking seems like a natural fit. A "life coach" may be certified by any of several organizations, and may or may not have any background in MI. Behavior change coaching has also been provided by licensed health professionals such as nurses (Bennett et al., 2005; Borrelli et al., 2005; Butterworth, Linden, McClay, & Leo, 2006) and psychologists (Passmore, 2007; Passmore & Whybrow, 2008).

The methods used for coaching, however, are as varied and often unspecified as those for counseling or psychotherapy. Certainly in its general intent—to assist people in making positive life changes—the enterprise of coaching has parallels with the communication style of MI (Antiss & Passmore, 2012; Lawson, Wolever, Donovan, & Greene, 2009; Mantler, Irwin, & Morrow, 2010; N. H. Miller, 2010; Newnham-Kanas, Morrow, & Irwin, 2010). Butterworth (2007) observed that "To date, motivational interviewing-based health coaching is the only technique to have been fully described and consistently demonstrated as causally and independently associated with positive behavioral outcomes" (p. 299).

More generally, coaches (including sports coaches and trainers) vary in style between directing and guiding. (Few athletic coaches would adopt a following style!) When coaching focuses more on guiding, bringing out the person's or team's own best performance, rather than a highly directing authoritarian style, there may be a role for MI. Good practice in teaching, coaching, and healing involves drawing out learning experiences from people in a manner often remarkably close to MI.

Education

Education is a more recent area in the application of MI, although there is a long history of person-centered and Socratic educational styles (Rogers, 1980b). Adaptations of MI have been described for preventing secondary school dropout (Atkinson & Woods, 2003) and depression (Connell & Dishion, 2008); reducing truancy (Enea & Dafinoiu, 2009); improving study habits and grade performance (Daugherty, 2009); addressing smoking (Bolger et al., 2010; Harris et al., 2010), alcohol (Baer, Kivlahan, Blume, McKnight, & Marlatt, 2001; Burke, Da Silva, Vaughan, & Knight, 2005; Scholl & Schmitt, 2009; Tevyaw et al., 2007), and marijuana use among students (Swan et al., 2008; Walker et al., 2006); preventing obesity (Flattum, Friend, Neumark-Sztainer, & Story, 2009); in classroom management (Reinke, Herman, & Sprick, 2001); and handling disciplinary referrals (Kelly & Lapworth, 2006; LaBrie, Lamb, Pedersen, & Quinlan, 2006).

You'll notice from the above list that these early efforts with MI in education have been slanted toward problem management of one kind or another. Yet to be fully explored is the striking compatibility between MI and good practice in nurturing achievement and emotional health more broadly. The potential for MI to inform everyday teaching practice is a promising avenue to traverse.

Opportunistic Intervention

Practitioners ask us, "Can you do MI in a few minutes?" It is in a way like asking, "Can you play the piano for 5 minutes?" It would not be enough time to perform a great concerto, but of course one can play an instrument or practice the style of MI in whatever amount of time is available. Perhaps the underlying question is whether it is possible to make a difference with a few minutes of MI. Not only is it possible, but if you have only a few minutes to discuss behavior change, MI is likely to be more effective than finger-wagging warnings (Soria et al., 2006). Examples of relatively brief MI consultations effecting behavior change have been reported in a wide variety of settings, including primary care (Aharonovich et al., 2006; Barkin, 2008; Bernstein et al., 2005; Butler et al., 1999; D'Amico, Miles, Stern, & Meredith, 2008; Hollis et al., 2005), psychiatry (Brown et al., 2009; Graeber, Moyers, Griffith, Guajardo, & Tonigan, 2003; Hulse & Tait, 2002), dentistry (Koerber, Crawford, & O'Connell, 2003; Weinstein, Harrison, & Benton, 2004), prenatal care (Handmaker & Wilbourne, 2001; Valanis et al., 2001), detoxification (Stotts et al., 2001), needle exchange (Stein, Charuvastra, Maksad, & Anderson, 2002), blood donation (Sinclair et al., 2010), emergency departments (Bernstein & Bernstein, 2008; Bernstein, Bernstein, & Levenson, 1997; Longabaugh et al., 2001; Monti et al., 1999; Neighbors, Barnett, Rohsenow, Colby, & Monti, 2010; Spirito et al., 2004), trauma centers (Monti et al., 2007; Schermer et al., 2006), and telephone consultation (Bell et al., 2005; Valanis et al., 2003). Although less explored, MI could also be offered as an opportunistic intervention in other service contexts such as social services, employee assistance programs, pharmacies, and legal services.

Corrections

Corrections is another area in which the use of MI has grown rapidly (McMurran, 2009; McMurran & Ward, 2004; Walters, Clark, Gingerich,

& Meltzer, 2007). Examples of applications have been described in probation and parole (Clark, 2005; Clark, Walters, Gingerich, & Meltzer, 2006; Harper & Hardy, 2000; Walters, Vader, Nguyen, Harris, & Eells, 2010), incarceration (Farbring & Johnson, 2008; Rosen, Hiller, Webster, Staton, & Leukefeld, 2004; Slavet et al., 2005; Stein et al., 2006), juvenile corrections and child welfare (Feldstein & Ginsburg, 2006; Hohman, 1998; Hohman & Matulich, 2010; Patel, Lambie, & Glover, 2008), and offender rehabilitation (Birgden, 2004; Dia, Simmons, Oliver, & Cooper, 2009; Easton, Swan, & Sinha, 2000; Kistenmacher & Weiss, 2008; LaChance et al., 2009; Mann & Rollnick, 1996), as well as in health promotion with police officers and firefighters (Anshel & Kang, 2008; Elliot et al., 2007).

Obviously behavior change is one important objective in correctional systems, so interventions that are effective in promoting change would be vital. Is there reason to expect that offenders as a group would respond differently than other people to change interventions? One consideration is that, by virtue of being deprived of prior freedoms, a higher than usual level of reactance might be present and an oppositional response could be anticipated to confrontational approaches that further challenge autonomy. Studies have supported a better response to MI than to a more directing style among people with higher reactance levels (Grodin, 2006; Karno & Longabaugh, 2005a, 2005b; Karno, Longabaugh, & Herbeck, 2009). From this perspective, MI may be a particularly appropriate style in working with offenders.

A contrary hypothesis is that antisocial individuals may not respond to MI because of their presumed inability to form therapeutic relationships. One study (Rosenblum et al., 2005) reported that cognitive-behavioral therapy was more effective than a motivational group treatment based on self-determination theory in a small sample of people with antisocial personality disorder. Other studies have not supported this prediction (Project MATCH Research Group, 1998b) and suggested that antisocial individuals may respond better to MI than to a more confrontational approach (Grant et al., 2009; Woodall, Delaney, Kunitz, Westerberg, & Zhao, 2007).

Professionals who work in correctional systems often have dual and potentially conflicting roles in relation to offenders (see Chapter 10). One is to promote behavior change, a role that may best be enacted in collaborative partnership with offenders. At the same time, professionals working with offenders often have enforcement or reporting requirements that could place them in an adversarial relationship. We believe that these roles are compatible when the professional's limitations and duties are clearly understood by both parties, and correction professionals can and do acquire skillfulness in MI (Hartzler & Espinosa, 2011). The if–then contingencies of an enforcement role are not incompatible with the message that "I want to do whatever I can to help you succeed and be free." As with other populations, the MI practitioner assumes that offenders have inherent motivations for positive change. Arguing for those changes may predictably evoke opposition or passive silence, whereas an MI approach seeks to find and strengthen the offender's own motivation for change. Early findings of decreased recidivism among offenders offered MI are encouraging (Antiss, Polaschek, & Wilson, 2011).

Organizations

As in corrections, it matters in organizations what *Menschenbild* managers have for those under their supervision. In his classic 1960 volume *The Human Side of Enterprise*, McGregor (2006) contrasted what he called Theory X and Theory Y about how to motivate people in the workplace. The first of these, Theory X, is that workers are ultimately lazy and unmotivated, dislike working, and will get away with doing as little as possible. Theory X managers therefore tend to be watchful, skeptical, and mistrustful of employees and rely heavily on threat, coercion, restrictive supervision, rewards, and punishment to make workers do what they would otherwise avoid. Theory Y, in contrast, is the view that workers have untapped talents and creativity, often enjoy their work, and are capable of self-control and self-direction. It is the Theory Y manager's job to provide such workers the right atmosphere to bring out their responsibility, motivation, and creative engagement in the workplace.

Both theories, it turns out, tend to be self-fulfilling prophecies, and successful businesses recognized long ago the advantages of a Theory Y organization to inspire productivity, creativity, and commitment. Although the ideas were early described by McGregor and Edwards Deming (Walton, 1986), they were most quickly accepted and implemented in Japan to transform its economy.

Managers, probation officers, or counselors who view their work within Theory X get engaged in a power struggle, a kind of wrestling match or cat-and-mouse game. You have to *make* the person see, comply, and change. Because human beings inherently dislike being controlled they naturally respond by complying as little as possible, avoiding, evading, and demonstrating their autonomy. This, in turn, simply confirms that Theory X is the correct view of human nature. In truth, it's not much fun being a Theory X supervisor, and burnout can be high. If you counsel people with Theory X in mind, they will tend to be defensive, resistant, angry, oppositional, and reluctant to come back or to change. If you counsel people with Theory Y in mind, they tend to be more open, exploring, motivated, comfortable, engaged, and prone to change.

MI has many similarities to Theory Y and to appreciative inquiry, a collaborative organizational change approach designed to evoke strengths and possibilities (Cooperrider & Whitney, 2005; Madsen, 2009). Rather than solutions coming from an outside expert they are elicited from the system itself, and good listening is key. MI also mirrors commonly used methods in mediation and dispute resolution, where engaging, focusing, evoking, and planning are familiar processes.

The same potential conflict of roles mentioned earlier in regard to corrections is also a consideration when using MI within organizations. Whose interests and welfare are being served? Trying to use MI in education, business, or corrections to make people more "manageable" is not consistent with the compassionate spirit of MI described in Chapter 2.

Religious Organizations

MI may be useful within religious organizations as well. Most world religions offer a model of what it means to live a good life and encourage people to mature toward certain principles and values (Kass & Lennox, 2005). Yet evidence-based methods for helping people to change may be neglected in these contexts, in part because of mutual suspicion between psychology and religion (Delaney, Miller, & Bisono, 2007; Miller & Martin, 1988). Within cultures where religion is central to personal and community identity, religious organizations can be a fruitful base through which to promote health behavior change (e.g., Resnicow et al., 2002, 2004). A person-centered communication style can certainly be practiced within religious contexts (Buber, 1971; Buber, Rogers, Anderson, & Cissna, 1997; Merton, 1960; Miller & Jackson, 1995), and MI is often compatible within a religious understanding of human nature (e.g., Martin & Sihn, 2009; Miller, 2000).

ADAPTING MOTIVATIONAL INTERVIEWING FOR SPECIAL POPULATIONS

Questions arise as to whether and how MI can be used with specific populations. For present purposes we consider two broad illustrative issues: the practice of MI with cognitively impaired people, and the cross-cultural adaptation of MI.

Cognitive Impairment

Can MI benefit brain-injured or stroke patients, people with schizophrenia or learning disabilities, or the cognitively impaired elderly? What are the specific needs of such groups? Do they struggle with motivation to change? What changes do they face, and how are these changes usually addressed in practice?

There is a tendency to rely on a highly directing style when working with people who are labeled as cognitively impaired: the greater the impairment, the greater the inclination to solve problems for them. Any journey through a sample of homes for the care of the elderly will testify to the institutional use of the righting reflex, well matched by heroic efforts of people to hang on to whatever dignity and autonomy they still have. People with cognitive impairment have needs and aspirations not so very different from those of other people. There's no shortage of well-justified calls to show such people at least the same respect and compassion afforded to those with less impairment. Champions abound for a more person-centered approach that attends to people's need for dignity and autonomy. Person-centered care is not equivalent to MI, but is an excellent foundation for it.

What role might MI play in helping people adapt to changed circumstances, difficult symptoms, and cognitive limitations? A literature is developing on the use of MI with different groups of people with various kinds of cognitive impairment. These studies have tended thus far to focus on people at the severe end of a spectrum, whereas much larger numbers experience more modest levels of impairment. Nevertheless, if MI proves beneficial even with greater impairment it is informative.

It is plausible that people with various kinds of cognitive impairment might not respond as well to MI as to more concrete approaches. Two broad kinds of evidence are relevant here. The first type of research examines cognitive impairment as a moderator of response to different treatments. Cognitive measures have not thus far been found to predict differential response to MI. In a large multisite trial clients were predicted to fare less well in MET than in two more intensive and structured comparison treatments if they (1) had more cognitive impairment, or (2) showed a lower (more concrete) conceptual level of cognitive functioning (Project MATCH Research Group, 1997a). Neither hypothesis was supported (Allen, 2001; Donovan, Kivlahan, Kadden, & Hill, 2001). Others have reported no relationship between cognitive functioning and MI outcomes (Aharonovich, Brooks, Nunes, & Hasin, 2008), although such studies examine main effects of cognitive impairment rather than a differential interaction with MI. Second, beyond studies of differential response based on cognitive functioning, MI has been specifically tested with a variety of cognitively impaired populations; we briefly discuss this research below.

There is also reason to anticipate that MI might be particularly helpful with the cognitively impaired, who commonly have difficulty in one or more of these areas: attention, speed of processing, memory, and executive functioning (including initiation or motivation, inhibition, flexible thinking, metacognition, and self-awareness). MI techniques can naturally help compensate for several of these common problems. Reflections and summaries provide repetition of key information and should facilitate attention and memory. Evoking change talk (as opposed to psychoeducational approaches) could also facilitate memory since the material comes from the patient and is processed more deeply. Reflections may also enhance metacognition and self-awareness and do it in a way that minimizes the opposition that is common after brain injury. Overall, MI explicitly seeks to improve motivation and action planning, which should benefit problems with initiation. For people who are quite concrete and have planning problems, more careful action planning (e.g., through the use of written specific goals and implementation intentions) may facilitate recall and follow-through. Finally, MI tends to be brief and focused. People with brain injury often struggle with fatigue, especially cognitive fatigue and overstimulation. MI may circumvent problems in those areas too.[1]

The literature thus far is certainly encouraging (Suarez, 2011). A randomized trial with 411 patients found that those given four sessions of MI soon after acute stroke were significantly less likely to be depressed or dead 1 year later (Watkins et al., 2007, 2011). Similarly, patients randomly assigned to receive a series of brief MI counseling telephone calls after acute treatment for traumatic brain injury showed significantly greater improvement in cognitive functioning, mood, and well-being through a year of follow-up (Bell et al., 2005; Bombardier et al., 2009). Alcohol abuse is also a common problem before and after traumatic brain injury, and in a cohort design MI significantly increased abstinence from drinking at 1 year postdischarge (Bombardier & Rimmele, 1999). Finally, in a small, uncontrolled pilot study with learning-disabled offenders, significant improvement was reported in motivation and self-efficacy for change following a three-session motivational group (Mendel & Hipkins, 2002).

Applications across Cultures

How well does motivational interviewing travel across cultures? We sometimes encounter comments that "people in our (or that) culture prefer straight talk and just need to be told what to do." Note the difference between "our" and "that" group. One perspective comes from within a culture, another from efforts to communicate across cultural differences. What unites them is often a hint of frustration or skepticism that MI might not work with a particular subgroup. Sometimes the concern is that listening and evoking seem too slow or subtle for a particular group. It's a testable question, of course, and is also a view that implies dubious dichotomies: that people within groups are homogeneous, and that the only alternatives are to tell people what to do (directing style) or leave them to make their minds up for themselves (following style). MI instead is founded on a guiding style that includes providing information and choices and helping people work out what might suit them best. It is certainly not about sitting back and letting the conversation go into freefall.

---

[1] Thanks to Charles Bombardier for these insights.

We find that the perceived need of a particular group to be told what to do comes more often from practitioners than from clients themselves. To be sure, clients differ in their preferences about directing, guiding, and following styles, and MI accommodates such preferences. The idea that all members of a particular group require or prefer one communication style underestimates within-group heterogeneity and itself smacks of stereotype. MI adapts to differences rather than assuming them.

> MI adapts to differences rather than assuming them.

A very simple resolution to the question of what individuals prefer is to ask them. What you will probably find is that this is less a personality or cultural trait and more likely depends on the context, including the seriousness of the problem being addressed and their faith in you as a practitioner.

The published research to date provides much encouragement and offers little to raise alarms about the cross-cultural transfer of MI. The clinical method of MI has been applied to challenges as diverse as promoting safe water practices in rural Zambian villages (Thevos et al., 2002; Thevos, Quick, & Yanduli, 2000), reducing unprotected sex (Golin et al., 2012), increasing fruit and vegetable intake through African American churches (Resnicow et al., 2001, 2005), encouraging HIV testing among Native Americans (Foley et al., 2005) and adherence to treatment for AIDS (Hill & Kavookjian, 2012), and prompting smoking cessation for the parents of sick children in Hong Kong (Chan et al., 2005). Such applications are some distance from the traditional counselor's consulting room, and are inspired by efforts to avoid the more commonly used top-down practice that typifies well-intentioned education worldwide: telling people what to do and why in hopes that they will change.

Further encouragement regarding the cross-cultural transferability of MI comes from the range of cultures and languages in which it is being practiced. Books about MI have been translated into at least 22 languages, and there are MI trainers speaking at least 45 different languages on six continents.

Processes for engaging do differ across cultures, but listening lies at the heart of nearly all of them. Good listening crosses cultures well. It stretches the imagination to think of people who don't appreciate being welcomed, heard, understood, affirmed, and recognized as autonomous human beings. In our experience these are universally valued. Within MI, people are recognized as experts on themselves, which is a far better way to counsel across cultural differences than presuming to know the other's identity. One meta-analysis of clinical trials found that the effect size of MI was twice as large when those being treated came predominantly from U.S. minority populations (primarily African American and Hispanic) in

> **BOX 25.1.** Motivational Interviewing through an Interpreter
>
> We have had the experience of practicing and teaching MI through an interpreter who translates back and forth between our English and another language. Some limitations are imposed simply by the interruption involved in translation. Empathic reflections normally come immediately after a client's statement. When working through an interpreter the client makes a statement, it is translated, then you make a response that is translated back. Even if the rendering is wholly accurate, this delay can add awkwardness to the conversation. There are further complications if the interpreter does not understand what you are doing. For example, hearing a perfectly good reflection an interpreter once chastised the practitioner: "She already said that!" If the interpreter does not understand the practitioner's intent in phrasing a question or in reflecting a particular aspect of the client's speech, MI can quickly go awry. For this reason if you have occasion to provide MI through a translator, it would be good to have one who is familiar with or even skilled in the style of MI.

comparison with the majority white population (Hettema et al., 2005; cf. Lasser et al., 2011). Native American participants in one trial showed significantly more change in an MI-based treatment than in two psychotherapies with which it was compared (Villanueva, Tonigan, & Miller, 2007).

There will be cultural nuances in many aspects of MI, for which counselors from the same context may be best prepared. Cultural norms of politeness may affect how and when one proceeds from engaging to focusing or from evoking to planning. The process of evoking is rooted in the language and folkways that people normally use with each other when asking for and negotiating about change. The co-creative process of planning will be affected by concepts of time, causation, and personal agency. For this reason, there may be an advantage when the person providing MI shares the client's ethnic background (Field & Caetano, 2010). Yet the core processes themselves cross cultures well and rely to a large extent on semantic universals.

WILL MOTIVATIONAL INTERVIEWING WORK WITH . . . ?

Even though MI has been used across quite an array of topics and contexts, it is still often the case that good research is sparse for the use of MI with a particular problem and population. From a scientific standpoint there is every reason for modesty with claims of efficacy in the absence of a solid research base. Yet the breadth of positive reports also suggests the potential fruitfulness of MI in still-untested areas. For practitioners our counsel is to "try it" rather than assume *a priori* that MI cannot be beneficial because of some client or cultural attribute. We were initially skeptical regarding the impact of MI with adolescents, people with schizophrenia or brain injury, or mothers in remote African villages. Try it. With compassion and thoughtfulness at the center of your efforts, you are unlikely to do any harm by exploring the potential of MI in helping people change.

And to this counsel of "try it" we add the reminder that developing skill in MI takes time. Hasty efforts with minimal training often fail to produce good results. Low-quality MI practice might be likened to half-doses of a vaccine or antibiotic: the right idea but insufficient strength.

KEY POINTS

✓ Beyond individual face-to-face consultation MI appears to be adaptable to delivery via telephone or televideo, with groups or families, and possibly through computer or print applications.

✓ MI can be combined or integrated with a variety of other active treatments, potentially enhancing the efficacy of both.

✓ MI has also been adapted to a variety of relational contexts including coaching, education, opportunistic intervention, corrections, and organizations.

✓ MI continues to be extended for use with special populations and across cultures.

CHAPTER 26

Integrating
Motivational Interviewing

Go alone, go faster; go together, go farther.
—Sotho-Tswana saying from Southern Africa

We must become the change we want to see in the world.
—MAHATMA GANDHI

How can MI be integrated into an ongoing service? The possibilities range all the way from its use by a few practitioners, through helping all willing staff to learn MI, to its broader application within a client-centered service. We do not mean this to be a sequence or an ideal, but simply a continuum of possibilities for using MI within a service system. The modest use of MI by a few practitioners might well suit the aspirations of your service. Helping all staff to learn MI can be achieved, but it requires far more than delivering doses of workshop training and assuming that the job has been done. A broader integration of MI would focus on clients' engagement and journey through a service and also on how colleagues exchange information and speak to each other about change. MI can find a home within services in any of these ways.

LIMITED IMPLEMENTATION WITH A FEW STAFF

Sometimes the first application of MI within a system is to address a particular concern or at a certain point in the flow of service delivery. For example, if an unacceptably high proportion of clients are being lost during an intake and initial assessment process it might be beneficial to integrate MI into the front end of services. Engagement and retention may be improved when clients experience high-quality MI at the outset of contact with a program. To install MI at such a particular point in service would require preparing those staff who conduct intake and initial assessment services to practice MI in the course of their duties. As discussed in Chapter 24 and later in this chapter, initial training is likely to be insufficient without ongoing ways to monitor and maintain quality.

Another modest option would be to train selected staff in MI. We believe it is better for a program to train several staff together so that they can work together to continue improving their skills. A trial approach would be to train up a particular team of practitioners in MI to determine whether it improves services and outcomes for the clients whom they serve. Good candidates for such training would be clinicians who are particularly interested in learning this approach, perhaps after participating in an introductory workshop. Remember that the effectiveness of MI depends on fidelity of practice, so client benefits would not be expected until staff have developed and are maintaining reasonable proficiency in delivering MI. Premature evaluation before staff have developed sufficient skill is unlikely to show benefit.

What we generally don't recommend is sending one or more staff to workshop-only training, which is unlikely to provide much return on investment of time and resources. A little training may convince staff that they can deliver MI (or were already doing so), but is unlikely to improve actual practice skills or benefit clients. We also don't recommend sending one staff member to initial training with the expectation that he or she will return and teach other staff because (1) workshop training alone is rarely enough to develop the trainee's own competence in and understanding of MI, let alone ability to teach it to others; and (2) he or she will have no similarly prepared on-site colleagues with whom to work in developing proficiency.

TOWARD TRAINING FOR ALL STAFF

Some programs and managers decide that it would be desirable for all their practitioners (and in some cases their entire staff) to develop skillfulness in MI. Although individuals will differ in their potential for proficiency in MI, the usual aim here is for staff to have this method within their clinical skill set.

While we were writing this book we were contacted by a government agency that planned to require MI training for all providers of certain mental health services. The intent, of course, was not merely that practitioners would complete some MI training event, but that they would develop skillfulness in practicing this approach that would improve their clients' outcomes. The initial plan had been that all providers would be required to complete two workshops: an introduction to MI and then an advanced workshop. With some time, effort, and cost it would be possible for all providers to attend such workshops and check off that they had done so, but would this accomplish the intended aim?

The Role of Workshops

Like most people who teach MI, we both began by offering clinical workshops of 1 to 2 days' duration. The assumption was that, having completed such a workshop, participants would be prepared to practice MI. On posttraining evaluation questionnaires our participants generally rated the workshops quite favorably and expressed confidence in their ability to use MI. As reported in Chapter 24, however, more careful evaluations of our own training based on pre- and postworkshop practice samples found that changes in skill were generally quite modest and unlikely to make much difference in client outcomes.

Workshop training is a good start but only a beginning. On average, what one can expect from a competent MI workshop is acquaintance with the purpose, spirit, and core concepts (to know something *about* MI), some sense of how MI sounds and feels in action, and a small increase in ability to recognize and practice relevant skills. The skill gains from workshop training are larger than those from self-study by reading books or viewing recordings about MI, but are modest (Miller et al., 2004). Perhaps a good analogy would be a classroom introduction to how to fly an airplane. Some useful knowledge can be gained and reflected in posttraining knowledge tests, but no one would care to be a passenger in a plane piloted by someone who had received only classroom or self-study instruction. It's just not enough to acquire or maintain proficiency.

> Workshop training is a good start, but only a beginning.

In Chapter 24 we described some content that we believe ought to be included in initial MI training. To this we add a few recommendations about the selection of trainers. First, we believe that anyone who aspires to help others learn MI should first be reasonably proficient in it themselves. An instructor teaching *about* MI within a college course might have only basic knowledge of it, but someone who professes to help people learn the practice of MI should be able to demonstrate it competently on the spot. It would be a rare violin teacher who cannot play the instrument competently. Second, to facilitate learning in others requires more than proficiency in practice. A brilliant guitarist does not necessarily have the skills or patience needed to teach others. The international Motivational Interviewing Network of Trainers (MINT) was designed to help trainers develop and continue to improve skills to facilitate the learning of MI (*www.motivationalinterviewing.org*). An experienced trainer does far more than talk about and demonstrate MI. We blush to remember our first training for MI trainers in 1993, in which we prescribed a fixed set and sequence of exercises without much regard for differences in trainees, practice contexts, and problem areas. It was a beginning, but skillful MI training requires the flexible use of a variety of learning strategies that blend "tell, show, and try" (describe, demonstrate, and provide ample opportunity to practice with feedback). Third, MI research and practice have been evolving quite quickly, and it is important for a competent trainer to keep up with current developments. A primary motivation for us to write this book was precisely this: the substantial new knowledge and evolutions in MI that have emerged since our second edition.

To be sure, learners differ in how readily they develop competence in practicing MI. As we noted in Chapter 24, a small minority do become proficient with only a workshop introduction. The key is to provide enough opportunities for learners to reach a criterion level of practice competence and then to maintain those skills over time. Workshops are rarely enough for this to happen. We no longer imply that people who attend our own workshops will be skilled at the end, but if we have done our work well they will know enough about what MI is to decide whether they want to learn it and to understand how they might do so.

Facilitate Ongoing Coaching and Peer Support

To the government agency mentioned earlier we recommended that they abandon their plan for all practitioners to take two workshops. The introductory workshops were already underway and that was fine, but we recommended that the resources that had been planned for advanced training workshops be used instead to help each provider program develop in-house MI expertise. Ideally, every program would have one or two people on staff with sufficient skills to help others learn and continue developing MI skills.

This is attractive for many reasons. On-site coaches have a more intimate understanding of the service than an outside trainer would, and can respond to ongoing learning needs and challenges. Even if an entire staff were well trained there will be turnover and new staff to train. Furthermore, learning MI is not a one-time affair but rather an ongoing process. An outside trainer delivers discrete events, but an in-house coach is there for the long run. Learning is also facilitated by the quality of engagement between trainers and trainees, and this is easier to achieve in ongoing collegial relationships. The imposition on staff of outside trainers can create struggles on both sides. This problem can be particularly acute in large systems where decisions are made in relative isolation from everyday practice, and well-intentioned efforts to train all staff can fail to have the intended impact. The glue that often binds the learning process is ongoing coaching and peer support.

How, then, can a program develop on-site expertise in MI? Instead of having an external trainer try to bring everyone up to a high standard of practice, resources are devoted to developing expertise of on-staff coaches. During initial phases of learning (such as introductory workshops) keep an eye out for individuals who seem to have a head start on learning MI themselves by virtue of existing skills (such as reflective listening), enthusiasm, understanding, and/or rapid gains. People who show such early aptitude for MI proficiency may be particularly good candidates to help other staff learn MI skills. Consideration can also be given to within-staff dynamics. Who among the clinical staff or supervisors are particularly respected and trusted? If such opinion leaders also show aptitude for learning MI they may become key resources in developing programwide expertise. Once they have developed reasonable proficiency in practice themselves they can be prepared to coach others in learning MI skills (Ball et al., 2006).

BOX 26.1. Personal Reflection: Shortcomings of a Top-Down Style in Training

Some years ago I readily joined forces with Carl Åke Farbring, who had a senior role in the criminal justice service across the whole of Sweden. We designed an elaborate MI training program starting with a small group of senior MI trainers and focusing mostly on how to train others. In turn, they provided training workshops throughout the correctional hierarchy, right down to prison staff working on the front lines. A few years later it became apparent that these top-down doses of workshop training had had little of the desired effect. In fact, it was difficult to find much evidence of MI in practice.

We set out, then, to train in a more collaborative manner, using coaches and staying close to the prison staff's daily challenges. Rather than trying to teach the method of MI per se, we focused on "everyday corridor conversations about change." We designed a software-driven, video-rich DVD to help all staff use more flexible communication styles when trying to promote change. These were viewed immediately before the staff gathered in a smaller seminar format to discuss how the material presented could be applied in their prison environment. Reports came back of enthusiasm and a much better atmosphere in one of the prisons. As Dr. Farbring reflected, "Officers noted that we were interested also in their own well-being, and that treating prisoners differently could also help them feel better about their work."

—SR

Another helpful resource within a demanding service environment is an ongoing context for constructive discussion about how to continue developing clinical skills and keep them robust. This might be led by an on-site coach or supervisor with expertise in MI, and it is also feasible as a relatively informal and organic small group of colleagues working together to strengthen their skills. Some services designate scheduled time for staff to work together on clinical challenges they face, a potentially ideal scenario for improving MI skills. The Family Nurse Partnership project in the United Kingdom, for example, provides continuity of learning from initial MI workshops through more frequent peer support sessions using a manual with case scenarios and guidelines for simulated practice. If such learning is included in ongoing clinical supervision groups it is important to protect time for skill building because such meetings are often consumed by discussion of administrative detail.

As discussed in Chapter 24 a key requisite for learning is the direct observation of practice, usually via recordings. Such observation can be provided by a supervisor or coach, and skill development is also promoted when clinicians can observe and learn from each other's practice within a supportive group, given sufficient MI training. Clinicians who have not been observed in practice for some time can understandably find the prospect threatening. It is important, therefore, to guide any discussion of observed practice in a way that facilitates learning and supports safety (see "Learning Communities" in Chapter 24). Building an atmosphere that fosters safety around exposing one's clinical skills to colleagues is an investment that bears much fruit. Simulated practice can also be used in supervisory sessions to build MI skillfulness, although the ability to demonstrate a skill in simulation does not guarantee that it is being used in actual practice.

IMPROVING SERVICEWIDE CONVERSATIONS ABOUT CHANGE

Beyond providing MI training for staff, some programs aspire to deliver services more generally in a person-centered way that is consistent with the underlying spirit described in Chapter 2. This extends not only to what happens within clinical consultations but also to what clients experience from the moment they contact the service: on the telephone or online, with reception and administrative staff, in any correspondence, even in the physical design of space. To what extent do all of these communicate respect, collaboration, and acceptance? Designing services that convey this spirit involves considering how staff members speak to clients as well as to each other. It matters how staff think about, talk to each other about, and commit to change, which is one reason why the top-down delivery of doses of training can fall far short of hoped-for impact. Without intending to step too far into the world of organizational change, a topic ably addressed by many others, we turn now to how communication within and outside of clinical consultations might be better aligned, thus allowing MI and other approaches to thrive in a service environment in which all participants approach change in a fruitful manner.

Life inside a clinical consultation is often an expression of forces outside of it. How people communicate with each other about change is a thread that runs through virtually all relationships. There can be a familiar ring to conversational styles across contexts, with parallel communication processes that run through different levels of the service. Consider, for example:

> Life inside a clinical consultation is often an expression of forces outside of it.

> *"What you need to do at this point is . . . "* (Is it a supervisor speaking to a counselor, or a counselor to a client?)
>
> *"I've told her this so many times before, but she just doesn't seem to listen."* (Is it someone speaking about a colleague or about a client?)
>
> *"Let me tell you how to get this done . . . "* (Is it a manager speaking to a staff member, or a clinician to a client?)
>
> *"That man is just impossible. He's being obstinate and won't cooperate."* (Is it about a colleague, a supervisor, or a client?)

Of course, it is sometimes essential to impart clear information both within clinical consultations and within a service at large, and managers do have a power relationship and responsibilities with the people they supervise. We also readily acknowledge the limitations of an MI style in operating a clinic, service, or system, and the necessity at times of a directing style. MI began as a clinical consultation approach, and the supervisor–staff relationship is not a therapeutic contract. There is a role for and the responsibility of directing. If, for example, a staff member were practicing in a manner likely to be ineffective or harmful for clients and is not responding to a guiding style, there is a supervisory duty for more directive intervention, as would be the case with those who oversee surgeons or airline pilots.

Nevertheless, there is typically room for improvement in the ways in which communication happens within a service. This was one of the initial inspirations for MI—to find a better way of having conversations about change. How might this and other features of MI inform interactions outside the context of clinical consultations?

Insight about Facilitating Change

A number of insights from MI might help inform conversations about change within a service at large. Here are a few:

1. How people talk about change matters. Beyond the specific content there are stylistic aspects of communication that have predictable effects on outcome and can promote discord or harmony.
2. Communications that evoke or exacerbate sustain talk and discord are unlikely to promote change.
3. One's first reflexive response to correct, fix, or make change happen may not be the best choice.
4. Listening is a powerful tool that in itself can facilitate change. Approaching people with respect and interest rather than an authoritarian-directing style is more likely to result in collaboration and change.
5. Ambivalence is common and normal. Staff as well as clients often feel ambivalent about changes that they face.
6. Engagement matters and is a foundation for all other collaborative communication.
7. People's own needs and motivations provide a foundation for ownership and better outcomes of change.
8. Binding this all together is the quality of interpersonal relationships. Improve communication about change and discord tends to decrease, ambivalence and ambiguity become more tolerable, and changes are more fruitfully accomplished.

These insights about interpersonal aspects of change do not arise uniquely from MI. They rest on a long-standing foundation of wisdom from fields including education, parenting, coaching, clinical practice, and management.

Consider these examples in Box 26.2 of parallel positive processes in communication to produce change. In each one of these scenarios change is being approached in a similar manner. The nurse's encouragement echoes the scaffolding skills described by the parent for helping her child learn self-regulation. Right across this list people are working collaboratively, viewing the other as a source of wisdom and insight, conveying respect for autonomy, drawing on strengths, and being restrained in stepping in with their own undoubted expertise, many of the qualities highlighted in Chapter 2 on the spirit of MI. Moreover, if these conversations were to continue, change talk is likely to emerge quite naturally. What effects might these attitudes toward change have if they were robust and widespread in a service setting?

BOX 26.2. Parallel Positive Communications across Roles

A young parent, talking about helping a child learn new puzzle-solving skills:	"I find that if I hold back from giving answers and allow him time and space to think about it, it's amazing: He comes up with a solution!"
A nurse talking to the young parent who is ambivalent about facing change:	"These challenges seem a bit daunting, yet you think you can probably get on top of them. How might you do that?"
A supervisor talking to the nurse about her work and workload:	"I've got some ideas, but I wonder what thoughts you have about how you could cope better with this kind of caseload."
A manager talking to a group of supervisors:	"It's not easy to see a way through these cutbacks. What kind of support could I provide that might help you?"
A program director writing to all staff:	"With the new year comes the chance to consider how we might improve our service in the year ahead. To that end I suggest that we spend a solid hour exploring this at our meeting on Friday. Bring some ideas that you have and I'll bring what I know about the budget."
A senior government official speaking at a conference for program directors:	"We need to speed up the process of entering assessment data into the system and we want to draw on your experience to help us think about how this might be accomplished."

Similarity in conversation styles inside and outside the consulting room is no coincidence. What is the service's normative view of human nature? If staff unite around the value of promoting autonomy, collaboration, and a belief in the strengths of the other to learn and change, MI will not seem foreign. The nurse and supervisor might not have learned MI, but they will probably be receptive to learning how to use conversational skills to bring out the best in their clients. In the course of everyday interactions people often discover that a collaborative approach is more successful than a demanding one in fostering long-term cooperation and change. Why, then, is this approach to change not more widely used in service settings?

Overuse of a Directing Style

A directing style is sometimes essential in managing a clinic and protecting client well-being. This style can be done with tact, clarity, and good timing, and can be offered within a broader context of support and collaboration, However, it can become overused and form the predominant interaction style within a service. It's not hard to imagine, for example, the scenarios in Box 26.2 being undermined by the use of a directing style and the righting reflex, perhaps driven by a desire to solve problems quickly and a feeling of being under pressure. The parent would be telling the child what to do, the nurse advising the parent how to manage life, the supervisor prescribing better caseload management practice, and so on up the ladder. How you approach change matters. Ask service providers what they like least about the introduction of change to their service, and a singular theme emerges: we often feel ambivalent about change, and we don't like being told "top-down" what to do. People want to have a say in changes that affect them and some time to absorb, reflect, and move on. Change without engagement often feels coercive and is likely to evoke discord.

Most services sit somewhere between the polarized scenarios of a directing "get it done" style and a guiding-collaborative style. We often hear tensions in balancing these styles from people who are learning MI. A practitioner told us:

> "It's really hard in the clinic. We're all so busy and we don't have much time to meet, let alone practice our skills. Then when I'm with clients, once I've completed the assessment that I must get through at the beginning, it's hard to fit in MI. Most of the time I'm just rushing through my job."

We consciously chose the verb "integrating" for this chapter to suggest a collaborative aligning of MI within a more broadly client-centered service. A top-down imposition approach to implementation clashes with the style and spirit of MI. One of our least favorite starting points in training is with a staff who have been told, "You're going to learn MI whether you like it or not." Rather, a meeting of minds across a service hierarchy is more likely to promote shared ownership and creative collaboration in implementation. Change sometimes must happen, as all managers well know, but like MI it is something best done with and for people, not on or to them.

Attention now turns to conceptual aids and practical things that might help to redress the overuse of a directing style, moving toward more constructive change conversations within the service at large and the better integration of MI in treating clients.

Three Areas for Improvement

The following three areas stand out as fertile foci for improving conversations about change inside and outside the consultation.

Two Feet Planted Firmly in the Guiding Style

In Chapter 1 we described the flexible use with clients of the direct–guide–follow continuum of communication styles. There are times when directing is needed and appropriate, whether it be in parenting, managing, teaching, or clinical consultations. Sometimes, too, a following style is best—just listening with no agenda beyond presence, support, and understanding. MI is grounded in the middle way, the guiding style, with ample use of following and restrained use of directing. One practitioner in MI training put it this way: "I keep my two feet planted firmly in the guiding style, and move to either side as needed." She was talking about her clinical work, but this stance can apply more broadly to improvement in a service at large.

Busyness is a double-edged sword in services settings. At best it is efficient and productive, at worst it is a stress-driven response to pressure. There is a tendency to believe that when change is needed and time is short, a directing style is essential in order "to get the job done." Although we understand the logic, we question the accuracy of this assumption that just telling people what to do is an efficient (let alone effective) way to promote change. Directing tends to evoke discord and reactance, and may actually decrease the likelihood that change will occur. Ironically, the use of a directing style is also sometimes justified as "doing my job."

> "My job as a social worker is to protect the children. I tell the parents what they have to do, and it's up to them to do it."

> "As a diabetes educator, I just have to get certain facts across to people and warn them about what happens if they don't keep good control of their sugar levels. I can't make them do it."

> "I tell my employees what is expected of them and the consequences of not following through. I'm the supervisor and if they don't like it they can work somewhere else."

It is as if there is a checklist of knowledge to be conveyed and things to tell people to do. (Sometimes there literally is such a checklist.) "When I've told them, then I've done my job." The question, of course, is whether one's job is to convey facts or to facilitate change. Lecturing is notoriously ineffective in changing established problem behaviors like excessive drinking (Miller, Wilbourne, & Hettema, 2003), and few training programs for skilled workers rely on conveying information alone. (Imagine: "I told him how the plane's controls work. Now it's up to him to fly it.") Whether as a clinician, parent, probation officer, teacher, or supervisor, one's job is to facilitate learning and change. Inflexible attachment to a directing style is usually ineffective if not detrimental for all involved. A practice implementation leader in government told us:

> "It's a real disappointment to me to see some managers speak with their clinical staff. They would be shocked if the clients were spoken to like that, so why talk to colleagues that way?"

If managers and supervisors mirror the proposed skillfulness of the practitioners, using particularly the guiding and following styles when resolving problems, the atmosphere in meetings and smaller conversations can improve. The same tolerance of ambivalence and restrained use of directing that is useful with clients can be marshalled to good effect outside of clinical consultations. Finessing communication in this way is not equivalent to learning or practicing MI, but a guiding style within a service can form the broad systemic platform upon which MI and client-centered practice flourish. One effect of using a guiding style in management could be stronger engagement between staff, a feeling of being appreciated and respected for the work they do.

> Tolerance of ambivalence and restrained use of directing can be marshalled to good effect outside of clinical consultations.

Engagement Improves Outcomes

Client engagement is often a thermometer of a well-functioning therapeutic relationship or service (S. D. Miller et al., 2005, 2006). Its flip side, well known to any practitioner, is the frustration of seeing clients drop out at various stages of their journey. Consider this example, which points to many areas for improvement in engagement:

> A young man enters a first counseling session angry and frustrated about how everything is blamed on him, on his use of drugs, and on his "bad behavior." He first came in for a scheduled afternoon appointment, agitated and overwhelmed, and waited for an hour in a seat facing other clients. The receptionist conducted a few abrupt transactions with him, then he briefly saw a social worker and the service coordinator. Now, on his second visit, the counselor conducts a routine assessment that takes 35 minutes, and then tries to talk to him about treatment goals like coming off drugs altogether. He remains resistant and angry.

If the first few moments of a meeting are critical, as many clinicians say that they are, then it's not hard to see how engagement could have been improved in the above scenario. How respectful was the experience of waiting an hour and facing others while in distress? How welcoming were all the people he met? How well was he listened to and how interested were staff in his own concerns? This is not merely a matter of better communication, but other things too: the waiting room experience might be changed, even the chairs rearranged.

Information Exchange Is an Art

One of the most fertile contributions of MI to service improvement could be in regard to how information is exchanged. Information overload can run through client and practitioner experiences. Memos, protocols, directives, algorithms, and assessment data can be written on the assumption that if people receive the data, and the content is accurate, all will be well. The clinical equivalent can be caricatured by the practitioner who believes that all they need to do is "lift the lid" of the patient's head, stuff it full with information, and change will follow in due course. How to give clients feedback about the results of assessment was one of the starting points of MI (Miller & Sovereign, 1989; Miller et al., 1988) and was the impetus for the elicit–provide–elicit framework described in Chapter 11, a skill set that could quite easily be acquired by managers and supervisors as well as service providers. Integration of information can be viewed as a process rather than an event, one that requires thoughtfulness on both sides.

This emphasis on the *how* of information exchange raises a challenge with clients; for example, how assessment can be integrated into an engaging conversation (see Chapter 9). In the wider service it calls for avoiding information "dumping" on staff, and a realization that both the written and spoken word have the power to promote change, or not. What we learned from MI was that providing information is a relational matter and not just a transaction to be traversed. Box 26.3 provides some suggestions for how to improve conversations about change as one aspect of culture change.

A BROADER VIEW

We have considered here specifically how MI might be used to improve conversations about change within a service. Obviously, there are much broader aspects of a service that can communicate partnership, acceptance, compassion, and a desire to evoke the insights and creativity of each person. What is the mission of the service, and what are the values that drive it? How are procedures determined and changed? What does the arrangement of physical space convey? The thread of communication runs through all of these service aspects.

MI is not a panacea or a comprehensive guide for organizational development, but it can be integrated into a service. As MI becomes part of good practice it may also inform communication within the service. Most services experience ongoing change, which can be as much of a challenge for staff as it is for the clients they serve. Insights from MI provide an alternative to overreliance on a directing style.

BOX 26.3. Examples for Improving Conversations about Change

	With clients	**With colleagues**
Two feet planted firmly in the guiding style	Use all three communication styles in response to your clients' stated needs. A guiding style often evokes change talk, and provides a good foundation for sharpening your MI skills.	Avoid overuse of directing, and use a following style before trying to solve problems. This enhances engagement and improves working relationships. Use guiding more than directing when trying to promote change in others.
Engagement improves outcomes	Consider the clients' journey through the service. How can engagement be improved? Consider every conversation, the design of procedures, and even things like the layout of the waiting area.	Consider how you might improve engagement with colleagues. Your relationships with them are the bedrock of the service and your own well-being. Respectful listening and an interest in understanding others' perspectives are key in fostering collaboration.
Information exchange is an art	Avoid conducting assessments before you have adequately engaged with clients. Consider creative ways of getting through assessment without a form dominating the conversation (see Chapter 9).	Avoid one-way information that is disengaged from colleagues. Consider how the elicit–provide–elicit strategy might help you in your communications with colleagues.

KEY POINTS

✓ MI can be integrated into a service in various ways, from training a few staff to implementing it in a particular aspect of service, through training of all staff, to diffusing a person-centered approach throughout the service.

✓ Workshops alone usually have little effect in changing practice; complex skills are typically learned with feedback and coaching.

✓ Services to promote change can benefit by shifting away from overreliance on directing toward a guiding style.

PART VII

EVALUATING
MOTIVATIONAL INTERVIEWING

In this final section we consider issues involved in evaluating the processes, outcomes, and quality of MI. A comprehensive review of the large body of clinical trials on MI is beyond the scope of this book, nor are we best skilled or positioned to provide an objective assessment of the evidence. Instead, in Chapter 27 we provide a brief history of the evolution of MI and the corresponding lines of research that have emerged. One clear finding is that the quality of MI practice matters, and in Chapter 28 we consider how to assess fidelity for quality assurance and improvement, and more generally what contributes to the effectiveness of motivational conversations.

Research Evidence
and the Evolution
of Motivational Interviewing

The facts are always friendly, every bit of evidence one can acquire,
in any area, leads one that much closer to what is true.
—CARL R. ROGERS

Learn to look at things familiar until they become unfamiliar again.
—G. K. CHESTERTON

No creator of a meaningful phrase, a useful invention or powerful
idea has the ability to control the uses to which his or her creation
is put. They cannot envision what the future may hold for the thing
they have put in motion.
—ANNETTE GORDON-REED

As we considered how best to summarize the research evidence on MI, we settled on a favorite device: to tell a story. The development of MI has been intertwined with emerging and sometimes surprising research findings from its inception. The story of how MI evolved is also the narrative of a lively dance between research and practice, and of how each informs the other. We thus begin with this emerging story and then conclude the chapter with our own perspective on the state of the evidence base to date. For convenience of storytelling, the narrative begins in first person singular (WRM).

THE EVOLUTION OF MOTIVATIONAL INTERVIEWING

Albuquerque

When I began my research career first at the University of Oregon and then in my faculty post at the University of New Mexico, my focus was on the treatment of problem drinking. My studies were not turning out as I had expected, and I wondered why. In my dissertation I had tested three different behavior therapies to help problem drinkers moderate their alcohol use (Miller, 1978). The least intensive (and intrusive) of these worked just as well as the most intensive, and there was also an unexpected finding regarding a self-help guidebook (Miller & Muñoz, 1976) that we distributed after treatment was over. Half of clients received the guidebook right away, while the other half (randomly chosen) did not receive it until the first follow-up interview 3 months later. To my surprise, those given the guidebook right away continued to decrease their drinking over the next 3 months, whereas for the others their drinking remained where it had been at the end of treatment.

This suggested the next study (Miller, Gribskov, & Mortell, 1981). How much better would people fare when treated by a counselor relative to working on their own with the self-help guidebook? The answer again was surprising: No better at all. Problem drinkers who came for a single consultation and went home with self-help materials decreased their alcohol use substantially and just as much on average as those given 10 outpatient sessions with a counselor. I so doubted the finding that we repeated the study with variations three more times in New Mexico, all yielding the same result (Harris & Miller, 1990; Miller & Taylor, 1980; Miller et al., 1980). Was therapy really no different from self-help?

Again a clue came from an unexpected source. In my training at the University of Oregon I had been exposed both to behavioral therapies and to the client-centered counseling style of Carl Rogers (1959, 1980b). The two seemed to me to fit together naturally, so in training therapists in New Mexico I had been teaching them both accurate empathy—the skillful listening style developed by Rogers—and behavioral techniques. The way in which we maintained treatment fidelity in these studies was to observe the therapists' sessions via one-way mirrors, and we documented not only adherence to behavior therapy procedures but also the quality of accurate empathy using a scale developed by Rogers's research group (Truax & Carkhuff, 1967). A particularly important collaborator at this time was an energetic undergraduate student named Cheryl Taylor, who helped to coordinate these studies. When our follow-up data had been collected, we examined the success rates for the nine therapists to whom clients had been randomly assigned (Miller et al., 1980). Even though all nine counselors were delivering the same structured and manual-guided behavior therapy, the percentage of their clients with successful outcomes varied widely. The therapist to whom clients had been assigned was by far the strongest influence on outcome. Then we lined up the therapists according to the extent to which they had been listening empathically to their clients, and this is what we saw:

PERCENT POSITIVE OUTCOMES BY THERAPIST

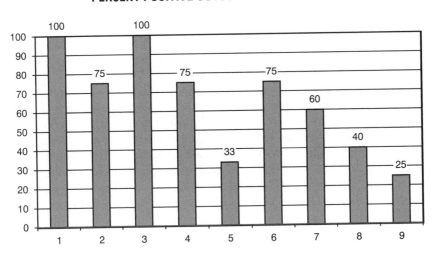

Of the clients who had worked with the therapist whom we all agreed had shown the highest level of empathic skill (#1), all had good success in managing their drinking. In contrast, only 25% of those working with the least empathic counselor had good outcomes. The correlation wasn't perfect, but it was quite strong (r = .82). We were able to predict two-thirds of the variation in clients' drinking outcomes at 6 months (the number of standard drink units they were consuming weekly) based on how well their counselor had *listened* to them! This effect was much larger than any other differences in treatments that we observed. Even at 1-year (r = .71) and 2-year follow-up (r = .51), we could still predict how much clients would be drinking from this one therapist skill: accurate empathy (Miller & Baca, 1983). An independent study published by another group a year later reported the same strong relationship between client drinking outcomes and therapists' skillfulness in client-centered counseling (Valle, 1981). Those working with therapists rated as low in client-centered skills had up to four times higher relapse rates compared to the clients of high-skill counselors in the same program.

It was with these puzzling findings in mind that I had embarked on sabbatical leave in 1982. They no doubt influenced my subsequent thinking about MI.

Norway

It began in a barbershop in Norway. In the fall of 1982 I was on sabbatical leave from the University of New Mexico, and my wife Kathy Jackson and

I lived where I was working, at the Hjellestad Clinic near Bergen. What had previously been the barber's headquarters was cleared out to provide a lovely corner office for me with windows on the forest. It was an idyllic 6 months with the only ways to reach me being by telephone or snail mail. My official duties involved lecturing on cognitive-behavioral methods for treating addiction, but the director of the clinic, Dr. Jon Laberg, asked if I might also be willing to meet regularly with their team of young psychologists, many of them recently graduated, to discuss research and treatment issues. I readily agreed, and these informal meetings turned out to be among the most important and productive experiences of my career.

With my fresh data on the importance of accurate empathy (Miller et al., 1980), I began teaching this group the skills of reflective listening. This melded into discussions and practical role play of how these skills might be applied in treating alcohol problems. The Norwegian psychologists would role-play clients whom they were seeing, posing clinical issues that they found particularly challenging, and I did my best to respond in a helpful way as I might in my own practice. They participated actively and reflectively, focusing on the processes occurring within these interactions. They would often stop me to ask analytic questions about the process.

"What are you *thinking* right now?"

"You just asked a question. Why did you ask that particular question?"

"You reflected what the client said. Of all the things you might have focused on, why did you reflect *that*, and why did you reflect rather than responding in some other way?"

In trying to understand why I was doing what I was doing clinically they required me to reflect on and verbalize it in greater depth. In the process I began to formulate some decision rules that I seemed to be using in practice, although I had not been consciously aware of them. For example, in contrast to common practice in addiction treatment at the time, I did not confront or disagree with "resistance" from the client but responded in a different manner (most often with reflective listening) in a way that seemed to diminish resistance. I also seemed to be arranging the conversation in a way that caused the client to make the arguments for change rather than doing so myself.

It is hard for me to separate what I brought to these conversations from the interactive contributions of my Norwegian colleagues. I certainly did not go to Hjellestad with any prior conception of this approach. Tom Barth, who was an important participant in this process, remembers his group bringing to the conversations the influence of the family therapy group at Palo Alto, California, from

MI was literally evoked from me.

which I had also benefitted during clinical internship there. Without question, what happened in the barbershop was highly interactive, ultimately yielding a process that I do not think any of us would have come up with on our own. There is a lovely resonance in the fact that MI was literally evoked from me.

Over the weeks of that autumn I took notes on these conversations and began to write down some clinical principles that were emerging from these role plays. About 3 months in, I put them into a working description that I called "motivational interviewing," which I distributed to the group and also sent to several colleagues for their comments (Moyers, 2004). I had no intention of publishing the paper; after all, we had no scientific evidence at all that it would work. It also was not derived from any particular psychological theory. It came purely from intuitive practice and reflection. One colleague to whom I sent the working paper was Ray Hodgson, who happened to be editing the British journal *Behavioural Psychotherapy*. To my surprise Ray wrote that he wanted to publish it as an article if I could reduce it in length by half. I did, and he did (Miller, 1983), and I thought that would probably be the last I heard of it.

The Transtheoretical Model of Change

During the 1980s the transtheoretical model (TTM) of change was also being developed and was gaining traction (Prochaska & DiClemente, 1984). The now-familiar TTM stages of change in psychotherapy (McConnaughy, Prochaska, & Velicer, 1983) highlighted the need for clinicians to be flexibly using methods appropriate to the client's current level of readiness for change. Most cognitive-behavioral therapies are designed for the action stage, when clients are ready for change, but what to do for clients who are at the earlier stages of precontemplation, contemplation, and preparation? MI as a clinical tool was conceptualized precisely for such "less ready" clients, a parallel that I drew in the original MI article (Miller, 1983). Subsequently the third International Conference on Treatment of Addictive Behaviors, convened in Scotland with the leadership of Nick Heather, was designed to introduce the TTM to an international audience and conceptualized clinical interventions according to the stage(s) at which they might be most applicable (Miller & Heather, 1986, 1998). There seemed to be a good conceptual fit with TTM, and MI provided a needed example of how to work with clients who are less ready to change.

The Drinker's Checkup

Would it be possible to evoke motivation for change from clients themselves, much as my colleagues had coaxed this idea of MI from me? What better source for motivation could there be? A first step was to explore what others had learned about motivation for treatment. Most of this reading I was able to complete during the latter half of my sabbatical leave at Stanford University in the spring of 1983. This was long before the era of electronic literature searches, and I was still writing on a typewriter, so I had the pleasure of roaming the Stanford stacks in search of journals and monographs, taking notes by hand at old wooden library desks. The resulting literature review (Miller, 1985b) persuaded me that the prevalent clinical focus on denial and motivation as client traits was misguided. Indeed, client motivation clearly was a dynamic process responding to a variety of interpersonal influences including advice, feedback, goal setting, contingencies, and perceived choice among alternatives.

Back at the University of New Mexico our group puzzled over how the clinical style of MI and the scientific literature on what influences motivation for treatment might be developed into a specific intervention that could be tested. My chief research assistant during this time, still prior to any grant funding, was another resourceful undergraduate named Gayle Benefield Sovereign. We developed the "Drinker's Checkup" (DCU) which was designed as a low-threshold brief intervention for problem drinkers. Our hope was that the DCU would increase the likelihood of seeking treatment for alcohol problems.

First described in 1988, the DCU consisted of a thorough assessment of alcohol use and potential related problems using measures sensitive to lower levels of impairment, plus a return visit to review findings in an MI-consistent style (Miller et al., 1988). It was advertised to the community as a free checkup for drinkers who would like to find out whether alcohol was harming them in any way. The announcement specified that it was not part of any treatment program, no one would be given diagnostic labels, and the result would be health information to use however they saw fit. The response was surprisingly large. Everyone who came for the DCU did have reason for concern, though most considered themselves to be "social drinkers" and had never sought help in relation to their alcohol use.

Contrary to our hopeful expectation, relatively few (14%) sought any help within 6 weeks of their feedback. Instead, participants as a whole showed a significant immediate reduction in their drinking that was retained at 18-month follow-up and confirmed by collateral reports (Miller et al., 1988). A second study of the DCU yielded similar results with still larger reductions in alcohol consumption, largely without additional treatment (Miller et al., 1993). Thus our expectation that the DCU would trigger help-seeking was not confirmed; rather, it appeared to motivate enduring self-change in drinking. Those randomly assigned to a waiting list in these studies showed little or no change at 6 weeks but a marked reduction after subsequently receiving the DCU. This converged with our earlier findings that problem drinkers responded well to an initial consultation and self-directed change, even over long periods of follow-up (Miller, Leckman, Delaney, & Tinkcom, 1992). Others had been reporting similar findings with brief interventions in other countries (Chick, Ritson, Connaughton, Stewart, & Chick, 1988; Edwards et al., 1977; Elvy, Wells, & Baird, 1988; Heather, Whitton, & Robertson, 1986; Kristenson, Ohlin, Hulten-Nosslin, Hood, & Trell, 1983). Our review of 32 controlled trials found that brief interventions for excessive drinking are more effective than no treatment and often similar in impact to more intensive interventions (Bien, Miller, & Tonigan, 1993). This review also pointed to six common components of effective brief treatment (cf. Miller & Sanchez, 1994), summarized by the acronym FRAMES:

Feedback of personal status relative to norms
Responsibility for personal change
Advice to change
Menu of options from which to choose in pursuing change
Empathic counselor style
Support for self-efficacy

What began as an interest in motivation for *treatment* had broadened now to focusing on motivation for *change*.

Australia

Armed with this information, Kathy and I departed in 1989 for a sabbatical year in Australia at the invitation of Nick Heather, then director of the National Drug and Alcohol Research Centre in Sydney. There, I had the good fortune of meeting Steve Rollnick, who was on leave from Wales and engaged in brief intervention research at the Centre. He was surprised to learn that I was the man who had written that 1983 article on MI, and I was surprised to learn that someone had actually read it. Steve proceeded to tell me that MI had become a popular method in addiction treatment in the United Kingdom and that he was responding to an increasing demand for MI training. "And I'm not even sure if I'm doing it right!" he told me. "You must write more about it."

It quickly became apparent not only that Steve practiced MI with the same set of mind and heart as I did, but also that he had developed helpful ways for teaching it to clinicians. There had been relatively little interest in such training in the United States, and I was fascinated to hear his ideas and experiences. We decided to write about MI together, and the result was the first edition of *Motivational Interviewing* (Miller & Rollnick, 1991). Because both of us had been developing MI to help people with alcohol problems, the book focused on addictions with some contributed chapters exploring its potential usefulness for other drug problems and with youth and offenders.

Project MATCH

While we were writing in Sydney, the U.S. National Institute on Alcohol Abuse and Alcoholism was launching what would become the largest randomized clinical trial of treatments for alcohol problems. Dubbed Project MATCH, it was specifically intended to determine how to match clients to the treatment approach that would work best for them (Project MATCH Research Group, 1993). An early task was to choose and standardize the three treatment methods that would be tested. Cognitive-behavioral therapy was a clear choice based on outcome data and the theoretical orientation of most of the researchers (Kadden et al., 1992). A clear contrast was provided by including a spiritually focused twelve-step facilitation therapy mirroring a highly popular treatment approach in the United States (Nowinski, Baker, & Carroll, 1992). Based on the brief intervention outcome research described above, the third chosen treatment was an adaptation of the Drinker's Checkup combining the clinical style of MI with structured assessment feedback. This provided a still different theoretical rationale and procedural approach from the other two and was given the name Motivational Enhancement Therapy (MET; Miller, Zweben, et al., 1992). To avoid too large a contrast of treatment doses (the other two treatments were 12 sessions in length), MET was lengthened from two to four sessions spaced over 12 weeks. Then came the process of specifying *a priori* hypotheses about which treatment should work best for whom and why (Longabaugh & Wirtz, 2001).

The results of Project MATCH have been extensively described and critiqued (Babor & Del Boca, 2003; Babor, Miller, DiClemente, & Longabaugh, 1999). We focus here on its role as the first multisite clinical trial of an MI-based intervention. No prediction had been made about differential performance of the three treatment methods, and indeed they did not differ on posttreatment outcome measures (Project MATCH Research Group, 1997a). Despite the discrepancy in treatment intensity (4 vs. 12 sessions) clients in all three groups showed large and enduring reductions in alcohol use and problems (Project MATCH Research Group, 1998a). Therapists differed significantly in their effectiveness in delivering MET after controlling for client factors (Project MATCH Research Group, 1998c). The most consistent matching effect was that angrier clients fared particularly well in MET compared with the other two treatments (Karno & Longabaugh, 2004, 2005a, 2005b; Waldron et al., 2001). People whose social networks lacked support for abstinence fared better in 12-step treatment than in MET, apparently because of the community support for abstinence that is found in AA (Longabaugh et al., 1998).

An Important Decision

In the 1990s we pondered whether to try to maintain control over the quality of practice and training in MI. Should we trademark the name "motivational interviewing" in order to restrict its use? A trusted colleague urged us to do so and cautioned that we would regret it if we did not exert quality control of its use, an increasingly common path with "brand-name" therapies. In this approach, in order to say that one practices or teaches Brand X therapy one must go through a prescribed course of training, perhaps meet various quality performance standards, and be certified or licensed by those who hold control of the brand name.

For better or worse we were very clear from the beginning that we did not want to be the MI police. To do so, in fact, seemed to us to be inconsistent with the spirit and style of MI. It would also imply that we alone are the arbiters of what constitutes proper MI practice and training. From its inception MI has been organic, emerging, and evolving through collaborative processes. How ironic it would be, then, to ossify it and require adherence to a fixed prescription! Our decision was to focus on promoting quality in MI practice and training rather than on preventing people from doing it "wrong."

> From its inception MI has been organic, emerging, and evolving.

There is, however, a dark side to our decision, as our colleague had warned. In 2007 someone else attempted to register "motivational interviewing" as a trademark for a different approach, offering to allow us also to use it. By this time, however, legal opinion was that the term was already in such general use that it could no longer be trademarked. Consequently, anyone can claim to be practicing or teaching MI without accountability. (The same is true, of course, of other approaches such as "behavioral," "cognitive," or "psychodynamic" psychotherapy.) We have encountered practice, descriptions, and training of "motivational interviewing" that bear little resemblance to the method as we understand it. We also know from experience and research that people can come away from a workshop convinced that they are now proficient in MI (or already were), when practice samples tell a very different story (Miller & Mount, 2001; Miller et al., 2004). In essence, there is little relationship between self-reported competence in MI and objective measures of skill based on observed practice. Obviously, this raises serious concerns regarding quality assurance.

As treatment systems have chosen to implement MI and government agencies have sought to promote the use of evidence-based practice, stakeholders properly ask, "How do we know that this provider can actually *do* MI or is really delivering it?" Without procedures for verifying competence and auditing practice, providers are only required to *say* that they are delivering an evidence-based practice (Miller & Meyers, 1995). We address this complex issue in Chapter 28.

Rapid Diffusion

Interest in clinical training in MI grew rapidly after publication of the first edition, and we soon decided to begin training other trainers to meet this demand. In Albuquerque in 1993 we offered the first Training for New Trainers (TNT), which has continued annually thereafter, varying between North America and Europe. Trainers who had completed the TNT began to ask whether they might get together informally to share training ideas and experiences in tandem with the annual TNT. The first such gathering happened in Malta in 1997 and grew into an international Motivational Interviewing Network of Trainers (MINT) that formally incorporated as a not-for-profit entity in 2008. As of this writing, more than 2,500 trainers have completed the TNT, teaching in at least 45 different languages.

During this time the use of MI was also diffusing rapidly into other fields of practice. Applications with addiction problems other than alcohol began early, particularly focusing on heroin, marijuana, cocaine and stimulant use, and pathological gambling. Successful trials of MI for the prevention of HIV infection soon generalized to its uses in public health efforts, spreading as far as the promotion of water purification practices in rural African villages (Thevos et al., 2002; Thevos, Quick, et al., 2000). It was a short step to applications in general medicine, particularly for medication adherence and behavior change in the management of chronic diseases. We were at first reluctant to call such brief applications "motivational interviewing" (Rollnick, Mason, & Butler, 1999), but it became apparent that it was the same spirit and method being applied in different contexts (Rollnick et al., 2008). Clinical trials proliferated to test various applications of MI in promoting health behavior change.

In what other areas do professionals hope for behavior change about which the people they serve are often reluctant? Societies' hope for correctional systems is that they will change criminal behavior, since the vast majority of offenders who are incarcerated do return to society and often soon. Substance use disorders are common among offenders, spurring the interest of probation, parole, and community correctional systems in MI (McMurran, 2009; Walters et al., 2007). Motivational barriers are often encountered when addressing family violence (Murphy & Maiuro, 2009), eating disorders (Schmidt & Treasure, 1997), and conduct problems among youth (Naar-King & Suarez, 2011). In educational systems the transition to a higher level of education often requires substantial behavior change (e.g., in study habits), frequently competing with the temptations of increased freedom. MI has been explored to promote study skills, address college alcohol/drug problems, and prevent dropout (Baer et al., 2001; Daugherty, 2009; Schaus, Sole, McCoy, Mullett, & O'Brien, 2009). Dental professionals puzzle over how to promote oral health practices (Almomani, Williams, Catley, & Brown, 2009; Weinstein, Harrison, & Benton, 2006; Yevlahova & Satur, 2009), dieticians and diabetes educators over facilitating healthy dietary changes (Bowen et al., 2002; VanWormer & Boucher, 2004). MI has been used successfully with health promotion goals as diverse as weight loss (Armstrong et al., 2011), reducing A1C levels in diabetes (Chen, Creedy, Lin, & Wollin, 2012; Maclean et al., 2012) and pain-related disability with cancer (Thomas et al., 2012), with physical therapy (Vong, Cheing, Chan, So, & Chan, 2011), and with parents to decrease the exposure of their children with asthma to secondary smoke (Borrelli, McQuaid, Novak, Hammond, & Becker, 2010) and their children's television viewing (Taveras et al., 2011). Social workers (Hohman, 2012), psychotherapists (Engle & Arkowitz, 2006; Westra, 2012), and those who work with youth (Jensen et al., 2011; Naar-King & Suarez, 2011) all meet client ambivalence as they seek to promote change.

Our second edition (Miller & Rollnick, 2002) therefore broadened the application of MI to behavior change more generally, no longer limited to addictive behaviors, where it was born (although that remains the largest clinical trial literature). As reflected in earlier chapters of this edition, we are now thinking of a still wider range of change where the issue is not necessarily "behavior" unless that term is interpreted so broadly as to encompass all of human experience. We are fascinated observers of this ever-broadening array of applications of MI, and not without some concern.

OUTCOME RESEARCH
ON MOTIVATIONAL INTERVIEWING

Since 1990, the number of scientific publications on MI has been doubling about every 3 years. There are currently more than 1,200 publications on this treatment method, including more than 200 randomized clinical trials reflecting a wide array of problems, professions, practice settings, and nations. Meta-analyses of MI research now comprise a literature of their own, and a bibliography of these can be found in Appendix B.

We do not propose to undertake a study-by-study review of this now immense literature on the efficacy and effectiveness of MI. Neither shall we pick and choose studies that cast a positive light on MI. What we offer here is our own perception of the state of clinical science on MI, with some observations about overall messages, methodological shortcomings, hopes for future research, and broader implications for psychotherapeutic research.

Meta-analyses focus on characterizing average effects, and the general conclusions to date have been that MI is associated with small to medium effect sizes across a variety of behavioral outcomes, with the strongest body of evidence being on addictive behaviors. We think it is fair to say after 200 clinical trials that something seems to be happening with the practice of MI that is often associated with beneficial outcomes when compared with no intervention or brief advice, or when added to other active treatment.

What is also clear is a very high degree of variability in effects across studies, sites, and clinicians. A number of clinical trials, including some of our own, have reported no meaningful effect of MI on *a priori* dependent measures (Carroll et al., 2006; Carroll, Libby, Sheehan, & Hyland, 2001; Miller, Yahne, & Tonigan, 2003). Within well-controlled trials of manual-guided, closely supervised MI interventions, substantial therapist effects remain (Miller et al., 1993; Project MATCH Research Group, 1998c). Multisite trials have also found site-by-treatment interaction effects, meaning that MI showed significant efficacy at some sites and not at others, sometimes with no overall significant effect when averaging across sites (Ball et al., 2007). This occurs even in controlled trials of medications where the contents of the capsule are fixed (Anton et al., 2006), but variability in effect size seems to be the norm rather than the exception in MI research. What all this suggests to us is that client response to MI is significantly influenced by clinician and contextual aspects of delivery, factors that are not adequately standardized by following a treatment manual. As mentioned earlier, one meta-analysis found that the average effect size of MI was smaller by half when the intervention was manual guided (Hettema et al., 2005).

One guess is that this variability is attributable in part to differences in clinician skill in delivering MI. Many early outcome studies included no measure of counselor MI fidelity at all. Others have relied solely on global adherence ratings (e.g., Chang et al., 2011; Nuro et al., 2005). Therapeutic process research has linked client outcomes to counselor skill on measures of MI fidelity (Daeppen et al., 2010; Gaume et al., 2009; Magill et al., 2010; Moyers, Miller, et al., 2005; Pollak et al., 2009, 2010; Smith, Hall, Jang, & Arndt, 2009; Vader et al., 2010), although other studies have failed to find such a relationship (e.g., Thrasher et al., 2006). It is also fair to say that we are just beginning to understand which aspects of MI practice most influence client outcomes. Miller and Rose (2009) concluded that both therapeutic relationship factors and specific proficiency in eliciting change talk contribute to the efficacy of MI, but it is likely that yet-unidentified aspects of practice are important as well. It is also unclear what level of MI fidelity is "good enough" to promote change. In any event, it is insufficient simply to claim that MI was provided in a clinical study. Outcomes are difficult to interpret apart from information about MI fidelity, for which a range of measures have already been developed and evaluated (Madson & Campbell, 2006; see Chapter 28).

> Both therapeutic relationship factors and specific proficiency contribute to the efficacy of MI.

MI occupies an interesting position within the ongoing discussion of the importance of "specific" factors in psychotherapy (APA Presidential Task Force on Evidence-Based Practice, 2006; Imel, Wampold, & Miller, 2008), precisely because of the hypothesized importance in MI of what are usually regarded to be "general" factors. The quality of therapeutic relationship, for example, has always been a central concern in MI, with empathy as a key construct. If such "nonspecific" or "common" factors are indeed important influences on treatment outcome, then they should be better understood, specified, and taught (Norcross & Wampold, 2011). That is what Carl Rogers and his students attempted to do in hypothesizing and measuring critical conditions for change (Rogers, 1959; Truax & Carkhuff, 1967). Across a broad range of clinical problems, settings, and cultures there seems to be something about this "way of being" with people that promotes positive change (Rogers, 1980b). Similarly, MI is intended to influence client factors that are associated with positive outcomes such as hope, self-efficacy, and active engagement (Bohart & Tallman, 1999; Hubble et al., 1999). It is not as simple, then, as a competition between "specific" effects of MI versus general factors. Our interest is in understanding better what it is about this way of being with people that promotes healthy change regardless of the label applied to it (cf. Wampold, 2007).

We suspect also that MI may benefit from a contrast effect. It is perhaps no accident that MI arose within the addiction field at a time when harsh, confrontational, even abusive treatment practices were acceptable, if not normative (White & Miller, 2007). Compared with such reprehensible treatment, a therapeutic approach that is empathic, compassionate, respectful, and supportive of human strengths and autonomy is likely to shine. MI has taken root in caring for some of the most neglected and rejected members of society. It also seems to take hold in systems that have relied too heavily on authoritarian directing. Even adding a single preparatory session with an empathic MI counselor who was not part of the regular treatment staff has been found to double favorable outcomes (Aubrey, 1998; Bien, Miller, & Boroughs, 1993; Brown & Miller, 1993). In contexts and populations where treatment is already more humane, MI may provide less of a stark contrast. As previously mentioned, a meta-analysis found that the effect size of MI was twice as large when those treated came primarily from U.S. minority groups rather than from the majority white populations (Hettema et al., 2005). Perhaps compassionate listening was a more unusual experience for those from minority backgrounds.

Relatedly, it is possible that training in MI improves outcomes if it suppresses counter-therapeutic responses. An early study found that when MI training yielded modest increases in MI-consistent counselor responses but no decrease in MI-inconsistent responses, the change was not large enough to make any difference in client response (Miller & Mount, 2001). It seems to take relatively few confrontive or directing responses to evoke client defensiveness and lack of change (Miller et al., 1993). One "active ingredient" in MI may simply be a decrease in unhelpful counselor responses.

Beyond these general (but measurable) factors, we also believe that the efficacy of MI is importantly linked to certain aspects of language. In multiple replications, prospective psycholinguistic studies have found that specific forms of client speech during treatment sessions (change talk) presage greater behavior change with MI (Amrhein et al., 2003; Baer et al., 2008; Gaume, Gmel, & Daeppen, 2008; Hodgins, Ching, & McEwen, 2009; Moyers et al., 2007; Moyers, Miller, et al., 2005; Strang & McCambridge, 2004) and in other therapies as well (Aharonovich, Amrhein, Bisaga, Nunes, & Hasin, 2008; Moyers et al., 2007). This could easily be dismissed as a client factor (e.g., that "motivated" clients get better) except that change talk (and its opposite) has been clearly linked to therapist behavior in correlational (Gaume, Bertholet, Faouzi, Gmel, & Daeppen, 2010; Miller et al., 1993), sequential (Moyers & Martin, 2006; Moyers et al., 2007) and experimental studies (Glynn & Moyers, 2010; Patterson & Forgatch, 1985; Vader et al., 2010). Therapists can learn to increase client change talk (Glynn & Moyers, 2010; Miller et al., 2004). When MI-consistent therapist practices facilitate client change talk, which in turn predicts client behavior change after treatment, a meditational link is being supported. There is also emerging evidence that this process is importantly facilitated by an empathic therapeutic relationship (Gaume et al., 2008; Moyers, Miller, et al., 2005). There is much still to be learned here, and we suspect that such processes underlie the efficacy not only of MI but of other "talk therapies" as well.

A number of studies including multisite trials have compared MI head-to-head with other more extensive treatments (rather than evaluating the additive value of each). Often such "horse race" comparisons have found similar overall efficacy despite the difference in treatment intensity. As such, MI may be a reasonable and specifiable "general factor" control against which to evaluate other active treatments.

As discussed earlier, there have been a number of published trials finding no effect of MI. In some of these there was no measurement of fidelity in treatment delivery. In others, the published quality assurance measures indicated a low level of clinician skill (or at least conscientiousness) in delivering MI. Often the pretrial training of MI providers has been too brief to expect proficiency. It is unsurprising that "MI" would be ineffective when delivered with low fidelity.

There have also been trials, however, where training and fidelity monitoring were done very well and yet no effect of MI was found. As discussed in Chapter 19, such a study conducted by Miller et al. (2003) yielded no trace of efficacy, and we concluded from retrospective process analyses (see Box 19.1) that we had been too restrictive in the therapist manual that was used, preventing the therapists from responding appropriately to client reluctance. If we as the progenitors of MI have inadvertenly made unwise decisions when crafting MI therapist manuals, it is likely that others have done so as well. This restriction of clinical flexibility may account for why the use of a therapist manual was associated with significantly lower effect sizes for MI (Hettema et al., 2005).

Another potential source of variation in the efficacy of MI is the nature of the treated sample. Three studies have reported not merely null but adverse outcomes of MI with clients who were ready for change prior to the intervention (Project Match Research Group, 1997a; Rohsenow et al., 2004; Stotts et al., 2001). Clients who enter treatment ready for change might not be expected to benefit from MI (or at least from the evoking process) since their ambivalence appears already to have been resolved. Null findings have also been reported with populations preselected for failed response to multiple prior intervention attempts (e.g., Kuchipudi, Hobein, Flickinger, & Iber, 1990; Welch, Zagarins, Feinberg, & Garb, 2011). Client characteristics may moderate the efficacy of MI (Ondersma, Winhusen, Erickson, Stine, & Wang, 2009).

Other puzzle pieces are provided by multisite trials. Those directly comparing MI-based interventions with longer or more elaborate treatments have often (Project MATCH Research Group, 1997a; UKATT Research Team, 2005), although not always (Marijuana Treatment Project Research Group, 2004), found no significant difference in efficacy. That is, the average outcomes of MI were as good as those from more intensive evidence-based treatments (cf. Bien, Miller, & Tonigan, 1993). No difference in efficacy has also been reported in several multisite trials in which MI or MET were competing with uncontrolled treatment as usual (Ball et al., 2007; Carroll et al., 2001, 2009; Westerberg, Miller, & Tonigan, 2000). This is in contrast to more positive findings when MI or MET has been *added to* treatment as usual (Hettema et al., 2005). As these large multisite trials with negative findings are incorporated into subsequent meta-analyses the result will be reduction in the computed average effect size of MI, perhaps to the extent of concluding no significant overall effect.

Did the efficacy of MI thus somehow disappear? There is indeed an old medical aphorism to "use new treatments while they still work," reflecting the nonspecific effect of enthusiasm when any novel treatment is introduced. One would then discontinue use of the no-longer-effective treatment and move on to a new "flavor of the month." While there is a kernel of truth in this aphorism, science progresses in a more cumulative way. MI has been found to be effective in many randomized clinical trials conducted by enough different investigators working in various nations and with very different problems to indicate that something significant is happening. The variability in its efficacy across therapists, sites, and studies tells us that we do not yet sufficiently understand what is happening to produce this change when it occurs.

So what about MI matters? There is research support for at least three hypotheses, as alluded to above. First, it seems evident that therapist empathy matters, the quality and nature of interpersonal relationship originally described by Rogers (1959, 1965) and often regarded to be a general or "nonspecific" factor. We have more broadly discussed the underlying spirit of MI (Miller & Rollnick, 2002; Rollnick & Miller, 1995), which tends to be strongly correlated with empathy. Level of counselor empathy predicts variation in client outcomes even when therapists are ostensibly delivering the "same" treatment. Even a manual-guided therapy is not the same treatment when delivered by different therapists (Miller et al., 1980; Project MATCH Research Group, 1998c).

Second, differences in the efficacy of MI may have to do with the concomitant level of MI-inconsistent therapist responses (Baer et al., 2012). Confrontive and directing responses can evoke defensiveness and sustain talk (Glynn & Moyers, 2010; Miller et al., 1993; Patterson & Forgatch, 1985) and can certainly be intermingled with MI-consistent responses. One thing that may be important in MI is not doing the wrong thing.

Third, we have reviewed literature linking MI fidelity to increased client change talk, which in turn predicts subsequent change. We have found that it is possible for counselors to learn and demonstrate substantial levels of MI proficiency without having any significant effect on client change talk (Miller et al., 2004). It is possible that MI is not effective unless and until the clinician is able to strengthen client change talk.

Some Recommendations for Outcome Research

With this background we offer for research colleagues a series of suggestions for future studies of the efficacy of MI. These may also be applicable in psychotherapy research more generally.

1. Train therapists to criterion proficiency before they provide MI in a clinical trial. There is no minimum or sufficient "dose" of training to guarantee competence in MI. The only way to document MI skillfulness is through observed practice. In Chapter 28 we suggest provisional thresholds for competence in MI practice, but as mentioned above it is an open question as to what level of proficiency on which skill measures is good enough. Establish a criterion performance level of proficiency for MI providers in a clinical trial and provide training, feedback, and coaching until each provider reaches it.

2. Document fidelity in the delivery of MI. Showing that clinicians can deliver MI proficiently does not mean that they actually do so in practice. Record all sessions and use a reliable coding instrument to monitor quality of delivery. This enables reporting of the actual level of MI fidelity within the trial.

3. Use ongoing quality assurance. Don't wait until the trial is well along before checking on MI quality. Fidelity monitoring should be immediate and ongoing. Providers who fall below a quality performance threshold can

be given feedback and a corrective action plan with close monitoring, or even decertified from treating further clients until they again demonstrate proficiency (Miller, Moyers, Arciniega, et al., 2005). Fidelity monitoring is discussed in Chapter 28.

4. It is possible to do fidelity monitoring by measuring only counselor responses (Hendrickson et al., 2004; Pierson et al., 2007), but this provides just part of the picture. If, for example, therapist efficacy depends on strengthening client change talk, this cannot be measured without also observing client responses. Coding systems that document both therapist and client responses allow one to do process as well as outcome analyses. An advantage of this is that if a trial fails to show an effect of MI it is possible to determine where the hypothesized causal chain broke down or alternatively why an intervention succeeded (Longabaugh & Wirtz, 2001; Moyers et al., 2009).

5. This leads in turn to a further recommendation: to formulate and then test *a priori* predictions about how and why an MI intervention should succeed or fail in influencing client outcomes. When this is added to an outcome trial, the study not only contributes a plus or minus to the bottom-line "box score" (or meta-analytic effect size) for a treatment, but also contributes to knowledge about how treatments influence outcomes.

6. Whenever possible, measure the endpoint outcome(s) that you care about. You may think that increased client motivation will lead to better retention in treatment, which in turn will trigger behavior change that facilitates better health outcomes, but if the last of these does not occur, do you really care about the rest? And if the desired outcome (in this case, improved health) occurs, does it matter if a paper-and-pencil measure of motivation didn't show change?

7. If you are comparing MI with an alternative intervention (including treatment-as-usual or a "placebo" condition), it is worthwhile to document MI fidelity and processes within both conditions. Change talk can occur in any form of treatment and its linkage to client outcome is not restricted to MI (Moyers et al., 2007). To what extent were therapeutic aspects of MI also present in and contributing to the outcomes of the condition(s) with which it was compared?

8. Be cautious if you use a manual to standardize the delivery of MI. Flexibility is key in the practice of MI, responding in the moment to whatever the client is offering. Manuals that tie the practitioner's hands regarding how and when to respond are unlikely to produce good practice. Therapists need discretion for when and whether to persist in delivering particular aspects of an intervention, depending on the client's responses. MI is foremost a clinical style, and not one amenable to formulaic presentation.

Throughout the development of MI we have sought, as Carl Rogers did, to subject our assumptions and interventions to scientific verification. Most of the important changes reflected in this volume are in response to evidence emerging from research published since our second edition. As often happens, research has provided not only some answers but also new and better questions. New clinical trials have continued to report positive effects of MI in promoting change in a widening array of areas. At the same time the wide variability of efficacy of MI has become clear, with effect size differing substantially across studies, therapists, and sites within multisite trials. The consensus use of a therapist manual to standardize practice may not be a good idea with MI, particularly if it limits the practitioner's ability to respond to clients flexibly.

We are confident that there are some powerful change catalysts operating within the domain that we have called MI. There is reasonable evidence to support a few of them, including empathic listening, strengthening change talk, and refraining from countertherapeutic responses that evoke defensiveness and inhibit change. We are also confident that most of what there is to know about MI and change is yet to be discovered. We believe that the therapeutic processes we have been observing and practicing are not unique to MI, and in a sense are more broadly about human nature. Yet, at least in part, they can be specified, learned, and applied to help people change. We are not particular about whether this is called MI. Our interest has always been in coming to a better understanding of why and how people change and in learning how to use that knowledge to alleviate human suffering.

KEY POINTS

✓ MI was not derived from a preexisting theory but emerged from clinical experience that generated testable hypotheses.

✓ The effectiveness of MI varies widely across counselors, studies, and sites within studies.

✓ Fidelity of delivery is an important consideration in understanding outcomes of MI and should be well documented in future studies using reliable observational codes.

CHAPTER 28

Evaluating
Motivational Conversations

> People cannot benefit from a treatment to which
> they are not exposed.
> —DEAN FIXSEN

> Doubt, doubt, and don't believe without experiment.
> —WILLIAM BLAKE

From the preceding chapters as well as the MI outcome research it is clear that there is no simple technique of MI that can be dispensed like the contents of a medication capsule. It matters very much how the conversation unfolds, and there is large variability in outcomes depending on the nature of the interaction.

In this final chapter we come full circle to the topic that first led us to MI: How best to have conversations about change. We have over the years become particularly fascinated with understanding the dynamics of such conversations. Our focus at this point in the book is on how to keep learning from experience, how to study the melodies and rhythms of the dance. While this is an appropriately broad topic with which to conclude, it also has direct implications for quality assurance and we will consider how to answer the practical question, "Is this good MI?"

THE DANCE

The beauty of a dance is influenced by many factors. Certainly the skill of each dancer matters, how their expertise blends to form a smooth flow or tell a good story. Each person brings something important to the dance. The music matters, as does the size and nature of the stage or hall that provide a context. There are also many different types of dances: the back and forth of a cha-cha, the smooth, fast-moving lines of a waltz, the structure of line dancing or square dancing. In a tango one person is clearly in charge and the other following. Disco and salsa are more free-form. In competition dancing the judges ask themselves, "What about this dance really worked (or didn't)?" We don't want to press this metaphor too far, but it does provide a loose structure for considering the contributions of the dancers, the context and the process of the dance itself, and for asking what kind of dance MI is.

Partner 1: The Client

People come to conversations about change with different starting points. By virtue of stage in life, some have more energy, perspective, or life experience than others. In many cultures men and women dance differently. In conversation style, for example, American men are on average more likely to interrupt and less likely to listen well as compared to women.

The urgency of change also matters. How severe are the problems and consequences of the status quo? A fundamental insight of the transtheoretical model is that people come to conversations about change with very different levels of readiness. Some arrive already decided and committed to change. Some are ambivalent and less ready, and still others see no reason for change and may even resent having the conversation at all. All of these starting points can influence the course of a conversation and the likelihood that it will lead to change. Yet if we have learned one thing along the way it is that the starting point is not destiny. It is not necessary to wait and hope for the person to come around to readiness.

> It is not necessary to wait and hope for the person to come around to readiness.

Partner 2: The Interviewer

Another large influence is the skill of the interviewer who might be thought of as a lead dancer. Leading need not be forceful. Indeed, a good dance should not look like a power struggle. How skillful is the interviewer in dancing with many different kinds of partners, in not stepping on toes, and in gently and enjoyably guiding the process of the dance? It is clear that the likelihood of a conversation leading to change has much to do with variations in interviewer skill.

The Context

Where and why is this conversation happening, and what music is playing? Heavy metal is not conducive to waltzing. Some professional contexts provide serious obstacles to having a constructive conversation about change. It may not be impossible, but at least it's more difficult. How much room is there to move? The client's own social context also matters. Who else is on the dance floor? How much support for change is there among the client's family, friends, and associates?

The Process

This is where we have devoted most of our attention: the dance itself, the process of conversations about change. Within whatever limits may be imposed by the context or the particular person, what can I do to help this go well? When all the elements come together—the dancers and the hall and the music—what worked (or didn't) about this particular dance? Within MI the convergence of client, clinician, and context shapes the process of the conversation (see Box 28.1).

In evaluating a motivational conversation it is clearly insufficient to wait outside the dance hall and ask Partner 2 how well they danced together. For a host of reasons people are not particularly reliable reporters of their own skillfulness in MI. There are things they miss in the busyness of the process. For people who are not depressed there is a natural human tendency to overestimate their own performance. Whether to judge the quality of the dance, to offer some helpful pointers, or just to enjoy the dance itself it is necessary to observe it. There is no substitute for seeing (or at least hearing) what actually transpired in a conversation. Such observation is also the only way to tell others (as in a clinical or scientific report) what actually transpired.

Yet raw observation itself has its shortcomings. It is easy to get caught up in the dance, in the content of a client's story, and miss important process

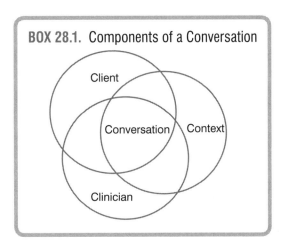

BOX 28.1. Components of a Conversation

details. People also have observational biases regarding what to attend to and what is important. We have found that it helps, therefore, also to have some structure to use when observing.

THE JOY OF CODING

Before we really got into it, we assumed that structured coding of clinical conversations would be deadly dull. In large doses it can be, and people vary in their dose tolerance, but we know no better way to get right inside what is happening in a conversation about change. Like anyone else we can enjoy just sitting back and appreciating the beauty and artful flow of a skillful conversation, but there is much more to learn beneath the surface. Here is some of what we and others have learned about how to document and learn from conversations.

The Raw Material

The most commonly used source material is probably audio recording. There is disagreement about how much video images add. On one hand, there are things that one can observe only from video recording: facial expressions, gestures, eye contact, and such. Sometimes the picture is also helpful in understanding what the words mean. On the other hand, some coders have found that the picture can be distracting and it is easier to focus on the words and sound of speech with audio alone. Audio and video recording also differ, of course, in obtrusiveness. Audio recording tends to be much simpler, and both clients and clinicians may be more nervous about video. A good external microphone tends to make speech more understandable than the built-in variety, although sound has improved greatly with more recent technology. Test it before you rely on it. Struggling to hear a poor recording is frustrating.

Transcribing a recorded conversation takes the raw material a step further. It is easier to follow a recorded conversation with a transcript in hand. A transcript also allows for more detailed step-by-step analysis of a conversation, and it is the only way to do certain kinds of coding reliably. We find transcripts very handy in helping people learn subtleties of MI.

A related question is how long a practice segment should be in order to have a representative sample of the conversation. Some consultations are necessarily brief, thus imposing an inherent length limit. Health behavior discussions within primary care are often of this kind—just a few minutes in duration (Rollnick, Miller, et al., 2008). When conversations are longer (like a 50-minute counseling session), how much of the interaction needs to be coded to get an adequate sample? This is a researchable question with no simple answer thus far. For shorter consultations the entire conversation can be coded. Coding of 20-minute clips within longer consultations can show reliable effects of training (Miller et al., 2004) but may miss crucial aspects of the interaction. In one study, for example, we chose the first 20 minutes of an MI session as our sample (Miller, Yahne, et al., 2003), but it turned out in later analysis of the entire sessions that client outcomes were predicted by what happened toward the end, not at the beginning of the conversation (Amrhein et al., 2003; cf. Bertholet, Faouzi, Gmel, Gaume & Daeppen, 2010; Campbell, Adamson, & Carter, 2010).

Another issue regards which practice samples to use. If clinicians select the sessions to be evaluated, they might naturally be expected to offer what they regard as their best performance. This would provide a best-case indication of the ability to demonstrate MI but not necessarily of the extent and quality of MI in regular practice. In clinical trials the common procedure is to record all consultations and evaluate a random or representative sample, with the clinician not knowing which sessions will be selected (Carroll et al., 1998; Miller, Moyers, Arciniega, Ernst, & Forcehimes, 2005). It can also happen that MI occupies only a portion of a session that includes other tasks as well, and it would make sense to focus on the segment where the intention was to provide MI.

Global Ratings

So what should you observe and how might it be recorded? Perhaps the easiest form of coding for a conversation is to do global ratings of quality, perhaps on a 1–5 Likert scale. For example, to what extent did the interviewer show accurate empathy, or more specifically, offer complex reflections? Such ratings might be done after listening to an entire interview or repeated at various intervals (e.g., every 5 or 10 minutes). Because global words like *empathy* and *reflection* can mean various things to different people it helps to have a clear, detailed description of the characteristics to be rated, a tradition in psychotherapy research that can be traced to Carl Rogers's own research group (Truax & Carkhuff, 1967). Having a clear definition can improve the reliability of ratings—the extent to which two independent raters will come up with the same answer. Box 28.2 provides an example of the level of detailed definition that is helpful in achieving reliable global ratings—in this case for counselor empathy.

Although they tend to be quick if not easy, global ratings also have some substantial disadvantages. Even with good definitions it is difficult to achieve interrater reliability with global scales. They require some accumulation of evidence across an entire conversation or segment—for example, as an average or as the highest level of skill demonstrated. Also, global ratings tend to be less useful than more specific feedback when it comes to helping people learn. Remember that global goals (e.g., "to be a better person") are harder to achieve or measure than more specific ones ("to give

BOX 28.2. An Operational Definition of Counselor Empathy

This scale measures the extent to which the clinician understands or makes an effort to grasp the client's perspective and feelings: literally, how much the clinician attempts to "try on" what the client feels or thinks. Empathy should not be confused with warmth, acceptance, genuineness, or client advocacy; these are independent of the empathy rating. Reflective listening is an important part of this characteristic, but this global rating is intended to capture all efforts that the clinician makes to understand the client's perspective and convey that understanding to the client.

Clinicians **low** in empathy show indifference or active dismissal of the client's perspective and experiences. They may probe for factual information or to pursue an agenda, but they do so to "build a case" for their point of view, rather than for the sole purpose of understanding the client's perspective. There is little effort to gain a deeper understanding of complex events and emotions, and questions asked reflect shallowness or impatience. They might express hostility toward the client's viewpoint or directly blame the client for negative outcomes.

Clinicians **high** in empathy approach the session as an opportunity to learn about the client. They are curious. They spend time exploring the client's opinions and ideas about the target behavior especially. Empathy is evident when providers show an active interest in understanding what the client is saying. It can also be apparent when the clinician accurately follows or perceives a complex story or statement by the client or probes gently to gain clarity.

Verbal Anchors for Ratings on the 1–5 Scale of Empathy

1. Clinician has no apparent interest in client's point of view. Gives little or no attention to the client's perspective.

   Examples:
   - Asking only information-seeking questions (often with an ulterior motive).
   - Probing for factual information with no attempt to understand the client's perspective.

2. Clinician makes sporadic efforts to explore the client's perspective. Clinicians' understanding may be inaccurate or may detract from the client's true meaning.

   Examples:
   - Clinician offers reflections but they misinterpret what the client had said.
   - Clinician displays shallow attempts to understand the client.

(cont.)

BOX 28.2. *(cont.)*

3. Clinician is actively trying to understand the client's perspective, with modest success.

   Examples:
   - Clinician displays average empathy to client.
   - Clinician may offer a few accurate reflections, but may miss the client's point.
   - Clinician makes an attempt to grasp the client's meaning throughout the session, but does so with mild success.

4. Clinician shows evidence of accurate understanding of client's worldview. Makes active and repeated efforts to understand client's point of view. Understanding mostly limited to explicit content.

   Examples:
   - Clinician conveys interest in the client's perspective or situation.
   - Clinician offers accurate reflections of what the client has said.
   - Clinician effectively communicates understanding of the client's viewpoint.

5. Clinician shows evidence of deep understanding of client's point of view, not just for what has been explicitly stated but what the client means and has not said.

   Examples:
   - Clinician effectively communicates an understanding of the client beyond what the client says in session.
   - Showing great interest in client's perspective or situation.
   - Attempting to "put self in client's shoes."
   - Often encouraging client to elaborate, beyond what is necessary to merely follow the story.
   - Using many accurate complex reflections.

   _____

   Note. Based on Hendrickson et al. (2004).

people more positive and less negative feedback"). Telling a learner that "you need to be more empathic" is less likely to be helpful than "Try using more reflections and fewer questions," or "Make a bit more of a guess when you reflect instead of just repeating what the person said." Global feedback doesn't really tell a learner what to do differently, nor does it help a coach remember what specifically to suggest. Global ratings are harder to compare across settings or studies because teams develop different

> Global feedback doesn't tell a learner what to do differently.

standards for their ratings. Finally, because it is difficult if not impossible to make objective self-ratings on global scales like these, they are not particularly useful when listening to one's own conversations. We therefore do not recommend relying on global rating scales alone to document fidelity.

More Specific Practice Measures

We tend to use more specific measures in addition to rather than instead of global ratings. Having both provides more information, although in giving feedback to learners we typically focus more on specifics, on what would be a good next step in developing skill.

A commonly used approach is to count something—how often it occurred. Here, too, you need a clear definition of what it is you're listening for in order to know it when you hear it and to improve interrater reliability. With a reliable measure two independent coders will come up with similar counts. An example definition of a countable interviewer response (reflection) is shown in Box 28.3. Detailed and tested behavioral definitions of this kind can be found in the Motivational Interviewing Treatment Integrity code (Bennett, Roberts, Vaughan, Gibbins, & Rouse, 2007; Forsberg, Berman, Källmén, Hermansson, & Helgason, 2008; Forsberg, Källmén,

---

BOX 28.3. An Operational Definition of a Reflection

Reflective listening statements are made by the clinician in response to client statements. A reflection may introduce new meaning or material, but it essentially captures and returns to clients something about what they have just said. Reflections are further categorized as simple or complex reflections.

Simple reflections typically convey understanding or facilitate client–clinician exchanges. These reflections add little or no meaning (or emphasis) to what clients have said. Simple reflections may mark very important or intense client emotions, but do not go far beyond the client's original intent in the statement.

Complex reflections typically add substantial meaning or emphasis to what the client has said. These reflections serve the purpose of conveying a deeper or more complex picture of what the client has said. Sometimes the clinician may choose to emphasize a particular part of what the client has said to make a point or take the conversation in a different direction. Clinicians may add subtle or very obvious content to the client's words, or they may combine statements from the client to form complex summaries.

When a coder cannot distinguish between a simple and complex reflection, the default category is simple reflection.

Note. Based on Hendrickson et al. (2004).

Hermansson, Berman, & Helgason, 2007; Moyers, Martin, et al., 2005), which can be downloaded from *www.motivationalinterviewing.org*.

Here are some specific interviewer responses based on material presented in earlier chapters. For learning purposes these can be counted "on the fly" while listening to a recorded conversation, although reliable coding for research purposes typically requires the use of transcripts.

Questions

One of the easier forms of speech to code is a question, a request for information. As discussed in Chapter 6, closed questions are those asking for specific information. Any question that can anticipate a "yes" or "no" answer is a closed question. So are those that request very specific information ("What is your mother's name?") or a numeric answer ("How many minutes of exercise did you do this week?"). In essence, closed questions tightly restrict the range of answers that the person can provide. Open questions, in contrast, allow for wider latitude in answering. ("What brings you here today?" or "How do you think you could do that?") "Tell me . . ." statements can also be open questions ("Tell me about how a typical day goes for you") even if your voice does not inflect up at the end. Any "reflection" where the voice inflects upward rather than downward at the end is a question ("You don't really think this is a problem?" vs. "You don't really think this is a problem").

So one thing that is easier to track in a conversation is how many questions were asked, and of those how many were open versus closed questions. The Open Question Percentage is the number of open questions asked divided by the total number questions (open plus closed).

Reflections

Reflections were thoroughly discussed in Chapter 5. They are always in response to something that the person has said. They essentially capture and reflect back to the person something about what he or she just said. Simple reflections add little or no meaning or emphasis beyond what the person said. They basically repeat the content, perhaps with some rewording, but there is not much of a guess involved as to what the person meant. Complex reflections, in contrast, do make a guess about meaning beyond the content that was spoken.

CLIENT: I had a really hard time sticking to my diet this week.

SIMPLE REFLECTION: It was difficult for you.

COMPLEX REFLECTION: You're wondering whether you'll be able to lose weight this way.

The number of reflections offered during a conversation can also be counted, dividing them into simple versus complex reflections. Two measures that we consider in conversations about change are the interviewer's percentage of complex reflections and the ratio of reflections to questions.

MI-Consistent and MI-Inconsistent Responses

Besides reflections and questions, it is possible to listen for other MI-consistent responses. Here are some examples from the Motivational Interviewing Treatment Integrity (MITI) code (Moyers, Martin, et al., 2005; Pierson et al., 2007):

- Asking permission before giving advice or information (Chapter 11).
- Affirming and supporting—saying something positive about the person (Chapter 6) or expressing compassion.
- Emphasizing the person's freedom of choice, autonomy, and control.

There are also certain responses that are generally inconsistent with an MI style and are mirror opposites of the above. These include:

- Giving advice or information without permission.
- Confronting the person by disagreeing, arguing, correcting, shaming, blaming, criticizing, labeling, ridiculing, or questioning the person's honesty (see Thomas Gordon's "roadblocks" in Chapter 5).
- Directing the person by giving orders, commands, or imperatives, or otherwise challenging the person's autonomy.

An index here is the percentage of MI consistency (number of MI-consistent divided by total MI-consistent + MI-inconsistent responses).

Coding Client Responses

A conversation, of course, involves language from both (or all) participants. Observational systems like the MITI that code only one side of the conversation (the interviewer's responses) can yield reliable estimates of MI proficiency that do predict client outcome, but they reflect only half of the picture. The original system for coding both interviewer and client responses within an MI conversation is the Motivational Interviewing Skill Code (MISC; Catley et al., 2006; de Jonge, Schippers, & Schaap, 2005; Gaume et al., 2010; Miller & Mount, 2001; Moyers et al., 2003).

To what client responses should one particularly attend within a conversation about change? From an MI perspective, especially important client speech would be change talk and sustain talk (Chapter 12), precisely because they presage and mediate change outcomes. The ratio of change talk to sustain talk appears to be a particularly promising index, and one that can be expected to change over the course of an MI session (Chapter 19).

It is also sensible to consider client change talk as an index of MI skillfulness. It appears to be easier to increase clinicians' MI-consistent responding (as measured by the MITI) than to teach them how to increase their clients' change talk (Miller & Mount, 2001; Miller et al., 2004). Yet if our understanding of how MI works is correct, the latter skill is particularly important. What does it matter whether clinicians practice in a more MI-consistent way if their clients don't respond any differently?

Sequential Analyses

A more fine-grained analysis examines sequential relationships within the conversation. For example, when a client offers change talk, what is this interviewer's next response likely to be (see Chapter 14)? What happens when an interviewer reflects sustain talk? What is the client likely to say next? Analysis at this level can yield even more specific suggestions for skill improvement (e.g., "When the client gives you change talk, try reflecting it more often") than might emerge from simple response counts (e.g., "Offer more reflections") or global ratings (e.g., "Be more empathic"). A well-developed tool for sequential analysis of conversations about change is the Motivational Interviewing Sequential Code for Observing Process Exchanges (MI-SCOPE; *casaa.unm.edu/download/scope.pdf*; Moyers & Martin, 2006; Moyers et al., 2007, 2009). Free software is also available for analyzing SCOPE data (Glynn et al., 2011; *casaa.unm.edu/dload.html*).

Proficiency and the Four Processes

Having introduced in this edition four processes that MI comprises, we briefly consider now how proficiency might be assessed in each of these processes.

Engaging as we understand it involves the use of client-centered counseling skills as described in Part II. These would be reflected in MITI global ratings for empathy, spirit, and collaboration. More specific practice skills would include OARS: open questions, affirmations, reflections, and summaries, the percentages of open questions and complex reflections, and the ratio of reflections to questions. These in turn should be reflected in client measures of working alliance, retention, and clinicians occupying less than 50% of talk time.

Focusing involves clarifying and then maintaining direction toward one or more identified change goals. Unless the client or context immediately define what the goal(s) should be, there would be an observable process of discussing the possible objectives of treatment. The MITI global measure of direction reflects the maintaining of a clear focus. Clients' working alliance ratings of goal agreement would also be pertinent to this dimension.

Evoking is the process that particularly characterizes MI and differentiates it from other approaches. It is difficult to obtain reliable ratings of a clinician response to "evoke change talk," precisely because there are so many different ways to do it and the rater must infer clinician intention. The evocation rating is a global evaluation of the extent to which this occurred. A straightforward client measure is the occurrence of change talk, which is the intended result of clinician evoking, and the ratio of client change talk to sustain talk. It is also possible within sequential coding to measure the extent to which clinicians recognize and respond appropriately to change talk by enumerating clinician behaviors that immediately follow occurrences of client change talk (OARS; see Chapter 14).

Planning is evident in clinician attempts to elicit and shape specific plans for how and when to implement change effects. A recapitulation and key question (see Chapter 19) is a discrete observable sequence, although planning can be initiated in many other ways. Open questions about *doing* (as opposed to DARN) tend to occur in planning. One possibility would be to code open questions in terms of the type of change talk they solicit, based on the verbs they contain; for example:

> "What would you *like* to be different?" [Desire]
> "What do you think you *could* do?" [Ability]
> "What would be some good *reasons* to make this change?" [Reasons]
> "How *important* is it for you to do this?" [Need]
> "So what do you think you *will* do?" [Commitment]
> "What are you *willing* to do?" [Activation]
> "What steps have you already taken?" [Taking steps]

If clinician responses can be identified that specifically demarcate each of the four processes it would become possible to code the extent to which each of the four processes occurred during a given conversation or segment of a session. It would not be expected, of course, that all four processes would occur within every MI session. Identified coding of the processes would permit study of the placement and extent of each over the course of one or more sessions and the relationship of processes to client outcomes.

Performance Thresholds in Motivational Interviewing

There is no predetermined adequate dose of training in MI. Learners have different levels of initial skillfulness and also vary in how quickly they develop proficiency in MI. It makes sense, therefore, to coach providers to criterion-based levels of skill rather than assuming that certain training experiences will be sufficient (Martino et al., 2011).

It remains an unresolved issue what level of MI competence is good enough. An immediate question is, "Good enough for what?" Once a particular objective is identified (e.g., to increase condom use in HIV-positive individuals through brief health care consultations), it is then an empirical question as to what level of MI skill is required. Is there a threshold proficiency level below which change is less likely to occur? And what are the most important benchmarks of the needed clinical skill? It is likely that sufficiency thresholds and key component skills will vary depending on the task at hand and the context.

As a provisional guideline we have suggested the following target criteria when developing skill in MI. Two levels of skill are described: (1) basic competency and (2) proficiency. We readily admit that we simply made these criteria up based on our experience, and they will surely need adjustment as more is learned about the skill levels needed for particular tasks and contexts. Whether these are "good enough" for a certain application we do not know, but here they are in Box 28.4. Every clinician is likely to vary on these indices from one interview or client to the next, so our guidelines represent averages. It is also the case that even very proficient clinicians would not hit every benchmark on every interview. These are meant as starting points to be improved with further research and experience.

As discussed above, another possible metric in learning MI is to track increases in client change talk. Because typical amounts of change talk vary substantially across clients and populations, the most appropriate reference for comparison may be with the learner's own pretraining levels.

Client Change

What does it matter if clinicians practice in a more MI-consistent manner *and* their clients offer more change talk but don't actually change? From the perspective of a treatment or funding agency what may matter most is the impact on client outcomes. Is there a significant improvement in client retention, adherence, and change as clinicians become more skilled with motivational conversations? Are there significant outcome differences among clinicians related to their skillfulness in MI?

This in turn raises the question of what is "significant," that is, how large an improvement matters. The usual standard in clinical research is statistical significance; for example, a change the magnitude of which would occur by chance only one time in twenty ($p < .05$), or a risk ratio with a confidence interval that does not overlap with 1.0. With large samples, however, it is possible to obtain statistical significance for relatively small effects. In fact, power analysis is used to determine how many participants should be included in a study in order to render the expected

---

BOX 28.4. Provisional Competency and Proficiency Thresholds

The following are performance indices based on the Motivational Interviewing Treatment Integrity (MITI) code:

Index	Computation	Basic competency	Proficiency
Global spirit ratings	Ratings on 1–5 scales	3.5 average	4.0 average
% complex reflections	Number of complex reflections divided by total reflections (simple + complex)	≥ 40%	≥ 50%
% open questions	Number of open questions divided by total questions (open + closed)	≥ 50%	≥ 70%
Reflection-to-question ratio	Number of reflections divided by number of questions	≥ 1.0	≥ 2.0
% MI consistent	Number of MI-consistent responses divided by number of MI-consistent and MI-inconsistent	≥ 90%	≥ 98%

---

effect statistically significant. A different question is whether a change of this magnitude would be regarded by clinicians as meaningful. Metrics of "clinical significance" are used to estimate meaningful change (e.g., the percentage of patients whose improvements fall within a range that physicians regard to be medically meaningful). It is possible to power studies to detect an effect size that is clinically (rather than just statistically) meaningful (Miller & Manuel, 2008).

A further consideration is *when* to look for change. In pharmacotherapy research the effect of a medication is expected during active treatment, but with a motivational conversation that is intended to affect subsequent behavior, its effect on health outcomes may not appear until later, which is sometimes called a sleeper effect. Such delayed effects would not be expected once a medication has been discontinued, but in psychotherapy research the standard for clinical significance has usually been whether change appears or endures during follow-up after treatment has been discontinued (Miller, LoCastro, Longabaugh, O'Malley, & Zweben, 2005). This would surely be true for brief interventions intended to affect motivation for change (e.g., Mason, Pate, Drapkin, & Sozinho, 2011). The effect on slower-moving outcome measures (e.g., weight loss or HbA1C levels in people with diabetes) would not be expected to appear immediately after the motivational conversation. Rather, the anticipated effect would be to increase health behaviors that over time will influence health outcomes. The average effects of MI on certain endpoints have been found to be larger at later rather than earlier follow-up points (Hettema et al., 2005).

Finally, we encourage meditational analyses when studying the impact of motivational conversations. Brief interventions of this kind are usually expected to affect certain client variables that in turn would lead to the hoped-for changes in outcome (Tevyaw & Monti, 2004). Causal chain analysis makes these implicit assumptions explicit by measuring each component in the anticipated sequence of effects (Longabaugh & Wirtz, 2001). When a beneficial effect is found it is possible to ascertain whether the intervention worked for the predicted reason. When the expected effect is not observed, one can determine where the causal chain failed.

SUMMING UP:
THE FAR SIDE OF COMPLEXITY

Motivational interviewing is a work in progress. We have sought in this third edition to convey our current understanding of the spirit, method, and skills involved and to reflect fairly what has been learned from the rapidly growing volume of research on MI. Three decades after its introduction, MI is a clinical intervention that is:

- *Evidence-based.* More than 200 randomized clinical trials have been published, with both positive and negative findings.
- *Relatively brief.* MI has been tested most often as an intervention of 1 to 4 sessions, and even with relatively brief consultation of 15 minutes or less.
- *Specifiable and verifiable.* Reliable and valid tools have been developed to measure the quality of MI being delivered (Madson & Campbell, 2006).
- *With testable mechanisms of action.* Several potential mediators of the effectiveness of motivational conversations have been evaluated, and no doubt others will be specified and tested.
- *Generalizable across problem areas.* Beneficial effects of MI have been observed across a broad range of change goals.

- *Complementary to other treatment methods.* MI is not a comprehensive treatment but was designed as a tool for addressing a particular clinical task: to resolve ambivalence in the direction of change. It is complementary to a variety of other therapeutic approaches.
- *Learnable by a broad range of providers.* MI appears to be learnable by providers from a wide variety of professional and educational backgrounds.

In summary, MI provides a somewhat structured and testable way to think about (and have) constructive conversations about change. Our own sense of this phenomenon of MI is not as something that we invented but rather like a rising wave on which we have been delighting in the ride, trying to stay on top of it, and eager to see where and how far it will go. If in a decade there is a fourth edition we cannot guess now how it will differ, any more than we anticipated the developments of the second and third editions from their predecessors.

MI began with some simple insights gleaned from clinical practice. The years have added layers of complexity in understanding the nature, practice, processes, and learning of MI, reflected now in dozens of books and translations and in many hundreds of articles and chapters. No doubt some of this complexity is superfluous and some current beliefs about MI will later be found to be at least in part inaccurate. Our hope is that out of complexity will emerge a greater simplicity.

> Out of complexity will emerge a greater simplicity.

While we hold a parental fondness for this growing child that we have nurtured, and entertain some worries for its future development, we have come far enough together to stand back in wonderment and curiosity to see what will happen next. We do not own it and do not wish to control its life course, nor could we. Motivational interviewing has ventured out into the world, and we hope that, whatever its course, it may contribute to the humanization of services and of conversations about change.

KEY POINTS

✓ Observation of actual practice is essential in quality assurance and in documenting fidelity of delivery.

✓ Global scales provide one way to rate practice but are not sufficient in themselves for measuring quality of delivery or providing useful feedback to clinicians who are learning MI.

✓ Behavioral measures facilitate comparison across studies and provide more specific information on which to base helpful feedback.

✓ Observational ratings should also track the occurrence of MI-inconsistent clinician responses such as confronting or giving advice without permission.

✓ Including behavioral measures of client as well as clinician responses permits analysis of therapeutic processes.

APPENDIX A

Glossary of Motivational Interviewing Terms

Ability—A form of client *preparatory change talk* that reflects perceived personal capability of making a change; typical words include *can*, *could*, and *able*.

Absolute Worth—One of four aspects of *acceptance* as a component of MI *spirit*, prizing the inherent value and potential of every human being.

Acceptance—One of four central components of the underlying *spirit* of MI by which the interviewer communicates *absolute worth*, *accurate empathy*, *affirmation*, and *autonomy support*.

Accurate Empathy—The skill of perceiving and reflecting back another person's meaning; one of four aspects of *acceptance* as a component of MI *spirit*.

Activation Language—A form of client *mobilizing change talk* that expresses disposition toward action, but falls short of *commitment language*; typical words include *ready*, *willing*, *considering*.

Affirmation—One of four aspects of *acceptance* as a component of MI *spirit*, by which the counselor accentuates the positive, seeking and acknowledging a person's strengths and efforts.

Affirming—An interviewer statement valuing a positive client attribute or behavior.

Agenda Mapping—A short *focusing* metaconversation in which you step back with the client to choose a *direction* from among several options.

Agreement with a Twist—A *reflection*, *affirmation*, or accord followed by a reframe.

Ambivalence—The simultaneous presence of competing motivations for and against change.

Amplified Reflection—A response in which the interviewer reflects back the client's content with greater intensity than the client had expressed; one form of response to client *sustain talk* or *discord*.

Apologizing—A way of responding to *discord* by taking partial responsibility.

Assessment Feedback—Providing a client with personal feedback of findings from an evaluation, often in relation to normative ranges; see *Motivational Enhancement Therapy*.

Assessment Trap—The clinical error of beginning consultation with expert information gathering at the cost of not listening to the client's concerns. See also *Question–Answer Trap*.

Autonomy Support—One of four aspects of *acceptance* as a component of MI *spirit*, by which the interviewer accepts and confirms the client's irrevocable right to self-determination and choice.

Blaming Trap—The clinical error of focusing on blame or fault-finding rather than change.

Bouquet—A particular kind of *summary* that collects and emphasizes the client's *change talk*.

Brainstorming—Generating options without initially critiquing them.

CATs—An acronym for three subtypes of client *mobilizing change talk*: Commitment, Activation, and *Taking Steps*.

Change Goal—A specific target for change in *motivational interviewing*; typically a particular behavior change, although it may also be a broader goal (e.g., glycemic control) toward which there are multiple avenues of approach.

Change Plan—A specific scheme to implement a *change goal*.

Change Ruler—A rating scale, usually 0–10, used to assess a client's motivation for a particular change; see *Confidence Ruler* and *Importance Ruler*.

Change Talk—Any client speech that favors movement toward a particular *change goal*.

Chat Trap—The clinical error of engaging in excessive small talk and informal chat that does not further the processes *of engaging, focusing, evoking*, and *planning*.

Client-centered Counseling—See *Person-centered Counseling*.

Closed Question—A question that asks for yes/no, a short answer, or specific information.

Coaching—The process of helping someone to acquire skill.

Collaboration—See *Partnership*.

Collecting Summary—A special form of *reflection* that pulls together a series of interrelated items that the person has offered. See also *Summary*.

Coming Alongside—A response to persistent *sustain talk* or *discord* in which the interviewer accepts and reflects the client's theme.

Commitment Language—A form of client *mobilizing change talk* that reflects intention or disposition to carry out change; common verbs include *will, do, going to*.

Compassion—One of four central components of the underlying *spirit* of MI by which the interviewer acts benevolently to promote the client's welfare, giving priority to the client's needs.

Complex Reflection—An interviewer *reflection* that adds additional or different meaning beyond what the client has just said; a guess as to what the client may have meant.

Confidence Ruler—A scale (typically 0–10) on which clients are asked to rate their level of confidence in their ability to make a particular change.

Confidence Talk—Change talk that particularly bespeaks *ability* to change.

Confront—(1) as a goal: to come face to face with one's current situation and experience; (2) as a practice: an MI-inconsistent interviewer response such as warning, disagreeing, or arguing.

Continuing the Paragraph—A method of *reflective listening* in which the counselor offers what might be the next (as yet unspoken) sentence in the client's paragraph.

DARN—An acronym for four subtypes of client preparatory change talk: *Desire, Ability, Reason*, and *Need*.

Decisional Balance—A choice-focused technique that can be used when counseling with neutrality, devoting equal exploration to the pros and cons of change or of a specific plan.

Depth of Reflection—The extent to which a *reflection* contains more than the literal content of what a person has already said. See also *Complex Reflection*.

Desire—A form of client *preparatory change talk* that reflects a preference for change; typical verbs include *want, wish*, and *like*.

Directing—A natural communication style that involves telling, leading, providing advice, information, or instruction.

Direction—The extent to which an interviewer maintains in-session momentum toward a *change goal*.

Discord—Interpersonal behavior that reflects dissonance in the working relationship; *sustain talk* does not in itself constitute *discord*; examples include arguing, interrupting, discounting, or ignoring.

Discrepancy—The distance between the *status quo* and one or more client *change goals*.

Docere—(Latin verb infinitive) To inform, in the sense of installing knowledge, wisdom, insight; etymologic root of *doctrine, indoctrinate, docent,* and *doctor.*

Double-Sided Reflection—An interviewer *reflection* that includes both client *sustain talk* and *change talk,* usually with the conjunction "and."

Ducere—(Latin verb infinitive) To elicit or draw out; a Socratic approach; etymologic root of education (*e ducere*); compare with *Docere.*

Elaboration—An interviewer response to client *change talk,* asking for additional detail, clarification, or example.

Elicit–provide–elicit—An information exchange process that begins and ends with exploring the client's own experience to frame whatever information is being provided to the client.

Empathy—The extent to which an interviewer communicates accurate understanding of the client's perspectives and experience; most commonly manifested as *reflection.*

Emphasizing Personal Control—An interviewer statement directly expressing *autonomy support,* acknowledging the client's ability for choice and self-determination.

Engaging—The first of four fundamental processes in MI, the process of establishing a mutually trusting and respectful helping relationship.

Envisioning—Client speech that reflects the client imagining having made a change.

Equipoise—The clinician's decision to counsel with neutrality in a way that consciously avoids guiding a client toward one particular choice or change and instead explores the available options equally.

Evocation—One of four central components of the underlying *spirit* of MI by which the interviewer elicits the client's own perspectives and motivation. See also *Ducere.*

Evocative Questions—Strategic open questions the natural answer to which is *change talk.*

Evoking—The third of four fundamental processes of MI, which involves eliciting the person's own motivation for a particular change.

Expert Trap—The clinical error of assuming and communicating that the counselor has the best answers to the client's problems.

Exploring Goals and Values—A strategy for evoking *change talk* by having people describe their most important life goals or values.

Focusing—The second of four fundamental processes of MI, which involves clarifying a particular goal or direction for change.

Following—A natural communication style that involves listening to and following along with the other's experience without inserting one's own material.

Formulation —Developing a shared picture or hypothesis regarding the client's situation and how it might be addressed.

FRAMES—An acronym summarizing six components commonly found in effective brief interventions for alcohol problems: *Feedback, Responsibility, Advice, Menu of options, Empathy,* and *Self-efficacy.*

Goal Attainment Scaling—A method originally developed by Thomas Kiresuk for evaluating treatment outcomes across a range of problem areas.

Goldilocks Principle—In order to be motivating, a discrepancy should be not too large or too small.

Guiding—A natural communication style for helping others find their way, combining some elements of both directing and following.

Implementation Intention—A stated intention or commitment to take a specific action.

Importance Ruler—A scale (typically 0–10) on which clients are asked to rate the importance of making a particular change.

Integrity—To behave in a manner that is consistent with and fulfills one's core values.

Intrinsic Motivation—The disposition and enactment of behavior for its consistency with personal goals and values.

Key Question—A particular form of question offered after a *recapitulation* at the transition from *evoking* to *planning,* that seeks to elicit *mobilizing change talk.*

Labeling Trap—The clinical error of engaging in unproductive struggles to persuade clients to accept a label or diagnosis.

Lagom—(Swedish) Just right; not too large, not too small. See also *Goldilocks Principle.*

Linking Summary—A special form of *reflection* that connects what the person has just said with something you remember from prior conversation. See also *Summary*.

Looking Back—A strategy for evoking client *change talk*, exploring a better time in the past.

Looking Forward—A strategy for evoking client *change talk*, exploring a possible better future that the client hopes for or imagines, or anticipating the future consequences of not changing.

Menschenbild (German)—One's fundamental view of human nature.

MET—An acronym for *Motivational Enhancement Therapy*.

MIA–STEP—A package of training materials for MI supervisors, produced by the U.S. Center for Substance Abuse Treatment.

MINT—The Motivational Interviewing Network of Trainers, founded in 1997 and incorporated in 2008 (*www.motivationalinterviewing.org*).

MISC—The Motivational Interviewing Skill Code, introduced by Miller and Mount as the first system for coding client and interviewer utterances within *motivational interviewing*.

MITI—The Motivational Interviewing Treatment Integrity coding system, simplified from the *MISC* and focusing only on interviewer responses, to document fidelity in MI delivery.

Mobilizing Change Talk—A subtype of client *change talk* that expresses or implies action to change; examples are *commitment*, *activation language*, and *taking steps*.

Motivational Enhancement Therapy (MET)—A combination of *motivational interviewing* with *assessment feedback*, originally developed and tested in Project MATCH.

Motivational Interviewing—
- Lay definition: A collaborative conversation style for strengthening a person's own motivation and commitment to change.
- Clinical definition: A person-centered counseling style for addressing the common problem of ambivalence about change.
- Technical definition: A collaborative, goal-oriented style of communication with particular attention to the language of change, designed to strengthen personal motivation for and commitment to a specific goal by eliciting and exploring the person's own reasons for change within an atmosphere of acceptance and compassion.

Need—A form of client *preparatory change talk* that expresses an imperative for change without specifying a particular reason. Common verbs include *need*, *have to, got to, must*.

OARS—An acronym for four basic client-centered communication skills: *Open question*, *Affirmation*, *Reflection*, and *Summary*.

Open Question—A question that offers the client broad latitude and choice in how to respond; compare with *Closed Question*.

Orienting—The process of finding a direction for change when the focus of consultation is unclear. See also *Focusing*.

Overshooting—A *reflection* that adds intensity to the content or emotion expressed by a client. See also *Amplified Reflection*.

Partnership—One of four central components of the underlying *spirit* of MI by which the interviewer functions as a partner or companion, collaborating with the client's own expertise.

Path Mapping—The process of choosing a *change plan* when there are several possible routes toward the goal.

Permission—Obtaining by the interviewer of client assent before providing advice or information.

Person-centered Counseling—A therapeutic approach introduced by psychologist Carl Rogers in which people explore their own experience within a supportive, empathic, and accepting relationship; also called *client-centered counseling*.

Phase 1—A term used in prior editions of *Motivational Interviewing* to describe the earlier "uphill" period of engaging, guiding, and evoking, in which the general goal is to elicit and strengthen client motivation for change.

Phase 2—A term used in prior editions of *Motivational Interviewing* to describe the latter "downhill" period of planning in which the general goal is to elicit and strengthen *commitment* to a *change goal* and to negotiate a specific *change plan*.

Planning—The fourth fundamental process of MI, which involves developing a specific *change plan* that the client is willing to implement.

Prefacing—A specific form of *permission* in which the interviewer does not directly ask the client's leave to provide information or advice, but instead precedes it with an *autonomy support* statement.

Premature Focus Trap—The clinical error of focusing before engaging, trying to direct before you have established a working collaboration and negotiated common goals.

Preparatory Change Talk—A subtype of client *change talk* that expresses motivations for change without stating or implying specific intent or commitment to do it; examples are *desire*, *ability*, *reason*, and *need*.

Q Sorting—A technique developed by William Stephenson, a colleague of Carl Rogers, in which a person sorts cards describing attributes into piles ranging from "not like me" to "very much like me."

Querying Extremes—A strategy for evoking *change talk* by asking clients to imagine best consequences of change or worst consequences of *status quo.*

Question–Answer Trap—The clinical error of asking too many questions, leaving the client in the passive role of answering them. See also *Assessment Trap.*

Reactance—The natural human tendency to reassert one's freedom when it appears to be threatened.

Readiness Ruler—See *Change Ruler.*

Reason—A form of client *preparatory change talk* that describes a specific if–then motive for change.

Recapitulation—A *bouquet* summary offered at the transition from *evoking* to *planning,* drawing together the client's *change talk.*

Reflective Listening—The skill of "active" listening whereby the counselor seeks to understand the client's subjective experience, offering *reflections* as guesses about the person's meaning. See also *Accurate Empathy.*

Reflection—An interviewer statement intended to mirror meaning (explicit or implicit) of preceding client speech. See also *Simple Reflection, Complex Reflection.*

Reframe—An interviewer statement that invites the client to consider a different interpretation of what has been said.

Resistance—A term previously used in MI, now deconstructed into its components: *sustain talk* and *discord.*

Righting Reflex—The natural desire of helpers to set things right, to prevent harm and promote client welfare.

Running Head Start—A strategy for eliciting client *change talk* in which the interviewer first explores perceived "good things" about the status quo, in order to then query the "not-so-good things."

Self-Actualization—The pursuit and realization of one's core values—becoming what one is meant to be. See also *Telos.*

Self-Disclosure—Sharing something of oneself that is true when there is good reason to expect that it will be helpful to the client.

Self-Efficacy—A client's perceived ability to successfully achieve a particular goal or perform a particular task; term introduced by Albert Bandura.

Self-Esteem—A client's general level of perceived worth.

Self-Motivational Statement—See *Change Talk*.

Self-Regulation—The ability to develop a plan of one's own and to implement behavior in order to carry it out.

Shifting Focus—A way of responding to *discord* by redirecting attention and discussion to a less contentious topic or perspective.

Simple Reflection—A *reflection* that contains little or no additional content beyond what the client has said.

Smoke Alarms—Interpersonal signals of *discord* in the working alliance.

Spirit—The underlying set of mind and heart within which MI is practiced, including *partnership*, *acceptance*, *compassion*, and *evocation*.

Stages of Change—Within the *transtheoretical model* of change, a sequence of steps through which people pass in the change process: precontemplation, contemplation, preparation, action, and maintenance.

Status Quo—The current state of affairs without change.

Summary—A *reflection* that draws together content from two or more prior client statements. See also *Collecting Summary, Linking Summary, Transitional Summary*.

Sustain Talk—Any client speech that favors *status quo* rather than movement toward a *change goal*.

Taking Steps—A form of client *mobilizing change talk* that describes an action or step already taken toward change.

Telos—(Greek) The natural, mature end state of an organism toward which it grows, given optimal conditions.

TNT—An acronym for a Training of New Trainers in *motivational interviewing*; begun in 1993.

Transitional Summary—A special form of *reflection* to wrap up a task or session by pulling together what seems important and signal a shift to something new.

Transtheoretical Model—A complex model of change developed by James Prochaska and Carlo DiClemente, one part of which describes *stages of change*.

Undershooting—A *reflection* that diminishes or understates the intensity of the content or emotion expressed by a client.

Values—A person's core goals or standards that provide meaning and direction in life.

Values Sorting—A technique used by Milton Rokeach and others, in which a person gives priority rankings to various values, for example, by sorting cards into piles ranging from "not at all important" to "most important."

Working Alliance—The quality of the collaborative relationship between client and counselor, which tends to predict client retention and outcome.

APPENDIX B

A Bibliography
of Motivational Interviewing

Christopher J. McLouth

Note: A full bibliography of more than 1,200 references, including outcome studies and clinical commentary arranged by topic, can be found at *www.guilford.com/p/miller2*.

BOOKS

Arkowitz, H., Westra, H. A., Miller, W. R., & Rollnick, S. (2008). *Motivational interviewing in the treatment of psychological problems*. New York: Guilford Press.

Botelho, R. (2004). *Motivational practice: Promoting healthy habits and self-care of chronic diseases* (2nd ed.). Rochester, NY: MHH Publications.

Dart, M. A. (2010). *Motivational interviewing in nursing practice: Empowering the patient*. Sudbury, MA: Jones & Bartlett.

Dimeff, L. A., Baer, J. S., Kivlahan, D. R., & Marlatt, G. A. (1999). *Brief alcohol screening and intervention for college students (BASICS): A harm reduction approach*. New York: Guilford Press.

Engle, D. E., & Arkowitz, H. (2006). *Ambivalence in psychotherapy: Facilitating readiness to change*. New York: Guilford Press.

Fields, A. E. (2004). *Curriculum-based motivation group: A five-session motivational interviewing group intervention*. Vancouver, WA: Hollifiend Associates.

Christopher J. McLouth is currently pursuing a PhD in clinical psychology at the University of New Mexico and also spends his time as a researcher at the university's Center on Alcoholism, Substance Abuse, and Addictions. His research interests include causal mechanisms for MI and the statistical modeling of behavior change.

Fields, A. E. (2006). *Enrolling our adult learners back into school: A five-session motivational interviewing engagement process.* Vancouver, WA: Hollifield Associates.

Fields, A. E. (2006). *Motivational enhancement therapy for problem and pathological gamblers: A five-session curriculum-based group intervention.* Vancouver, WA: Hollifield Associates.

Fields, A. E. (2006). *Paradigm shifts and corporate change—All on board?: Motivational interviewing in the business world.* Vancouver, WA: Hollifield Associates.

Fields, A. E. (2006). *Resolving patient ambivalence: A five-session motivational interviewing intervention.* Vancouver, WA: Hollifield Associates.

Fuller, C., & Taylor, P. (2008). *A toolkit of motivational skills: Encouraging and supporting change in individuals* (2nd ed.). New York: Wiley.

Hibbard, J., Lawson, K., Moore, M., & Wolever, R. (2010). *Three pillars of health coaching: Patient activation motivational interviewing and positive psychology.* Manasquan, NJ: Healthcare Intelligence Network.

Hohman, M. (2012). *Motivational interviewing in social work practice.* New York: Guilford Press.

Lawson, K., Wolever, R., Donovan, P., & Greene, L. M. (2009). *Health coaching for behavior change: Motivational interviewing methods and practice.* Manasquan, NJ: Healthcare Intelligence Network.

Levounis, P., & Arnaout, B. (2010). *Handbook of motivation and change: A practical guide for clinicians.* Arlington, VA: American Psychiatric.

Maiuro, R. D., & Murphy, C. (2002). *Motivational interviewing and stages of change in intimate partner violence.* New York: Springer.

Mason, P. G., & Butler, C. C. (2010). *Health behavior change: A guide for practitioners* (2nd ed.). Edinburgh, Scotland: Churchill Livingstone.

Matulich, B. (2010). *How to do motivational interviewing: A guidebook for beginners.* Kindle Edition: *www.amazon.com.*

McMurran, M. (2002). *Motivating offenders to change: A guide to enhancing engagement in therapy.* West Sussex, UK: Wiley.

McNamara, E. (2009). *Motivational interviewing: Theory, practice and applications with children and young people.* Ainsdale, UK: Positive Behaviour Management.

Miller, W. R., & Rollnick, S. (1991). *Motivational interviewing: Preparing people to change addictive behavior.* New York: Guilford Press.

Miller, W. R., & Rollnick, S. (2002). *Motivational interviewing: Preparing people for change* (2nd ed.). New York: Guilford Press.

Murphy, C. M., & Maiuro, R. D. (2009). *Motivational interviewing and stages of change in intimate partner violence.* New York: Springer.

Naar-King, S., & Suarez, M. (2010). *Motivational interviewing with adolescents and young adults.* New York: Guilford Press.

Reinke, K., Herman, K. C., & Sprick, R. (2011). *Motivational interviewing for effective classroom management: The classroom check-up.* New York: Guilford Press.

Rollnick, S., Mason, P. G., & Butler, C. C. (1999). *Health behavior change: A guide for practitioners.* London: Churchill Livingstone.

Rollnick, S., Miller, W. R., & Butler, C. C. (2008). *Motivational interviewing in health care: Helping patients change behavior.* New York: Guilford Press.

Rosengren, D. B. (2009). *Building motivational interviewing skills: A practitioner workbook.* New York: Guilford Press.

Schmidt, U., & Treasure, J. (1997). *Clinician's guide to getting better bit(e) by bit(e): A survival kit for sufferers of bulimia nervosa and binge eating disorders.* Hove, UK: Psychology Press.

Tober, G., & Raistrick, D. (2007). *Motivational dialogue: Preparing addiction professionals for motivational interviewing practice.* New York: Routledge.

Tomlin, K. M., & Richardson, R. (2004). *Motivational interviewing and stages of change: Integrating best practices for substance abuse professionals.* Center City, MN: Hazelden.

Walters, S. T., & Baer, J. S. (2005). *Talking with college students about alcohol: Motivational strategies for reducing abuse.* New York: Guilford Press.

Walters, S. T., Clark, M. D., Gingerich, R., & Meltzer, M. L. (2007). *Motivating offenders to change: A guide for probation and parole.* Washington, DC: National Institute of Corrections, U.S. Dept. of Justice.

Weinstein, P. (2002). *Motivate your dental patients: A workbook.* Seattle, University of Washington. Available from the author: *philw@u.washington.edu.*

Wolf, S. (2009). *Retaining addicted and HIV infected clients in treatment services.* Saärbrucken, Germany: VDM Verlag.

SYSTEMATIC REVIEWS

† Indicates studies that include a statistical meta-analysis.

† Apodaca, T. R., & Longabaugh, R. (2009). Mechanisms of change in motivational interviewing: A review and preliminary evaluation of the evidence. *Addiction, 104*(5), 705–715.

† Armstrong, M. J., Mottershead, T. A., Ronksley, P. E., Sigal, R. J., Campbell, T. S., & Hemmelgarn, B. R. (2011). Motivational interviewing to improve weight loss in overweight and/or obese patients: A systematic review and meta-analysis of randomized controlled trials. *Obesity Reviews, 12*(9), 709–723.

Baker, A., & Hambridge, J. (2002). Motivational interviewing: Enhancing engagement in treatment for mental health problems. *Behaviour Change, 19*(3), 138–145.

Baker, A., & Lee, N. K. (2003). A review of psychosocial interventions for amphetamine use. *Drug and Alcohol Review, 22*(3), 323–335.

Baker, A., Turner, A., Kay-Lambkin, F. J., & Lewin, T. J. (2009). The long and the short of treatments for alcohol or cannabis misuse among people with severe mental disorders. *Addictive Behaviors, 34*(10), 852–858.

Barkhof, E., De Haan, L., Meijer, C. J., Fouwels, A. J., Keet, I. P. M., Hulstijn, K. P., et al. (2006). Motivational interviewing in psychotic disorders. *Current Psychiatry Reviews, 2*(2), 207–213.

Barnett, N. P., Tevyaw, T. O'L., Fromme, K., Borsari, B., Carey, K. B., Corbin, W.

R., et al. (2004). Brief alcohol interventions with mandated or adjudicated college students. *Alcoholism: Clinical and Experimental Research, 28*(6), 966–975.

Bechdolf, A., Pohlmann, B., Geyer, C., Ferber, C., Klosterkotter, J., & Gouzoulis-Mayfrank, E. (2005). [Motivational interviewing for patients with comorbid schizophrenia and substance abuse disorders: A review]. *Fortschritte der Neurologie-Psychiatrie, 73*(12), 728–735.

Bernstein, E., & Bernstein, J. (2008). Effectiveness of alcohol screening and brief motivational intervention in the emergency department setting. *Annals of Emergency Medicine, 51*(6), 751–754.

Bien, T. H., Miller, W. R., & Tonigan, J. S. (1993). Brief interventions for alcohol problems: A review. *Addiction, 88*(3), 315–335.

Branscum, P., & Sharma, M. (2010). A review of motivational interviewing-based interventions targeting problematic drinking among college students. *Alcoholism Treatment Quarterly, 28*(1), 63–77.

Britt, E., Blampied, N., & Hudson, S. (2003). Motivational interviewing: A review. *Australian Psychologist, 38*(3), 193–201.

Britt, E., Hudson, S. M., & Blampied, N. M. (2004). Motivational interviewing in health settings: A review. *Patient Education and Counseling, 53*(2), 147–155.

Burke, B. L. (2011). What can motivational interviewing do for you? *Cognitive and Behavioral Practice, 18*(1), 74–81.

† Burke, B. L., Arkowitz, H., & Menchola, M. (2003). The efficacy of motivational interviewing: A meta-analysis of controlled clinical trials. *Journal of Consulting and Clinical Psychology, 71*(5), 843–861.

† Burke, B. L., Dunn, C. W., Atkins, D. C., & Phelps, J. S. (2004). The emerging evidence base for motivational interviewing: A meta-analytic and qualitative inquiry. *Journal of Cognitive Psychotherapy, 18*(4), 309–322.

Bux, D. A., Jr., & Irwin, T. W. (2006). Combining motivational interviewing and cognitive-behavioral skills training for the treatment of crystal methamphetamine abuse/dependence. *Journal of Gay and Lesbian Psychotherapy, 10*(3–4), 143–152.

Carroll, K. M. (2005). Recent advances in the psychotherapy of addictive disorders. *Current Psychiatry Reports, 7*(5), 329–336.

Chambless, D. L., & Ollendick, T. H. (2001). Empirically supported psychological interventions: Controversies and evidence. *Annual Review of Psychology, 52*, 685–716.

Chanut, F., Brown, T. G., & Dongier, M. (2005). Motivational interviewing and clinical psychiatry. *Canadian Journal of Psychiatry, 50*(9), 548–554.

Chanut, F., Brown, T. G., & Donguier, M. (2005). Motivational interviewing and clinical psychiatry. *Canadian Journal of Psychiatry, 50*(11), 715–721.

Cleary, M., Hunt, G. E., Matheson, S., & Walter, G. (2009). Psychosocial treatments for people with co-occurring severe mental illness and substance misuse: Systematic review. *Journal of Advanced Nursing, 65*(2), 238–258.

† Cleary, M., Hunt, G. E., Matheson, S. L., Siegfried, N., & Walter, G. (2008). Psychosocial interventions for people with both severe mental illness and substance misuse. *Cochrane Database of Systematic Reviews* (1).

Cloud, R. N., Besel, K., Bledsoe, L., Golder, S., McKiernan, P., Patterson, D., et al. (2006). Adapting motivational interviewing strategies to increase posttreatment 12-step meeting attendance. *Alcoholism Treatment Quarterly, 24*(3), 31–53.

Cooperman, N. A., & Arnsten, J. H. (2005). Motivational interviewing for improving adherence to antiretroviral medications. *Current HIV/AIDS Reports, 2*(4), 159–164.

Cummings, S. M., Cooper, R. L., & Cassie, K. M. (2009). Motivational interviewing to affect behavioral change in older adults. *Research on Social Work Practice, 19*(2), 195–204.

Deas, D. (2008). Evidence-cased treatments for alcohol use disorders in adolescents. *Pediatrics, 121*, S348–S354.

Deas, D., & Clark, A. (2009). Current state of treatment for alcohol and other drug use disorders in adolescents. *Alcohol Research and Health, 32*(1), 76–82.

Demmel, R. (2001). Motivational Interviewing: Ein Literaturüberblick. *Sucht: Zeitschrift für Wissenschaft und Praxis, 47*(3), 171–188.

DiClemente, C. C., Marinilli, A. S., Singh, M., & Bellino, L. E. (2001). The role of feedback in the process of health behavior change. *American Journal of Health Behavior, 25*(3), 217–227.

† DiRosa, L. C. (2010). *Motivational interviewing to treat overweight/obesity: A meta-analysis of relevant research.* Unpublished doctoral dissertation, Wilmington University, New Castle, Delaware.

Drymalski, W. M., & Campbell, T. C. (2009). A review of motivational interviewing to enhance adherence to antipsychotic medication in patients with schizophrenia: Evidence and recommendations. *Journal of Mental Health, 18*(1), 6–15.

Dunn, C. (2003). Brief motivational interviewing interventions targeting substance abuse in the acute care medical setting. *Seminars in Clinical Neuropsychiatry, 8*(3), 188–196.

† Dunn, C., Deroo, L., & Rivara, F. P. (2001). The use of brief interventions adapted from motivational interviewing across behavioral domains: A systematic review. *Addiction, 96*(12), 1725–1742.

Duran, L. S. (2003). Motivating health: Strategies for the nurse practitioner. *Journal of the American Academy of Nurse Practitioners, 15*(5), 200–205.

Erickson, S. J., Gerstle, M., & Feldstein, S. W. (2005). Brief interventions and motivational interviewing with children, adolescents, and their parents in pediatric health care settings: A review. *Archives of Pediatrics and Adolescent Medicine, 159*(12), 1173–1180.

Feldstein, S. W., & Ginsburg, J. I. D. (2006). Motivational interviewing with dually diagnosed adolescents in juvenile justice settings. *Brief Treatment and Crisis Intervention, 6*(3), 218–233.

† Gooding, P., & Tarrier, N. (2009). A systematic review and meta-analysis of cognitive-behavioural interventions to reduce problem gambling: Hedging our bets? *Behaviour Research and Therapy, 47*(7), 592–607.

Grenard, J. L., Ames, S. L., Pentz, M. A., & Sussman, S. (2006). Motivational interviewing with adolescents and young adults for drug-related problems. *International Journal of Adolescent Medicine and Health, 18*(1), 53–67.

† Grimshaw, G. M., & Stanton, A. (2006). Tobacco cessation interventions for young people. *Cochrane Database of Systematic Reviews* (4), CD003289.

Handmaker, N. S., & Wilbourne, P. (2001). Motivational interventions in prenatal clinics. *Alcohol Research and Health, 25*(3), 219–229.

† Hettema, J., Steele, J., & Miller, W. R. (2005). Motivational interviewing. *Annual Review of Clinical Psychology, 1*, 91–111.

† Hettema, J. E. (2007). *A meta-analysis of motivational interviewing across behavioral domains.* Unpublished doctoral dissertation, University of New Mexico, Albuquerque.

Hjorthøj, C., Fohlmann, A., & Nordentoft, M. (2009). Treatment of cannabis use disorders in people with schizophrenia spectrum disorders—A systematic review. *Addictive Behaviors, 34*(6–7), 520–525.

Horsfall, J., Cleary, M., Hunt, G. E., & Walter, G. (2009). Psychosocial treatments for people with co-occurring severe mental illnesses and substance use disorders (dual diagnosis): A review of empirical evidence. *Harvard Review of Psychiatry, 17*(1), 24–34.

Ilott, R. (2005). Does compliance therapy improve use of antipsychotic medication? *British Journal of Community Nursing, 10*(11), 514–519.

† Jensen, C. D., Cushing, C. C., Aylward, B. S., Craig, J. T., Sorell, D. M., & Steele, R. G. (2011). Effectiveness of motivational interviewing interventions for adolescent substance use behavior change: A meta-analytic review. *Journal of Consulting and Clinical Psychology, 79*(4), 433–440.

Julius, R. J., Novitsky, M. A., Jr., & Dubin, W. R. (2009). Medication adherence: A review of the literature and implications for clinical practice. *Journal of Psychiatric Practice, 15*(1), 34–44.

Kaplan, A. S. (2002). Psychological treatments for anorexia nervosa: A review of published studies and promising new directions. *Canadian Journal of Psychiatry, 47*(3), 235–242.

† Kelly, T. M., Daley, D. C., & Douaihy, A. B. (2011). Treatment of substance abusing patients with comorbid psychiatric disorders. *Addictive Behaviors, 37*(1), 11–24.

Kienast, T., & Heinz, A. (2005). Therapy and supportive care of alcoholics: Guidelines for practitioners. *Digestive Diseases, 23*(3–4), 304–309.

Knight, K. M., McGowan, L., Dickens, C., & Bundy, C. (2006). A systematic review of motivational interviewing in physical health care settings. *British Journal of Health Psychology, 11*(2), 319–332.

Laker, C. J. (2007). How reliable is the current evidence looking at the efficacy of harm reduction and motivational interviewing interventions in the treatment of patients with a dual diagnosis? *Journal of Psychiatric and Mental Health Nursing, 14*(8), 720–726.

Larimer, M. E., & Cronce, J. M. (2007). Identification, prevention, and treatment revisited: Individual-focused college drinking prevention strategies 1999–2006. *Addictive Behaviors, 32*(11), 2439–2468.

Lawendowski, L. A. (1998). A motivational intervention for adolescent smokers. *Preventive Medicine, 27*(5, Pt. 2), A39–A46.

Lewis, S. W., Tarrier, N., & Drake, R. J. (2005). Integrating non-drug treatments in early schizophrenia. *British Journal of Psychiatry, 187*(Suppl. 48), s65–s71.

Lewis, T. F., & Osborn, C. J. (2004). Solution-focused counseling and motivational interviewing: A consideration of confluence. *Journal of Counseling and Development, 82*(1), 38–48.

† Lopez, L. M., Tolley, E. E., Grimes, D. A., & Chen-Mok, M. (2009). Theory-based interventions for contraception. *Cochrane Database of Systematic Reviews* (1), CD007249.

Lopez-Bushnell, K., & Fassler, C. (2004). Nursing care of hospitalized medical patients with addictions. *Journal of Addictions Nursing, 15*(4), 177–182.

† Lundahl, B., & Burke, B. L. (2009). The effectiveness and applicability of motivational interviewing: A practice-friendly review of four meta-analyses. *Journal of Clinical Psychology, 65*(11), 1232–1245.

† Lundahl, B. W., Kunz, C., Brownell, C., Tollefson, D., & Burke, B. L. (2010). A meta-analysis of motivational interviewing: Twenty-five years of empirical studies. *Research on Social Work Practice, 20*(2), 137–160.

Macgowan, M. J., & Engle, B. (2010). Evidence for optimism: Behavior therapies and motivational interviewing in adolescent substance abuse treatment. *Child and Adolescent Psychiatric Clinics of North America, 19*(3), 527–545.

Madson, M. B., & Campbell, T. C. (2006). Measures of fidelity in motivational enhancement: A systematic review. *Journal of Substance Abuse Treatment, 31*(1), 67–73.

Madson, M. B., Loignon, A. C., & Lane, C. (2009). Training in motivational interviewing: A systematic review. *Journal of Substance Abuse Treatment, 36*(1), 101–109.

Martins, R. K., & McNeil, D. W. (2009). Review of motivational interviewing in promoting health behaviors. *Clinical Psychology Review, 29*(4), 283–293.

McCollum, E. E., Trepper, T. S., & Smock, S. (2003). Solution-focused group therapy for substance abuse: Extending competency-based models. *Journal of Family Psychotherapy, 14*(4), 27–42.

McMurran, M. (2009). Motivational interviewing with offenders: A systematic review. *Legal and Criminological Psychology, 14*(1), 83–100.

Miller, W. R. (1985). Motivation for treatment: A review with special emphasis on alcoholism. *Psychological Bulletin, 98*(1), 84–107.

Miller, W. R. (1996). Motivational interviewing: Research, practice, and puzzles. *Addictive Behaviors, 21*(6), 835–842.

Miller, W. R. (2000). Rediscovering fire: Small interventions, large effects. *Psychology of Addictive Behaviors, 14*(1), 6–18.

Miller, W. R. (2004). Motivational interviewing in service to health promotion. *American Journal of Health Promotion, 18*(3), 1–10.

Miller, W. R. (2005). Motivational interviewing and the incredible shrinking treatment effect. *Addiction, 100*(4), 421.

Miller, W. R., & Wilbourne, P. L. (2002). Mesa Grande: A methodological analysis of clinical trials of treatments for alcohol use disorders. *Addiction, 97*(3), 265–277.

Noonan, W. C., & Moyers, T. B. (1997). Motivational interviewing. *Journal of Substance Misuse: For Nursing, Health and Social Care, 2*(1), 8–16.

† Osborn, L. D. (2007). *A meta-analysis of controlled clinical trials of the efficacy of motivational interviewing in a dual-diagnosis population.* Unpublished doctoral dissertation, The Wright Institute, Berkeley, California.

Perney, P., Rigole, H., & Blanc, F. (2008). [Alcohol dependence: Diagnosis and treatment]. *Revue de Medecine Interne, 29*(4), 297–304.

RachBeisel, J., Scott, J., & Dixon, L. (1999). Co-occurring severe mental illness and substance use disorders: A review of recent research. *Psychiatric Services*, 50(11), 1427–1434.

Resnicow, K., DiIorio, C., Soet, J. E., Borrelli, B., Hecht, J., & Ernst, D. (2002). Motivational interviewing in health promotion: It sounds like something is changing. *Health Psychology*, 21(5), 444–451.

Rollnick, S., & Miller, W. R. (1995). What is motivational interviewing? *Behavioural and Cognitive Psychotherapy*, 23(4), 325–334.

† Rubak, S., Sandbaek, A., Lauritzen, T., & Christensen, B. (2005). Motivational interviewing: A systematic review and meta-analysis. *British Journal of General Practice*, 55(513), 305–312.

Rush, B. R., Dennis, M. L., Scott, C. K., Castel, S., & Funk, R. R. (2008). The interaction of co-occurring mental disorders and recovery management checkups on substance abuse treatment participation and recovery. *Evaluation Review*, 32(1), 7–38.

Ryder, D. (1999). Deciding to change: Enhancing client motivation to change behaviour. *Behaviour Change*, 16(3), 165–174.

Schmidt, P., Kohler, J., & Soyka, M. (2008). [Evidence-based treatments in the inpatient rehabilitation of alcoholics]. *Fortschr Neurol Psychiatr*, 76(2), 86–90.

Sindelar, H. A., Abrantes, A. M., Hart, C., Lewander, W., & Spirito, A. (2004). Motivational interviewing in pediatric practice. *Current Problems in Pediatric and Adolescent Health Care*, 34(9), 322–339.

† Smedslund, G., Berg, R. C., Hammerstrom, K. T., Steiro, A., Leiknes, K. A., Dahl, H. M., et al. (2011). Motivational interviewing for substance abuse. *Cochrane Database of Systematic Reviews* (5).

Smith, A. J., Shepherd, J. P., & Hodgson, R. J. (1998). Brief interventions for patients with alcohol-related trauma. *British Journal of Oral and Maxillofacial Surgery*, 36(6), 408–415.

Söderlund, L. L., Madson, M. B., Rubak, S., & Nilsen, P. (2011). A systematic review of motivational interviewing training for general health care practitioners. *Patient Education and Counseling*, 84(1), 16–26.

† Tait, R. J., & Hulse, G. K. (2003). A systematic review of the effectiveness of brief interventions with substance using adolescents by type of drug. *Drug and Alcohol Review*, 22(3), 337–346.

Tevyaw, T. O'L., & Monti, P. M. (2004). Motivational enhancement and other brief interventions for adolescent substance abuse: Foundations, applications, and evaluations. *Addiction*, 99(Suppl. 2), 63–75.

Thompson, D. R., Chair, S. Y., Chan, S. W., Astin, F., Davidson, P. M., & Ski, C. F. (2011). Motivational interviewing: A useful approach to improving cardiovascular health? *Journal of Clinical Nursing*, 20(9/10), 1236–1244.

VanWormer, J. J., & Boucher, J. L. (2004). Motivational interviewing and diet modification: A review of the evidence. *The Diabetes Educator*, 30(3), 404–406, 408–410, 414–406, passim.

† Vasilaki, E. I., Hosier, S. G., & Cox, W. M. (2006). The efficacy of motivational interviewing as a brief intervention for excessive drinking: A meta-analytic review. *Alcohol and Alcoholism*, 41(3), 328–335.

Wagner, C. C., & McMahon, B. T. (2004). Motivational interviewing and rehabilitation counseling practice. *Rehabilitation Counseling Bulletin, 47*(3), 152–161.

† Wilbourne, P. L. (2005). *An empirical basis for the treatment of alcohol problems.* Unpublished doctoral dissertation, University of New Mexico, Albuquerque.

Yevlahova, D., & Satur, J. (2009). Models for individual oral health promotion and their effectiveness: A systematic review. *Australian Dental Journal, 54*(3), 190–197.

Zygmunt, A., Olfson, M., Boyer, C. A., & Mechanic, D. (2002). Interventions to improve medication adherence in schizophrenia. *American Journal of Psychiatry, 159*(10), 1653–1664.

TRAINING

Adams, J., & Madson, M. (2007). Reflection and outlook for the future of addictions treatment and training: An interview with William R. Miller. *Journal of Teaching in the Addictions, 5*(1), 95–109.

Ager, R., Roahen-Harrison, S., Toriello, P. J., Kissinger, P., Morse, P., Morse, E., et al. (2011). Predictors of adopting motivational enhancement therapy. *Research on Social Work Practice, 21*(1), 65–76.

Alexander, M., VanBenschoten, S. W., & Walters, S. T. (2008). Motivational interviewing training in criminal justice: Development of a model plan. *Federal Probation, 72*(2), 61–66.

Amrhein, P. C., Miller, W. R., Yahne, C., Knupsky, A., & Hochstein, D. (2004). Strength of client commitment language improves with therapist training in motivational interviewing. *Alcoholism: Clinical and Experimental Research, 28*(5), 74A.

Arthur, D. (1999). Assessing nursing students' basic communication and interviewing skills: The development and testing of a rating scale. *Journal of Advanced Nursing, 29*(3), 658–665.

Baer, J. S., Rosengren, D. B., Dunn, C. W., Wells, E. A., Ogle, R. L., & Hartzler, B. (2004). An evaluation of workshop training in motivational interviewing for addiction and mental health clinicians. *Drug and Alcohol Dependence, 73*(1), 99–106.

Baer, J. S., Wells, E. A., Rosengren, D. B., Hartzler, B., Beadnell, B., & Dunn, C. (2009). Agency context and tailored training in technology transfer: A pilot evaluation of motivational interviewing training for community counselors. *Journal of Substance Abuse Treatment, 37*(2), 191–202.

Ball, S., Bachrach, K., DeCarlo, J., Farentinos, C., Keen, M., McSherry, T., et al. (2002). Characteristics, beliefs and practices of community clinicians trained to provide manual-guided therapy for substance abusers. *Journal of Substance Abuse Treatment, 23*(4), 309–318.

Bell, K., & Cole, B. A. (2008). Improving medical students' success in promoting health behavior change: A curriculum evaluation. *Journal of General Internal Medicine, 23*(9), 1503–1506.

Bennett, G. A., Moore, J., Vaughan, T., Rouse, L., Gibbins, J. A., Thomas, P., et al. (2007). Strengthening motivational interviewing skills following initial training: A randomized trial of workplace-based reflective practice. *Addictive Behaviors*, 32(12), 2963–2975.

Britt, E., & Blampied, N. M. (2010). Motivational interviewing training: A pilot study of the effects on practitioner and patient behaviour. *Behavioural and Cognitive Psychotherapy*, 38(2), 239–244.

Broers, S., Smets, E., Bindels, P., Evertsz, F. B., Calff, M., & de Haes, H. (2005). Training general practitioners in behavior change counseling to improve asthma medication adherence. *Patient Education and Counseling*, 58(3), 279–287.

Brown, R. L., & Oriel, K. (1998). Teaching motivational interviewing to first-year students. *Academic Medicine*, 73(5), 589–590.

Brown, R. L., Pfeifer, J. M., Gjerde, C. L., Seibert, C. S., & Haq, C. L. (2004). Teaching patient-centered tobacco intervention to first-year medical students. *Journal of General Internal Medicine*, 19(5), 534–539.

Burke, P. J., Da Silva, J. D., Vaughan, B. L., & Knight, J. R. (2005). Training high school counselors on the use of motivational interviewing to screen for substance abuse. *Substance Abuse*, 26(3–4), 31–34.

Carise, D., Brooks, A., Alterman, A., McLellan, A. T., Hoover, V., & Forman, R. (2009). Implementing evidence-based practices in community treatment programs: Initial feasibility of a counselor "toolkit." *Substance Abuse*, 30(3), 239–243.

Carpenter, K. M., Watson, J. M., Raffety, B., & Chabal, C. (2003). Teaching brief interventions for smoking cessations via an interactive computer-based tutorial. *Journal of Health Psychology*, 8(1), 149–160.

Casey, D. (2007). Using action research to change health-promoting practice. *Nursing and Health Sciences*, 9(1), 5–13.

D'Ambrosio, R., Laws, K. E., Gabriel, R. M., Hromco, J., & Kelly, P. (2006). Implementing motivational interviewing in a non-MI world: A MI knowledge adoption study. *Journal of Teaching in the Addictions*, 5(2), 21–37.

Doherty, Y., Hall, D., James, P. T., Roberts, S. H., & Simpson, J. (2000). Change counselling in diabetes: The development of a training programme for the diabetes team. *Patient Education and Counseling*, 40(3), 263–278.

Evangeli, M., Engelbrecht, S.-K., Swartz, L., Turner, K., Forsberg, L., & Soka, N. (2009). An evaluation of a brief motivational interviewing training course for HIV/AIDS counsellors in Western Cape Province, South Africa. *AIDS Care*, 21(2), 189–196.

Fitzgerald, N., Watson, H., McCaig, D., & Stewart, D. (2009). Developing and evaluating training for community pharmacists to deliver interventions on alcohol issues. *Pharmacy World and Science*, 31(2), 149–153.

Forrester, D., McCambridge, J., Waissbein, C., Emlyn-Jones, R., & Rollnick, S. (2008). Child risk and parental resistance: Can motivational interviewing improve the practice of child and family social workers in working with parental alcohol misuse? *British Journal of Social Work*, 38(7), 1302–1319.

Forsberg, L., Ernst, D., & Farbring, C. (2011). Learning motivational interviewing in a real-life setting: A randomised controlled trial in the Swedish Prison Service. *Criminal Behaviour and Mental Health*, 21(3), 177–188.

Forsberg, L., Forsberg, L. G., Lindqvist, H., & Helgason, A. R. (2010). Clinician acquisition and retention of motivational interviewing skills: A two-and-a-half-year exploratory study. *Substance Abuse Treatment, Prevention, and Policy, 5*(8).

Goggin, K., Hawes, S. M., Duval, E. R., Spresser, C. D., Martinez, D. A., Lynam, I., et al. (2010). A motivational interviewing course for pharmacy students. *American Journal of Pharmaceutical Education, 74*(4).

Haeseler, F., Fortin, A. H., Pfeiffer, C., Walters, C., & Martino, S. (2011). Assessment of a motivational interviewing curriculum for year 3 medical students using a standardized patient case. *Patient Education and Counseling, 84*(1), 27–30.

Handmaker, N. S., Hester, R. K., & Delaney, H. D. (1999). Videotaped training in alcohol counseling for obstetric care practitioners: A randomized controlled trial. *Obstetrics and Gynecology, 93*(2), 213–218.

Hartzler, B., Beadnell, B., Rosengren, D. B., Dunn, C., & Baer, J. S. (2010). Deconstructing proficiency in motivational interviewing: Mechanics of skillful practitioner delivery during brief simulated encounters. *Behavioural and Cognitive Psychotherapy, 38*(5), 611–628.

Hohman, M., Doran, N., & Koutsenok, I. (2009). Motivational interviewing training for juvenile correctional staff in California: One year initial outcomes. *Journal of Offender Rehabilitation, 48*(7), 635–648.

Koerber, A., Crawford, J., & O'Connell, K. (2003). The effects of teaching dental students brief motivational interviewing for smoking-cessation counseling: A pilot study. *Journal of Dental Education, 67*(4), 439–447.

Kralikova, E., Bonevski, B., Stepankova, L., Pohlova, L., & Mladkova, N. (2009). Postgraduate medical education on tobacco and smoking cessation in Europe. *Drug and Alcohol Review, 28*(5), 474–483.

Lane, C., Hood, K., & Rollnick, S. (2008). Teaching motivational interviewing: Using role play is as effective as using simulated patients. *Medical Education, 42*(6), 637–644.

Lane, C., Johnson, S., Rollnick, S., Edwards, K., & Lyons, M. (2003). Consulting about lifestyle change: Evaluation of a training course for specialist diabetes nurses. *Practical Diabetes International, 20*(6), 204–208.

Lozano, P., McPhillips, H. A., Hartzler, B., Robertson, A. S., Runkle, C., Scholz, K. A., et al. (2010). Randomized trial of teaching brief motivational interviewing to pediatric trainees to promote healthy behaviors in families. *Archives of Pediatrics and Adolescent Medicine, 164*(6), 561–566.

MacLeod, J. B. A., Hungerford, D. W., Dunn, C., & Hartzler, B. (2008). Evaluation of training of surgery interns to perform brief alcohol interventions for trauma patients. *Journal of the American College of Surgeons, 207*(5), 639–645.

Madson, M. B., Loignon, A. C., & Lane, C. (2009). Training in motivational interviewing: A systematic review. *Journal of Substance Abuse Treatment, 36*(1), 101–109.

Martino, S., Ball, S. A., Nich, C., Canning-Ball, M., Rounsaville, B. J., & Carroll, K. M. (2011). Teaching community program clinicians motivational interviewing using expert and train-the-trainer strategies. *Addiction, 106*(2), 428–441.

Martino, S., Canning-Ball, M., Carroll, K. M., & Rounsaville, B. J. (2011). A criterion-based stepwise approach for training counselors in motivational interviewing. *Journal of Substance Abuse Treatment, 40*(4), 357–365.

Martino, S., Haeseler, F., Belitsky, R., Pantalon, M., & Fortin, A. H., IV. (2007). Teaching brief motivational interviewing to year three medical students. *Medical Education, 41*(2), 160–167.

Mastroleo, N. R., Turrisi, R., Carney, J. V., Ray, A. E., & Larimer, M. E. (2010). Examination of posttraining supervision of peer counselors in a motivational enhancement intervention to reduce drinking in a sample of heavy-drinking college students. *Journal of Substance Abuse Treatment, 39*(3), 289–297.

Miller, W. R., & Mount, K. A. (2001). A small study of training in motivational interviewing: Does one workshop change clinician and client behavior? *Behavioural and Cognitive Psychotherapy, 29*(4), 457–471.

Miller, W. R., & Moyers, T. B. (2006). Eight stages in learning motivational interviewing. *Journal of Teaching in the Addictions, 5*(1), 3–17.

Miller, W. R., Moyers, T. B., Arciniega, L., Ernst, D., & Forcehimes, A. A. (2005). Training, supervision and quality monitoring of the COMBINE study behavioral interventions. *Journal of Studies on Alcohol, 66*(Suppl. 15), S188–S195.

Miller, W. R., Yahne, C. E., Moyers, T. B., Martinez, J., & Pirritano, M. (2004). A randomized trial of methods to help clinicians learn motivational interviewing. *Journal of Consulting and Clinical Psychology, 72*(6), 1050–1062.

Mitcheson, L., Bhavsar, K., & McCambridge, J. (2009). Randomized trial of training and supervision in motivational interviewing with adolescent drug treatment practitioners. *Journal of Substance Abuse Treatment, 37*(1), 73–78.

Mounsey, A. L., Bovbjerg, V., White, L., & Gazewood, J. (2006). Do students develop better motivational interviewing skills through role-play with standardized patients or with student colleagues? *Medical Education, 40*(8), 775–780.

Moyers, T. B., Manuel, J. K., Wilson, P. G., Hendrickson, S. M. L., Talcott, W., & Durand, P. (2008). A randomized trial investigating training in motivational interviewing for behavioral health providers. *Behavioural and Cognitive Psychotherapy, 36*(2), 149–162.

Moyers, T. B., Martin, T., Manuel, J. K., Hendrickson, S. M., & Miller, W. R. (2005). Assessing competence in the use of motivational interviewing. *Journal of Substance Abuse Treatment, 28*(1), 19–26.

Opheim, A., Andreasson, S., Eklund, A. B., & Prescott, P. (2009). The effects of training medical students in motivational interviewing. *Health Education Journal, 68*(3), 170–178.

Periasamy, S. (2005). *The relationship between the fidelity of motivational interviewing and nutritional outcomes in African American church populations.* Unpublished doctoral dissertation, Georgia State University, Atlanta.

Poirier, M. K., Clark, M. M., Cerhan, J. H., Pruthi, S., Geda, Y. E., & Dale, L. C. (2004). Teaching motivational interviewing to first-year medical students to improve counseling skills in health behavior change. *Mayo Clinic Proceedings, 79*(3), 327–331.

Rollnick, S., Kinnersley, P., & Butler, C. (2002). Context-bound communication skills training: Development of a new method. *Medical Education, 36*(4), 377–383.

Roman, B., Borges, N., & Morrison, A. K. (2011). Teaching motivational interviewing skills to third-year psychiatry clerkship students. *Academic Psychiatry, 35*(1), 51–53.

Rubak, S., Sandbaek, A., Lauritzen, T., Borch-Johnsen, K., & Christensen, B. (2006). An education and training course in motivational interviewing influence: GPs' professional behaviour—ADDITION Denmark. *British Journal of General Practice, 56*(527), 429–436.

Rubel, E. C., Sobell, L. C., & Miller, W. R. (2000). Do continuing education workshops improve participants' skills? Effects of a motivational interviewing workshop on substance-abuse counselors' skills and knowledge. *Behavior Therapist, 23*(4), 73–77, 90.

Runkle, C., Osterholm, A., Hoban, R., McAdam, E., & Tull, R. (2000). Brief negotiation program for promoting behavior change: The Kaiser Permanente approach to continuing professional development. *Education for Health, 13*(3), 377–386.

Scal, P., Hennrikus, D., Ehrlich, L., Ireland, M., & Borowsky, I. (2004). Preparing residents to counsel about smoking. *Clinical Pediatrics, 43*(8), 703–708.

Schoener, E. P., Madeja, C. L., Henderson, M. J., Ondersma, S. J., & Janisse, J. J. (2006). Effects of motivational interviewing training on mental health therapist behavior. *Drug and Alcohol Dependence, 82*(3), 269–275.

Schumacher, J. A., Madson, M. B., & Norquist, G. S. (2011). Using telehealth technology to enhance motivational interviewing training for rural substance abuse treatment providers: A services improvement project. *Behavior Therapist, 34*(4), 64–70.

Sepulveda, A. R., Lopez, C., Macdonald, P., & Treasure, J. (2008). Feasibility and acceptability of DVD and telephone coaching-based skills training for carers of people with an eating disorder. *International Journal of Eating Disorders, 41*(4), 318–325.

Shafer, M. S., Rhode, R., & Chong, J. (2004). Using distance education to promote the transfer of motivational interviewing skills among behavioral health professionals. *Journal of Substance Abuse Treatment, 26*(2), 141–148.

Smith, J. L., Amrhein, P. C., Brooks, A. C., Carpenter, K. M., Levin, D., Schreiber, E. A., et al. (2007). Providing live supervision via teleconferencing improves acquisition of motivational interviewing skills after workshop attendance. *American Journal of Drug and Alcohol Abuse, 33*(1), 163–168.

Sobell, L. C., Manor, H. L., Sobell, M. B., & Dum, M. (2008). Self-critiques of audiotaped therapy sessions: A motivational procedure for facilitating feedback during supervision. *Training and Education in Professional Psychology, 2*(3), 151–155.

Söderlund, L. L. (2008). Learning motivational interviewing: Exploring primary health care nurses' training and counselling experiences. *Health Education Journal, 67*(2), 102–109.

Söderlund, L. L., Madson, M. B., Rubak, S., & Nilsen, P. (2011). A systematic review of motivational interviewing training for general health care practitioners. *Patient Education and Counseling, 84*(1), 16–26.

Söderlund, L. L., & Nilsen, P. (2009). Feasibility of using motivational interviewing in a Swedish pharmacy setting. *International Journal of Pharmacy Practice, 17*(3), 143–149.

Stott, N. C. H., Rees, M., Rollnick, S., Pill, R. M., & Hackett, P. (1996).

Professional responses to innovation in clinical method: Diabetes care and negotiating skills. *Patient Education and Counseling, 29*(1), 67–73.

Tober, G., Godfrey, C., Parrott, S., Copello, A., Farrin, A., Hodgson, R., et al. (2005). Setting standards for training and competence: The UK alcohol treatment trial. *Alcohol and Alcoholism, 40*(5), 413–418.

van Eijk-Hustings, Y. J., Daemen, L., Schaper, N. C., & Vrijhoef, H. J. (2011). Implementation of motivational interviewing in a diabetes care management initiative in the Netherlands. *Patient Education and Counseling, 84*(1), 10–15.

Velasquez, M. M., Hecht, J., Quinn, V. P., Emmons, K. M., DiClemente, C. C., & Dolan-Mullen, P. (2000). Application of motivational interviewing to prenatal smoking cessation: Training and implementation issues. *Tobacco Control, 9*(Suppl. 3), iii36–iii40.

Villaume, W. A., Berger, B. A., & Barker, B. N. (2006). Learning motivational interviewing: Scripting a virtual patient. *American Journal of Pharmaceutical Education, 70*(2), 33.

White, L. L., Gazewood, J. D., & Mounsey, A. L. (2007). Teaching students behavior change skills: Description and assessment of a new motivational interviewing curriculum. *Medical Teacher, 29*(4), e67–e71.

Wilson, G. T., & Schlam, T. R. (2004). The transtheoretical model and motivational interviewing in the treatment of eating and weight disorders. *Clinical Psychology Review, 24*(3), 361–378.

PROCESS RESEARCH

Amrhein, P. C., Miller, W. R., Yahne, C., Knupsky, A., & Hochstein, D. (2004). Strength of client commitment language improves with therapist training in motivational interviewing. *Alcoholism: Clinical and Experimental Research, 28*(5), 74A.

Amrhein, P. C., Miller, W. R., Yahne, C. E., Palmer, M., & Fulcher, L. (2003). Client commitment language during motivational interviewing predicts drug use outcomes. *Journal of Consulting and Clinical Psychology, 71*(5), 862–878.

Baer, J. S., Beadnell, B., Garrett, S. B., Hartzler, B., Wells, E. A., & Peterson, P. L. (2008). Adolescent change language within a brief motivational intervention and substance use outcomes. *Psychology of Addictive Behaviors, 22*(4), 570–575.

Barsky, A., & Coleman, H. (2001). Evaluating skill acquisition in motivational interviewing: The development of an instrument to measure practice skills. *Journal of Drug Education, 31*(1), 69–82.

Boardman, T., Catley, D., Grobe, J. E., Little, T. D., & Ahluwalia, J. S. (2006). Using motivational interviewing with smokers: Do therapist behaviors relate to engagement and therapeutic alliance? *Journal of Substance Abuse Treatment, 31*(4), 329–339.

Campbell, S. D., Adamson, S. J., & Carter, J. D. (2010). Client language during motivational enhancement therapy and alcohol use outcome. *Behavioural and Cognitive Psychotherapy, 38*(4), 399–415.

Catley, D., Harris, K. J., Mayo, M. S., Hall, S., Okuyemi, K. S., Boardman, T., et al.

(2006). Adherence to principles of motivational interviewing and client within-session behavior. *Behavioural and Cognitive Psychotherapy*, 34(1), 43–56.

Collins, S. E., Carey, K. B., & Smyth, J. (2005). Relationships of linguistic and motivation variables with drinking outcomes following two mailed brief interventions. *Journal of Studies on Alcohol*, 66(4), 526–535.

Dunn, C., Droesch, R. M., Johnston, B. D., & Rivara, F. P. (2004). Motivational interviewing with injured adolescents in the emergency department: In-session predictors of change. *Behavioural and Cognitive Psychotherapy*, 32(1), 113–116.

Ernst, D. B. (2008). *Motivational interviewing and health coaching: A quantitative and qualitative exploration of integration.* Unpublished doctoral dissertation, University of New Mexico, Albuquerque.

Faris, A. S. (2007). *Examining process variables in a motivational intervention for college student drinkers.* Unpublished doctoral dissertation, University of Arkansas, Fayetteville.

Flores-Ferrán, N. (2010). An examination of mitigation strategies used in Spanish psychotherapeutic discourse. *Journal of Pragmatics*, 42(7), 1964–1981.

Forrester, D., Kershaw, S., Moss, H., & Hughes, L. (2008). Communication skills in child protection: How do social workers talk to parents? *Child and Family Social Work*, 13(1), 41–51.

Gaume, J., Bertholet, N., Faouzi, M., Gmel, G., & Daeppen, J.-B. (2010). Counselor motivational interviewing skills and young adult change talk articulation during brief motivational interventions. *Journal of Substance Abuse Treatment*, 39(3), 272–281.

Gaume, J., Gmel, G., & Daeppen, J.-B. (2008). Brief alcohol interventions: Do counsellors' and patients' communication characteristics predict change? *Alcohol and Alcoholism*, 43(1), 62–62.

Gaume, J., Gmel, G., Faouzi, M., & Daeppen, J.-B. (2008). Counsellor behaviours and patient language during brief motivational interventions: A sequential analysis of speech. *Addiction*, 103(11), 1793–1800.

Gaume, J., Gmel, G., Faouzi, M., & Daeppen, J. B. (2009). Counselor skill influences outcomes of brief motivational interventions. *Journal of Substance Abuse Treatment*, 37(2), 151–159.

Glynn, L. H., & Moyers, T. B. (2010). Chasing change talk: The clinician's role in evoking client language about change. *Journal of Substance Abuse Treatment*, 39(1), 65–70.

Hallgren, K. A., & Moyers, T. B. (2011). Does readiness to change predict in-session motivational language? Correspondence between two conceptualizations of client motivation. *Addiction*, 106(7), 1261–1269.

Hodgins, D. C., Ching, L. E., & McEwen, J. (2009). Strength of commitment language in motivational interviewing and gambling outcomes. *Psychology of Addictive Behaviors*, 23(1), 122–130.

Imel, Z. E., Baer, J. S., Martino, S., Ball, S. A., & Carroll, K. M. (2011). Mutual influence in therapist competence and adherence to motivational enhancement therapy. *Drug and Alcohol Dependence*, 115(3), 229–236.

Karno, M. P., & Longabaugh, R. (2005). Less directiveness by therapists improves drinking outcomes of reactant clients in alcoholism treatment. *Journal of Consulting and Clinical Psychology*, 73(2), 262–267.

Karno, M. P., Longabaugh, R., & Herbeck, D. (2009). Patient reactance as a moderator of the effect of therapist structure on posttreatment alcohol use. *Journal of Studies on Alcohol and Drugs*, 70(6), 929–936.

Karno, M. P., Longabaugh, R., & Herbeck, D. (2010). What explains the relationship between the therapist structure × patient reactance interaction and drinking outcome? An examination of potential mediators. *Psychology of Addictive Behaviors*, 24(4), 600–607.

Lee, C. S., Baird, J., Longabaugh, R., Nirenberg, T. D., Mello, M. J., & Woolard, R. (2010). Change plan as an active ingredient of brief motivational interventions for reducing negative consequences of drinking in hazardous drinking emergency-department patients. *Journal of Studies on Alcohol and Drugs*, 71(5), 726–733.

Martin, T., Christopher, P. J., Houck, J. M., & Moyers, T. B. (2011). The structure of client language and drinking outcomes in project match. *Psychology of Addictive Behaviors*, 25(3), 439–445.

Martino, S., Ball, S. A., Nich, C., Frankforter, T. L., & Carroll, K. M. (2008). Community program therapist adherence and competence in motivational enhancement therapy. *Drug and Alcohol Dependence*, 96(1–2), 37–48.

McCambridge, J., Day, M., Thomas, B. A., & Strang, J. (2011). Fidelity to motivational interviewing and subsequent cannabis cessation among adolescents. *Addictive Behaviors*, 36(7), 749–754.

Moyers, T. B., & Martin, T. (2006). Therapist influence on client language during motivational interviewing sessions. *Journal of Substance Abuse Treatment*, 30(3), 245–251.

Moyers, T. B., Martin, T., Christopher, P. J., Houck, J. M., Tonigan, J. S., & Amrhein, P. C. (2007). Client language as a mediator of motivational interviewing efficacy: Where is the evidence? *Alcoholism: Clinical and Experimental Research*, 31(Suppl. S3), 40S–47S.

Moyers, T. B., Martin, T., Houck, J. M., Christopher, P. J., & Tonigan, J. S. (2009). From in-session behaviors to drinking outcomes: A causal chain for motivational interviewing. *Journal of Consulting and Clinical Psychology*, 77(6), 1113–1124.

Moyers, T. B., Miller, W. R., & Hendrickson, S. M. (2005). How does motivational interviewing work?: Therapist interpersonal skill predicts client involvement within motivational interviewing sessions. *Journal of Consulting and Clinical Psychology*, 73(4), 590–598.

Naar-King, S., Outlaw, A., Green-Jones, M., Wright, K., & Parsons, J. T. (2009). Motivational interviewing by peer outreach workers: A pilot randomized clinical trial to retain adolescents and young adults in HIV care. *AIDS Care*, 21(7), 868–873.

Pierson, H. M., Hayes, S. C., Gifford, E. V., Roget, N., Padilla, M., Bissett, R., et al. (2007). An examination of the motivational interviewing treatment integrity code. *Journal of Substance Abuse Treatment*, 32(1), 11–17.

Pollak, K. I., Alexander, S. C., Coffman, C. J., Tulsky, J. A., Lyna, P., Dolor, R. J., et al. (2010). Physician communication techniques and weight loss in adults: Project CHAT. *American Journal of Preventive Medicine*, 39(4), 321–328.

Pollak, K. I., Alexander, S. C., Østbye, T., Lyna, P., Tulsky, J. A., Dolor, R. J., et al. (2009). Primary care physicians' discussions of weight-related topics with overweight and obese adolescents: Results from the Teen CHAT Pilot Study. *Journal of Adolescent Health, 45*(2), 205–207.

Pollak, K. I., Østbye, T., Alexander, S. C., Gradison, M., Bastian, L. A., Brouwer, R. J. N., et al. (2007). Empathy goes a long way in weight loss discussions. *Journal of Family Practice, 56*(12), 1031–1036.

Santa Ana, E. J., Carroll, K. M., Anez, L., Paris, M., Jr., Ball, S. A., Nich, C., et al. (2009). Evaluating motivational enhancement therapy adherence and competence among Spanish-speaking therapists. *Drug and Alcohol Dependence, 103*(1–2), 44–51.

Strang, J., & McCambridge, J. (2004). Can the practitioner correctly predict outcome in motivational interviewing? *Journal of Substance Abuse Treatment, 27*(1), 83–88.

Tappin, D. M., McKay, C., McIntyre, D., Gilmour, W. H., Cowan, S., Crawford, F., et al. (2000). A practical instrument to document the process of motivational interviewing. *Behavioural and Cognitive Psychotherapy, 28*(1), 17–32.

Thrasher, A. D., Golin, C. E., Earp, J. A. L., Tien, H., Porter, C., & Howie, L. (2006). Motivational interviewing to support antiretroviral therapy adherence: The role of quality counseling. *Patient Education and Counseling, 62*(1), 64–71.

Thyrian, J. R., Freyer-Adam, J., Hannover, W., Roske, K., Mentzel, F., Kufeld, C., et al. (2007). Adherence to the principles of motivational interviewing, clients' characteristics and behavior outcome in a smoking cessation and relapse prevention trial in women postpartum. *Addictive Behaviors, 32*(10), 2297–2303.

Tollison, S. J., Lee, C. M., Neighbors, C., Neil, T. A., Olson, N. D., & Larimer, M. E. (2008). Questions and reflections: The use of motivational interviewing microskills in a peer-led brief alcohol intervention for college students. *Behavior Therapy, 39*(2), 183–194.

Vader, A. M., Walters, S. T., Prabhu, G. C., Houck, J. M., & Field, C. A. (2010). The language of motivational interviewing and feedback: Counselor language, client language, and client drinking outcomes. *Psychology of Addictive Behaviors, 24*(2), 190–197.

Walker, D., Stephens, R., Rowland, J., & Roffman, R. (2011). The influence of client behavior during motivational interviewing on marijuana treatment outcome. *Addictive Behaviors, 36*(6), 669–673.

THEORETICAL COMMENTARY

Amrhein, P. C. (2004). How does motivational interviewing work? What client talk reveals. *Journal of Cognitive Psychotherapy, 18*(4), 323–336.

Bricker, J., & Tollison, S. (2011). Comparison of motivational interviewing with acceptance and commitment therapy: A conceptual and clinical review. *Behavioural and Cognitive Psychotherapy, 39*(5), 541–559.

Britton, P. C., Patrick, H., Wenzel, A., & Williams, G. C. (2011). Integrating motivational interviewing and self-determination theory with cognitive behavioral therapy to prevent suicide. *Cognitive and Behavioral Practice, 18*(1), 16–27.

Cheng, M. K. S. (2007). New approaches for creating the therapeutic alliance:

Solution-focused interviewing, motivational interviewing, and the medication interest model. *Psychiatric Clinics of North America*, *30*(2), 157–166.

Christopher, P. J., & Dougher, M. J. (2009). A behavior-analytic account of motivational interviewing. *Behavior Analyst*, *32*(1), 149–161.

Draycott, S., & Dabbs, A. (1998). Cognitive dissonance. 2: A theoretical grounding of motivational interviewing. *British Journal of Clinical Psychology*, *37*(3), 355–364.

Faris, A. S., Cavell, T. A., Fishburne, J. W., & Britton, P. C. (2009). Examining motivational interviewing from a client agency perspective. *Journal of Clinical Psychology*, *65*(9), 955–970.

Frankel, Z. e., & Levitt, H. (2006). Postmodern strategies for working with resistance: Problem resolution or self-revolution? *Journal of Constructivist Psychology*, *19*(3), 219–250.

Gache, P., Fortini, C., Meynard, A., Reiner Meylan, M., & Sommer, J. (2006). [Motivational interviewing: Some theoretical aspects and some practical exercises]. *Revue Medicale Suisse*, *2*(80), 2154, 2156–2162.

Gerber, S., & Basham, A. (1999). Responsive therapy and motivational interviewing: Postmodernist paradigms. *Journal of Counseling and Development*, *77*(4), 418–422.

Leffingwell, T. R., Neumann, C. A., Babitzke, A. C., Leedy, M. J., & Walters, S. T. (2007). Social psychology and motivational interviewing: A review of relevant principles and recommendations for research and practice. *Behavioural and Cognitive Psychotherapy*, *35*(1), 31–45.

Markland, D., Ryan, R. M., Tobin, V. J., & Rollnick, S. (2005). Motivational interviewing and self-determination theory. *Journal of Social and Clinical Psychology*, *24*(6), 811–831.

Miller, J. H., & Moyers, T. B. (2002). Motivational interviewing in substance abuse: Applications for occupational medicine. *Occupational Medicine*, *17*(1), 51–65.

Miller, W. R. (1983). Motivational interviewing with problem drinkers. *Behavioural Psychotherapy*, *11*(2), 147–172.

Miller, W. R. (1994). Motivational interviewing: III. On the ethics of motivational intervention. *Behavioural and Cognitive Psychotherapy*, *22*(2), 111–123.

Miller, W. R. (1995). The ethics of motivational interviewing revisited. *Behavioural and Cognitive Psychotherapy*, *23*(4), 345–348.

Miller, W. R. (2000). Motivational interviewing: IV. Some parallels with horse whispering. *Behavioural and Cognitive Psychotherapy*, *28*(3), 285–292.

Miller, W. R., & Rollnick, S. (2004). Talking oneself into change: Motivational interviewing, stages of change, and therapeutic process. *Journal of Cognitive Psychotherapy*, *18*(4), 299–308.

Miller, W. R., & Rose, G. S. (2009). Toward a theory of motivational interviewing. *American Psychologist*, *64*(6), 527–537.

Moos, R. H. (2007). Theory-based active ingredients of effective treatments for substance use disorders. *Drug and Alcohol Dependence*, *88*(2–3), 109–121.

Moyers, T. B. (2004). History and happenstance: How motivational interviewing got its start. *Journal of Cognitive Psychotherapy*, *18*(4), 291–298.

Moyers, T. B., & Rollnick, S. (2002). A motivational interviewing perspective on resistance in psychotherapy. *Journal of Clinical Psychology*, *58*(2), 185–193.

Muscat, A. C. (2005). Ready, set, go: The transtheoretical model of change and motivational interviewing for "fringe" clients. *Journal of Employment Counseling, 42*(4), 179–192.

Newnham-Kanas, C., Morrow, D., & Irwin, J. D. (2010). Motivational coaching: A functional juxtaposition of three methods for health behaviour change: Motivational interviewing, coaching, and skilled helping. *International Journal of Evidence Based Coaching and Mentoring, 8*(2), 27–48.

Putnam, S. M. (2002). Changing health behaviors through the medical interview. *Epidemiologia e Psichiatria Sociale, 11*(4), 218–225.

Ryan, R. M., Lynch, M. F., Vansteenkiste, M., & Deci, E. L. (2011). Motivation and autonomy in counseling, psychotherapy, and behavior change: A look at theory and practice. *Counseling Psychologist, 39*(2), 193–260.

Scheel, M. J. (2011). Client common factors represented by client motivation and autonomy. *Counseling Psychologist, 39*(2), 276–285.

Seager, M. (1995). Healing psychology's own motivational conflicts: A comment on Miller's "Ethics of Motivational Intervention." *Behavioural and Cognitive Psychotherapy, 23*(4), 341–343.

Sheldon, K. M. (2003). Reconciling humanistic ideals and scientific clinical practice. *Clinical Psychology: Science and Practice, 10*(3), 302.

Stanton, M. (2010). Motivational interviewing and the social context. *American Psychologist, 65*(4), 297–298.

Vansteenkiste, M., & Sheldon, K. M. (2006). There's nothing more practical than a good theory: Integrating motivational interviewing and self-determination theory. *British Journal of Clinical Psychology, 45*(1), 63–82.

Velasquez, M., von Sternberg, K., Dodrill, C., Kan, L., & Parsons, J. (2005). The transtheoretical model as a framework for developing substance abuse interventions. *Journal of Addictions Nursing, 16*(1), 31–40.

Wagner, C. C., & Ingersoll, K. S. (2008). Beyond cognition: Broadening the emotional base of motivational interviewing. *Journal of Psychotherapy Integration, 18*(2), 191–206.

Weegmann, M. (2002). Motivational interviewing and addiction: A psychodynamic appreciation. *Psychodynamic Practice: Individuals, Groups and Organisations, 8*(2), 179–195.

References

Agostinelli, G., Brown, J. M., & Miller, W. R. (1995). Effects of normative feedback on consumption among heavy drinking college students. *Journal of Drug Education, 25*, 31–40.

Aharonovich, E., Amrhein, P. C., Bisaga, A., Nunes, E. V., & Hasin, D. S. (2008). Cognition, commitment language, and behavioral change among cocaine-dependent patients. *Psychology of Addictive Behaviors, 22*, 557–562.

Aharonovich, E., Brooks, A. C., Nunes, E. V., & Hasin, D. S. (2008). Cognitive deficits in marijuana users: Effects on motivational enhancement therapy plus cognitive behavioral therapy treatment outcome. *Drug and Alcohol Dependence, 95*(3), 279–283.

Aharonovich, E., Hatzenbuehler, M. L., Johnston, B., O'Leary, A., Morgenstern, J., Wainberg, M. L., et al. (2006). A low-cost, sustainable intervention for drinking reduction in the HIV primary care setting. *AIDS Care, 18*(6), 561–568.

Ajzen, I. (1985). From intentions to actions: A theory of planned behavior. In J. Kuhl & J. Beckmann (Eds.), *Action control: From cognition to behavior* (pp. 11–39). Berlin: Springer-Verlag.

Ajzen, I. (1991). The theory of planned behavior. *Organizational Behavior and Human Decision Processes, 50*, 179–211.

Ali, N., Hagshenas, L., Reza, M. R., Ira, B., & Maryam, F. (2011). Comparing the effectiveness of group cognitive behavior therapy and its integration with motivational interviewing on symptoms of patients with obsessive–compulsive disorder. *Journal of Research in Behavioural Sciences, 9*(1 (17), 13–23.

Allen, J. P. (2001). Prospects for matching clients to alcoholism treatments based on conceptual level. In R. Longabaugh & P. W. Wirtz (Eds.), *Project MATCH hypotheses: Results and causal chain analyses* (pp. 149–153). Bethesda, MD: National Institute on Alcohol Abuse and Alcoholism.

Allport, G. W. (1961). *Pattern and growth in personality.* New York: Holt, Rinehart & Winston.

Almomani, F., Williams, K., Catley, D., & Brown, C. (2009). Effects of an oral health promotion program in people with mental illness. *Journal of Dental Research*, 88(7), 648–652.

Amrhein, P. C., Miller, W. R., Yahne, C. E., Palmer, M., & Fulcher, L. (2003). Client commitment language during motivational interviewing predicts drug use outcomes. *Journal of Consulting and Clinical Psychology*, 71(5), 862–878.

Ang, D., Kesavalu, R., Lydon, J. R., Lane, K. A., & Bigatti, S. (2007). Exercise-based motivational interviewing for female patients with fibromyalgia: A case series. *Clinical Rheumatology*, 26(11), 1843–1849.

Anshel, M. H., & Kang, M. (2008). Effectiveness of motivational interviewing on changes in fitness, blood lipids, and exercise adherence of police officers: An outcome-based action study. *Journal of Correctional Health Care*, 14(1), 48–62.

Antiss, B., Polaschek, D. L. L., & Wilson, M. (2011). A brief motivational interviewing intervention with prisoners: When you lead a horse to water, can it drink for itself? *Psychology, Crime and Law*, 17(8), 689–710.

Antiss, T., & Passmore, J. (2012). Motivational interviewing coaching. In J. Passmore, D. Peterson, & T. Freire (Eds.), *The Wiley–Blackwell handbook of the psychology of coaching and mentoring*. Chichester, UK: Wiley–Blackwell.

Anton, R. F., Moak, D. H., Latham, P., Waid, L. R., Myrick, H., Voronin, K., et al. (2005). Naltrexone combined with either cognitive behavioral or motivational enhancement therapy for alcohol dependence. *Journal of Clinical Psychopharmacology*, 25(4), 349–357.

Anton, R. F., O'Malley, S. S., Ciraulo, D. A., Couper, D., Donovan, D. M., Gastfriend, D. R., et al. (2006). Combined pharmacotherapies and behavioral interventions for alcohol dependence. The COMBINE study: A randomized controlled trial. *Journal of the American Medical Association*, 295, 2003–2017.

APA Presidential Task Force on Evidence-Based Practice. (2006). Evidence-based practice in psychology. *American Psychologist*, 61(4), 271–285.

Arkowitz, H., & Westra, H. A. (2004). Integrating motivational interviewing and cognitive behavioral therapy in the treatment of depression and anxiety. *Journal of Cognitive Psychotherapy*, 18(4), 337–350.

Arkowitz, H., Westra, H. A., Miller, W. R., & Rollnick, S. (Eds.). (2008). *Motivational interviewing in the treatment of psychological problems*. New York: Guilford Press.

Armstrong, M. J., Mottershead, T. A., Ronksley, P. E., Sigal, R. J., Campbell, T. S., & Hemmelgarn, B. R. (2011). Motivational interviewing to improve weight loss in overweight and/or obese patients: A systematic review and meta-analysis of randomized controlled trials. *Obesity Reviews*, 12(9), 709–723.

Atkinson, C., & Woods, K. (2003). Motivational interviewing strategies for disaffected secondary school students: A case example. *Educational Psychology in Practice*, 19(1), 49–64.

Aubrey, L. L. (1998). *Motivational interviewing with adolescents presenting for outpatient substance abuse treatment*. Unpublished doctoral dissertation, University of New Mexico, Albuquerque.

Azrin, N. H., Sisson, R. W., Meyers, R. J., & Godley, M. (1982). Alcoholism treatment by disulfiram and community reinforcement therapy. *Journal of Behavior Therapy and Experimental Psychiatry*, 13, 105–112.

Babor, T. F., & Del Boca, F. K. (Eds.). (2003). *Treatment matching in alcoholism.* Cambridge, UK: Cambridge University Press.

Babor, T. F., Miller, W. R., DiClemente, C. C., & Longabaugh, R. (1999). A study to remember: Response of the Project MATCH Research Group. *Addiction, 94*, 66–69.

Baca, C. T., & Manuel, J. K. (2007). Satisfaction with long-distance motivational interviewing for problem drinking. *Addictive Disorders and Their Treatment, 6*, 39–41.

Baer, J., Kaufman, J. C., & Baumeister, R. F. (Eds.). (2008). *Are we free?: Psychology and free will.* New York: Oxford University Press.

Baer, J. S., Beadnell, B., Garrett, J. A., Hartzler, B., Wells, E. A., & Peterson, P. L. (2008). Adolescent change language within a brief motivational intervention and substance use outcomes. *Psychology of Addictive Behaviors, 22*, 570–575.

Baer, J. S., Carpenter, K. M., Beadnell, B., Stoner, S. A., Ingalsbe, M. H., Hartzler, B., et al. (2012). Computer assessment of simulated patient interviews (CASPI): Psychometric properties of a web-based system for the assessment of motivational interviewing skills. *Journal of Studies on Alcohol and Drugs, 73*(1), 154–164.

Baer, J. S., Kivlahan, D. R., Blume, A. W., McKnight, P., & Marlatt, G. A. (2001). Brief intervention for heavy-drinking college students: 4-year follow-up and natural history. *American Journal of Public Health, 91*(8), 1310–1316.

Baer, J. S., Rosengren, D. B., Dunn, C. W., Wells, W. A., Ogle, R. L., & Hartzler, B. (2004). An evaluation of workshop training in motivational interviewing for addiction and mental health clinicians. *Drug and Alcohol Dependence, 73*(1), 99–106.

Bailey, K. A., Baker, A. L., Webster, R. A., & Lewin, T. J. (2004). Pilot randomized controlled trial of a brief alcohol intervention group for adolescents. *Drug and Alcohol Review, 23*(2), 157–166.

Baker, A., & Hambridge, J. (2002). Motivational interviewing: Enhancing engagement in treatment for mental health problems. *Behaviour Change, 19*(3), 138–145.

Ball, S., Hamilton, J., Martino, S., Carroll, K. M., Gallon, S. L., Coperich, S., et al. (2006). *Motivational interviewing assessment: Supervisory tools for enhancing proficiency (MIA:STEP).* Salem, OR: Northwest Frontier Addiction Technology Transfer Center.

Ball, S. A., Martino, S., Nich, C., Frankforter, T. L., Van Horn, D., Crits-Christoph, P., et al. (2007). Site matters: Multisite randomized trial of motivational enhancement therapy in community drug abuse clinics. *Journal of Consulting and Clinical Psychology, 75*(4), 556–567.

Bamatter, W., Carroll, K. M., Añez, L. M., Paris, M. J., Ball, S. A., Nich, C., et al. (2010). Informal discussions in substance abuse treatment sessions with Spanish-speaking clients. *Journal of Substance Abuse Treatment, 39*(4), 353–363.

Bandura, A. (1982). Self-efficacy mechanism in human agency. *American Psychologist, 37*, 122–147.

Bandura, A. (1997). *Self-efficacy: The exercise of control.* New York: Freeman.

Barber, J. G., & Crisp, B. R. (1995). Social support and prevention of relapse following treatment for alcohol abuse. *Research on Social Work Practice, 5*(3), 283–296.

Bargh, J. A., & Chartrand, T. L. (1999). The unbearable automaticity of being. *American Psychologist, 54,* 462–479.

Bargh, J. A., & Ferguson, M. J. (2000). Beyond behaviorism: On the automaticity of higher mental processes. *Psychological Bulletin, 126,* 925–945.

Barkin, S. L. (2008). Is office-based counseling about media use, timeouts, and firearm storage effective?: Results from a cluster-randomized, controlled trial. *Pediatrics, 122*(1), e15–e25.

Barnet, B., Liu, J., DeVoe, M., Duggan, A. K., Gold, M. A., & Pecukonis, E. (2009). Motivational intervention to reduce rapid subsequent births to adolescent mothers: A community-based randomized trial. *Annals of Family Medicine, 7*(5), 436–445.

Baumeister, R. F. (1994). The crystallization of discontent in the process of major life change. In T. F. Heatherton & J. L. Weinberger (Eds.), *Can personality change?* (pp. 281–297). Washington, DC: American Psychological Association.

Baumeister, R. F. (2005). Self and volition. In W. R. Miller & H. D. Delaney (Eds.), *Judeo-Christian perspectives on psychology: Human nature, motivation, and change.* Washington, DC: American Psychological Association.

Baumeister, R. F., Heatherton, T. F., & Tice, D. M. (1994). *Losing control: How and why people fail at self-regulation.* New York: Academic Press.

Beach, M. C., Inui, T., & the Relationship-Centered Care Research Network. (2006). Relationship-centered care: A constructive reframing. *Journal of General Internal Medicine, 21*(S1), S3–S8.

Beauchamp, T. L., & Childress, J. F. (2001). *Principles of biomedical ethics* (5th ed.). New York: Oxford University Press.

Bell, K. R., Temkin, N. R., Esselman, P. C., Doctor, J. N., Bombardier, C. H., Fraser, R. T., et al. (2005). The effect of a scheduled telephone intervention on outcome after moderate to severe traumatic brain injury: A randomized trial. *Archives of Physical Medicine and Rehabilitation, 86*(5), 851–856.

Bellg, A. J. (2003). Maintenance of health behavior change in preventive cardiology: Internalization and self-regulation of new behaviors. *Behavior Modification, 27*(1), 103–131.

Bem, D. J. (1967). Self-perception: An alternative interpretation of cognitive dissonance phenomena. *Psychological Review, 74,* 183–200.

Bem, D. J. (1972). Self-perception theory. In L. Berkowitz (Ed.), *Advances in experimental social psychology* (Vol. 6, pp. 1–62). New York: Academic Press.

Bennett, G. A., Roberts, H. A., Vaughan, T. E., Gibbins, J. A., & Rouse, L. (2007). Evaluating a method of assessing competence in Motivational Interviewing: A study using simulated patients in the United Kingdom. *Addictive Behaviors, 32*(1), 69–79.

Bennett, J. A., Lyons, K. S., Winters-Stone, K., Nail, L. M., & Scherer, J. (2007). Motivational interviewing to increase physical activity in long-term cancer survivors: A randomized controlled trial. *Nursing Research, 56*(1), 18–27.

Bennett, J. A., Perrin, N. A., Hanson, G., Bennett, D., Gaynor, W., Flaherty-Robb, M., et al. (2005). Healthy aging demonstration project: Nurse coaching for behavior change in older adults. *Research in Nursing and Health, 28*(3), 187–197.

Berger, B. A., Liang, H., & Hudmon, K. S. (2005). Evaluation of software-based telephone counseling to enhance medication persistency among patients with multiple sclerosis. *Journal of the American Pharmacists Association, 45*(4), 466–472.

Bergin, A. E. (1980). Psychotherapy and religious values. *Journal of Consulting and Clinical Psychology, 48,* 95–105.

Bernstein, E., & Bernstein, J. (2008). Effectiveness of alcohol screening and brief motivational intervention in the emergency department setting. *Annals of Emergency Medicine, 51*(6), 751–754.

Bernstein, E., Bernstein, J., & Levenson, S. (1997). Project ASSERT: An ED-based intervention to increase access to primary care, preventive services, and the substance abuse treatment system. *Annals of Emergency Medicine, 30*(2), 181–189.

Bernstein, J., Bernstein, E., Tassiopoulos, K., Heeren, T., Levenson, S., & Hingson, R. (2005). Brief motivational intervention at a clinic visit reduces cocaine and heroin use. *Drug and Alcohol Dependence, 77*(1), 49–59.

Bertholet, N., Faouzi, M., Gmel, G., Gaume, J., & Daeppen, J. B. (2010). Change talk sequence during brief motivational intervention, towards or away from drinking. *Addiction, 105,* 2016–2112.

Bien, T. H., Miller, W. R., & Boroughs, J. M. (1993). Motivational interviewing with alcohol outpatients. *Behavioural and Cognitive Psychotherapy, 21,* 347–356.

Bien, T. H., Miller, W. R., & Tonigan, J. S. (1993). Brief interventions for alcohol problems: A review. *Addiction, 88,* 315–336.

Birgden, A. (2004). Therapeutic jurisprudence and responsivity: Finding the will and the way in offender rehabilitation. *Psychology, Crime and Law, 10*(3), 283–295.

Blanchard, K. H., & Johnson, S. (1982). *The one-minute manager.* New York: William Morrow.

Bohart, A. C., Elliott, R., Greenberg, L. S., & Watson, J. C. (2002). Empathy. In J. C. Norcross (Ed.), *Psychotherapy relationships that work* (pp. 89–108). New York: Oxford University Press.

Bohart, A. C., & Tallman, K. (1999). *How clients make therapy work: The process of active self-healing.* Washington, DC: American Psychological Association.

Bolger, K., Carter, K., Curtin, L., Martz, D. M., Gagnon, S. G., & Michael, K. D. (2010). Motivational interviewing for smoking cessation among college students. *Journal of College Student Psychotherapy, 24*(2), 116–129.

Bombardier, C. H., Bell, K. R., Temkin, N. R., Fann, J. R., Hoffman, J., & Dikmen, S. (2009). The efficacy of a scheduled telephone intervention for ameliorating depressive symptoms during the first year after traumatic brain injury. *Journal of Head Trauma Rehabilitation, 24*(4), 230–238.

Bombardier, C. H., & Rimmele, C. T. (1999). Motivational interviewing to prevent alcohol abuse after traumatic brain injury: A case series. *Rehabilitation Psychology, 44*(1), 52–67.

Bordin, E. S. (1979). The generalizability of the psychoanalytic concept of the working alliance. *Psychotherapy: Theory, Research and Practice, 16,* 252–260.

Borrelli, B., McQuaid, E. L., Novak, S. P., Hammond, S. K., & Becker, B. (2010). Motivating Latino caregivers of children with asthma to quit smoking: A randomized trial. *Journal of Consulting and Clinical Psychology, 78*(1), 34–43.

Borrelli, B., Novak, S., Hecht, J., Emmons, K., Papandonatos, G., & Abrams, D. (2005). Home health care nurses as a new channel for smoking cessation treatment: Outcomes from Project CARES (Community-nurse Assisted Research and Education on Smoking). *Preventive Medicine, 41*, 815–821.

Borrelli, B., Riekert, K. A., Weinstein, A., & Rathier, L. (2007). Brief motivational interviewing as a clinical strategy to promote asthma medication adherence. *Journal of Allergy and Clinical Immunology, 120*(5), 1023–1030.

Bowen, D., Ehret, C., Pedersen, M., Snetselaar, L., Johnson, M., Tinker, L., et al. (2002). Results of an adjunct dietary intervention program in the women's health initiative. *Journal of the American Dietetic Association, 102*(11), 1631–1637.

Boyatzis, R. E., Passarelli, A. M., Koenig, K., Lowe, M., Mathew, B., Stoller, J. K., et al. (2012). Examination of the neural substrates activated in memories of experiences with resonant and dissonant leaders. *Leadership Quarterly, 23*(2), 259–272.

Braithwaite, V. A., & Law, H. G. (1985). Structure of human values: Testing the adequacy of the Rokeach Value Survey. *Journal of Personality and Social Psychology, 49*(1), 250–263.

Brehm, S. S., & Brehm, J. W. (1981). *Psychological reactance: A theory of freedom and control.* New York: Academic Press.

Brown, J. M. (1998). Self-regulation and the addictive behaviors. In W. R. Miller & N. Heather (Eds.), *Treating addictive behaviors* (2nd ed., pp. 61–74). New York: Plenum Press.

Brown, J. M., & Miller, W. R. (1993). Impact of motivational interviewing on participation and outcome in residential alcoholism treatment. *Psychology of Addictive Behaviors, 7*, 211–218.

Brown, R. A., Strong, D. R., Abrantes, A. M., Myers, M. G., Ramsey, S. E., & Kahler, C. W. (2009). Effects on substance use outcomes in adolescents receiving motivational interviewing for smoking cessation during psychiatric hospitalization. *Addictive Behaviors, 34*(10), 887–891.

Brown, T. G., Dongier, M., Latimer, E., Legault, L., Seraganian, P., Kokin, M., et al. (2007). Group-delivered brief intervention versus standard care for mixed alcohol/other drug problems. *Alcoholism Treatment Quarterly, 24*(4), 23–40.

Buber, M. (1971). *I and thou.* New York: Free Press.

Buber, M., Rogers, C. R., Anderson, R., & Cissna, K. N. (1997). *The Martin Buber–Carl Rogers dialogue: A new transcript with commentary.* Albany: State University of New York Press.

Buckner, J. D., & Schmidt, N. B. (2009). A randomized pilot study of motivation enhancement therapy to increase utilization of cognitive-behavioral therapy for social anxiety. *Behavior Research and Therapy, 47*(8), 710–715.

Burke, B. L., Vassilev, G., Kantchelov, A., & Zweben, A. (2002). Motivational interviewing with couples. In W. R. Miller & S. Rollnick (Eds.), *Motivational interviewing: Preparing people for change* (2nd ed., pp. 347–361). New York: Guilford Press.

Burke, P. J., Da Silva, J. D., Vaughan, B. L., & Knight, J. R. (2005). Training high school counselors on the use of motivational interviewing to screen for substance abuse. *Substance Abuse, 26*(3–4), 31–34.

Butler, C. C., Rollnick, S., Cohen, D., Bachmann, M., Russell, I., & Stott, N. (1999). Motivational consulting versus brief advice for smokers in general practice: A randomized trial. *British Journal of General Practice, 49*(445), 611–616.

Butterworth, S. (2007). Health coaching as an intervention in health management programs. *Disease Management and Health Outcomes, 15*(5), 299–307.

Butterworth, S., Linden, A., McClay, W., & Leo, M. C. (2006). Effect of motivational interviewing-based health coaching on employees' physical and mental health status. *Journal of Occupational Health Psychology, 11*(4), 358–365.

Campbell, M. K., Carr, C., DeVellis, B., Switzer, B., Biddle, A., Amamoo, M. A., et al. (2009). A randomized trial of tailoring and motivational interviewing to promote fruit and vegetable consumption for cancer prevention and control. *Annals of Behavioral Medicine, 38*(2), 71–85.

Campbell, S. D., Adamson, S. J., & Carter, J. D. (2010). Client language during motivational enhancement therapy and alcohol use outcomes. *Behavioural and Cognitive Psychotherapy, 38*, 399–415.

Carey, K. B., Maisto, S. A., Carey, M. P., & Purnine, D. M. (2001). Measuring readiness-to-change substance misuse among psychiatric outpatients: I. Reliability and validity of self-report measures. *Journal of Studies on Alcohol, 62*(1), 79–88.

Carr, S. (2011). *Scripting addiction: The politics of therapeutic talk and American sobriety.* Princeton, NJ: Princeton University Press.

Carroll, K. M., Ball, S. A., Nich, C., Martino, S., Frankforter, T. L., Farentinos, C., et al. (2006). Motivational interviewing to improve treatment engagement and outcome in individuals seeking treatment for substance abuse: A multisite effectiveness study. *Drug and Alcohol Dependence, 81*, 301–312.

Carroll, K. M., Connors, G. J., Cooney, N. L., DiClemente, C. C., Donovan, D. M., Kadden, R. R., et al. (1998). Internal validity of Project Match treatments: Discriminability and integrity. *Journal of Consulting and Clinical Psychology, 66*(2), 290–303.

Carroll, K. M., Libby, B., Sheehan, J., & Hyland, N. (2001). Motivational interviewing to enhance treatment initiation in substance abusers: An effectiveness study. *American Journal on Addictions, 10*(4), 335–339.

Carroll, K. M., Martino, S., Ball, S. A., Nich, C., Frankforter, T., Anez, L. M., et al. (2009). A multisite randomized effectiveness trial of motivational enhancement therapy for Spanish-speaking substance users. *Journal of Consulting and Clinical Psychology, 77*(5), 993–999.

Catley, D., Harris, K. J., Mayo, M. S., Hall, S., Okuyemi, K. S., Boardman, T., et al. (2006). Adherence to principles of motivational interviewing and client within-session behavior. *Behavioural and Cognitive Psychotherapy, 34*(1), 43–56.

Chan, S. C., Lam, T. H., Salili, F., Leung, G. M., Wong, D. C. N., Botelho, R. J., et al. (2005). A randomized controlled trial of an individualized motivational intervention on smoking cessation for parents of sick children: A pilot study. *Applied Nursing Research, 18*(3), 178–181.

Chang, G., Fisher, N. D. L., Hornstein, M. D., Jones, J. A., Jauke, S. H., Niamkey, N., et al. (2011). Brief intervention for women with risky drinking and medical diagnoses: A randomized controlled trial. *Journal of Substance Abuse Treatment, 41*(2), 105–114.

Chariyeva, Z., Golin, C. F., Earp, J. A., Maman, S., Suchindran, C., & Zimmer, C. (in press). The role of self-efficacy and motivation to explain the effect of motivational interviewing time on changes in risky sexual behavior among people living with HIV: A mediation analysis. *AIDS and Behavior.* doi:10.1007/ s10461-0115-8.

Charles, C., & Whelan, T. (1997). Shared decision making in the medical encounter: What does it mean? (or it takes at least two to tango). *Social Science and Medicine, 44*(5), 681–692.

Chen, S. M., Creedy, D., Lin, H-S., & Wollin, J. (2012). Effects of motivational interviewing intervention on self-management, psychological and glycemic outcomes in type 2 diabetes: A randomized controlled trial. *International Journal of Nursing.* Posted online December 30, 2011 at *dx.doi.org/10.1016/j. ijnurstu.2011.11.011.*

Chick, J., Ritson, B., Connaughton, J., Stewart, A., & Chick, J. (1988). Advice versus extended treatment for alcoholism: A controlled study. *British Journal of Addiction, 83,* 159–170.

Childress, C. A. (1999). Interactive e-mail journals: A model for providing psychotherapeutic interventions using the internet. *CyberPsychology and Behavior, 2*(3), 213–221.

Christensen, A., Miller, W. R., & Muñoz, R. F. (1978). Expanding mental health service delivery. *Professional Psychology, 9,* 249–270.

Cialdini, R. B. (2007). *Influence: The psychology of persuasion.* New York: Collins Business.

Clark, M. D. (2005). Motivational interviewing for probation staff: Increasing the readiness to change. *Federal Probation, 69*(2), 22–28.

Clark, M. D., Walters, S., Gingerich, R., & Meltzer, M. (2006). Motivational interviewing for probation officers: Tipping the balance toward change. *Federal Probation, 70*(1), 38–44.

Connell, A. M., & Dishion, T. J. (2008). Reducing depression among at-risk early adolescents: Three-year effects of a family-centered intervention embedded within schools. *Journal of Family Psychology, 22*(4), 574–585.

Cook, P. F., Emiliozzi, S., Waters, C., & El Hajj, D. (2008). Effects of telephone counseling on antipsychotic adherence and emergency department utilization. *American Journal of Managed Care, 14*(12), 841–846.

Cooperrider, D. L., & Whitney, D. (2005). *Appreciative inquiry: A positive revolution in change.* San Francisco: Berrett-Koehler Publishers.

Cordova, J. V., Warren, L. Z., & Gee, C. B. (2001). Motivational interviewing as an intervention for at-risk couples. *Journal of Marital and Family Therapy, 27*(3), 315–326.

Cozby, P. C. (1973). Self-disclosure: A literature review. *Psychological Bulletin, 79*(2), 73–91.

Critcher, C. R., Dunning, D., & Armor, D. A. (2010). When self-affirmations reduce defensiveness: Timing is key. *Personality and Social Psychology Bulletin, 36*(7), 947–959.

Crits-Christoph, P., Hamilton, J. L., Ring-Kurtz, S. R. G., McClure, B., Kulaga, A., & Rotrosen, J. (2011). Program, counselor, and patient variability in the alliance: A multilevel study of the alliance in relation to substance use outcomes. *Journal of Substance Abuse Treatment, 40*(4), 405–413.

Cummings, C. C., Gordon, J. R., & Marlatt, G. A. (1980). Relapse: Prevention and prediction. In W. R. Miller (Ed.), *The addictive behaviors: Treatment of alcoholism, drug abuses, smoking and obesity* (pp. 291–321). New York: Pergamon Press.

D'Amico, E. J., Miles, J. N. V., Stern, S. A., & Meredith, L. S. (2008). Brief motivational interviewing for teens at risk of substance use consequences: A randomized pilot study in a primary care clinic. *Journal of Substance Abuse Treatment, 35*(1), 53–61.

Daeppen, J.-B., Bertholet, N., Gmel, G., & Gaume, J. (2007). Communication during brief intervention, intention to change, and outcome. *Substance Abuse, 28*(3), 43–51.

Daeppen, J.-B., Bertholet, N., & Gaume, J. (2010). What process research tells us about brief intervention efficacy. *Drug and Alcohol Review, 29*, 612–616.

Daley, D. C., Salloum, I. M., Suckoff, A., Kirisci, L., & Thase, M. E. (1998). Increasing treatment adherence among outpatients with depression and cocaine dependence: Results of a pilot study. *American Journal of Psychiatry, 155*, 1611–1613.

Daugherty, M. D. (2009). *A randomized trial of motivational interviewing with college students for academic success.* Doctoral dissertation, University of New Mexico, Albuquerque. Retrieved from *http://libproxy.unm.edu/login?url=http://search.ebscohost.com/login.aspx?direct=true&db=psyh&AN=2009-99060-447&login.asp&site=ehost-live&scope=site.*

Davidson, D., Gulliver, S. B., Longabaugh, R., Wirtz, P. W., & Swift, R. (2007). Building better cognitive-behavioral therapy: Is broad-spectrum treatment more effective than motivational enhancement therapy for alcohol-dependent patients treated with naltrexone? *Journal of Studies on Alcohol and Drugs, 68*(2), 238–247.

Davis, T. M., Baer, J. S., Saxon, A. J., & Kivlahan, D. R. (2003). Brief motivational feedback improves post-incarceration treatment contact among veterans with substance use disorders. *Drug and Alcohol Dependence, 69*, 197–203.

de Jonge, J. M., Schippers, G. M., & Schaap, C. P. D. R. (2005). The motivational interviewing skill code: Reliability and a critical appraisal. *Behavioural and Cognitive Psychotherapy, 33*(3), 285–298.

Deci, E. L., & Ryan, R. M. (1985). *Intrinsic motivation and self-determination in human behavior.* New York: Plenum Press.

Delaney, H. D., Miller, W. R., & Bisono, A. M. (2007). Religiosity and spirituality among psychologists: A survey of clinician members of the American Psychological Association. *Professional Psychology: Research and Practice, 38*, 538–546.

DeShazer, S., Dolan, Y., Korman, H., Trepper, T., McCollum, E., & Berg, I. K. (2007). *More than miracles: The state of the art of solution-focused brief therapy.* Binghamton, NY: Haworth Press.

Dia, D. A., Simmons, C. A., Oliver, M. A., & Cooper, R. L. (2009). Motivational interviewing for perpetrators of intimate partner violence. In P. Lehmann &

C. A. Simmons (Eds.), *Strengths-based batterer intervention: A new paradigm in ending family violence* (pp. 87–111). New York: Springer.

Diaz, R. M., & Berk, L. E. (Eds.). (1992). *Private speech: From social interaction to self-regulation.* Hillsdale, NJ: Erlbaum.

Diaz, R. M., & Fruhauf, A. G. (1991). The origins and development of self-regulation: A developmental model on the risk for addictive behaviours. In N. Heather, W. R. Miller, & J. Greeley (Eds.), *Self-control and the addictive behaviours* (pp. 83–106). Sydney: Maxwell Macmillan Publishing Australia.

Diaz, R. M., Neal, C. J., & Amaya-Williams, M. (1990). The social origins of self-regulation. In L. C. Moll (Ed.), *Vygotsky and education: Instructional implications and applications of sociohistorical psychology* (pp. 127–154). New York: Cambridge University Press.

Diaz, R. M., Winsler, A., Atencio, D. J., & Harbors, K. (1992). Mediation of self-regulation through the use of private speech. *International Journal of Cognitive Education and Mediated Learning, 2,* 155–167.

DiClemente, C. C. (2003). *Addiction and change: How addictions develop and addicted people recover.* New York: Guilford Press.

DiClemente, C. C., & Velasquez, M. M. (2002). Motivational Interviewing and the stages of change. In W. R. Miller & S. Rollnick (Eds.), *Motivational interviewing: Preparing people for change.* (2nd ed., pp. 201–216). New York: Guilford Press.

DiLillo, V., Siegfried, N. J., & West, D. S. (2003). Incorporating motivational interviewing into behavioral obesity treatment. *Cognitive and Behavioral Practice, 10*(2), 120–130.

Dillard, J. P., & Shen, L. (2005). On the nature of reactance and its role in persuasive health communication. *Communication Monographs, 72*(2), 144–168.

Donnelly, D. A., & Murray, E. J. (1991). Cognitive and emotional changes in written essays and therapy interviews. *Journal of Social and Clinical Psychology, 10,* 334–350.

Donovan, D. M., Kivlahan, D. R., Kadden, R. M., & Hill, D. (2001). Cognitive impairment as a client–treatment matching hypothesis. In R. Longabaugh & P. W. Wirtz (Eds.), *Project MATCH hypotheses: Results and causal chain analyses* (pp. 62–81). Bethesda, MD: National Institute on Alcohol Abuse and Alcoholism.

Easton, C., Swan, S., & Sinha, R. (2000). Motivation to change substance use among offenders of domestic violence. *Journal of Substance Abuse Treatment, 19*(1), 1–5.

Edwards, G., Orford, J., Egert, S., Guthrie, S., Hawker, A., Hensman, C., et al. (1977). Alcoholism: A controlled trial of "treatment" and "advice." *Journal of Studies on Alcohol, 38,* 1004–1031.

Elliot, D. L., Goldberg, L., Kuehl, K. S., Moe, E. L., Breger, R. K., & Pickering, M. A. (2007). The PHLAME (Promoting Healthy Lifestyles: Alternative Models' Effects) firefighter study: Outcomes of two models of behavior change. *Journal of Occupational and Environmental Medicine, 49*(2), 204–213.

Ellis, A., & MacLaren, C. (2005). *Rational emotive behavior therapy: A therapist's guide* (2nd ed.). Atascadero, CA: Impact.

Elvy, G., Wells, J., & Baird, K. (1988). Attempted referral as intervention for problem drinking in the general hospital. *British Journal of Addiction, 83,* 83–89.

Elwyn, G., Edwards, A., Kinnersley, P., & Grol, R. (2000). Shared decision making and the concept of equipoise: The competences of involving patients in healthcare choices. *British Journal of General Practice, 50*(460), 892–899.

Enea, V., & Dafinoiu, I. (2009). Motivational/solution-focused intervention for reducing school truancy among adolescents. *Journal of Cognitive and Behavioral Psychotherapies, 9*(2), 185–198.

Engle, D. E., & Arkowitz, H. (2006). *Ambivalence in psychotherapy: Facilitating readiness to change.* New York: Guilford Press.

Erickson, S. J., Gerstle, M., & Feldstein, S. W. (2005). Brief interventions and motivational interviewing with children, adolescents, and their parents in pediatric health settings: A review. *Archives of Pediatrics and Adolescent Medicine, 159,* 1173–1180.

Erol, S., & Erdogan, S. (2008). Application of a stage based motivational interviewing approach to adolescent smoking cessation: The transtheoretical model-based study. *Patient Education and Counseling, 72*(1), 42–48.

Evans, C. C., Sherer, M., Nakase-Richardson, R., Mani, T., & Irby, J. W., Jr. (2008). Evaluation of an interdisciplinary team intervention to improve therapeutic alliance in post-acute brain injury rehabilitation. *Journal of Head Trauma Rehabilitation, 23*(5), 329–338.

Farbring, C. Å., & Johnson, W. R. (2008). Motivational interviewing in the correctional system: An attempt to implement motivational interviewing in criminal justice. In H. Arkowitz, H. A. Westra, W. R. Miller, & S. Rollnick (Eds.), *Motivational interviewing in the treatment of psychological problems* (pp. 304–323). New York: Guilford Press.

Feldstein, S. W., & Ginsburg, J. I. D. (2006). Motivational interviewing with dually diagnosed adolescents in juvenile justice settings. *Brief Treatment and Crisis Intervention, 6*(3), 218–233.

Feldstein Ewing, S. W., Filbey, F. M., Sabbineni, A., Chandler, L. D., & Hutchinson, K. E. (2011). How psychological alcohol interventions work: A preliminary look at what fMRI can tell us. *Alcoholism: Clinical and Experimental Research, 35*(4), 643–651.

Festinger, L. (1957). *A theory of cognitive dissonance.* Stanford, CA: Stanford University Press.

Field, C., & Caetano, R. (2010). The role of ethnic matching between patient and provider on the effectiveness of brief alcohol interventions with Hispanics. *Alcoholism: Clinical and Experimental Research, 34*(2), 262–271.

Fixsen, D. L., Naoom, S. F., Blase, K. A., Friedman, R. M., & Wallace, F. (2005). *Implementation research: A synthesis of the literature.* Tampa, FL: National Implementation Research Network.

Flattum, C., Friend, S., Neumark-Sztainer, D., & Story, M. (2009). Motivational interviewing as a component of a school-based obesity prevention program for adolescent girls. *Journal of the American Dietetic Association, 109*(1), 91–94.

Foley, K., Duran, B., Morris, P., Lucero, J., Jiang, Y., Baxter, B., et al. (2005).

Using motivational interviewing to promote HIV testing at an American Indian substance abuse treatment facility. *Journal of Psychoactive Drugs*, 37(3), 321–329.

Ford, M. E. (1992). *Motivating humans: Goals, emotions, and personal agency beliefs*. Newbury Park, CA: Sage.

Forsberg, L., Berman, A. H., Källmén, H., Hermansson, U., & Helgason, A. R. (2008). A test of the validity of the motivational interviewing treatment integrity code. *Cognitive Behaviour Therapy*, 37(3), 1–9.

Forsberg, L., Källmén, H., Hermansson, U., Berman, A. H., & Helgason, Á. R. (2007). Coding counsellor behaviour in motivational interviewing sessions: Inter-rater reliability for the Swedish motivational interviewing treatment integrity code (MITI). *Cognitive Behaviour Therapy*, 36(3), 162–169.

Frank, J. D., & Frank, J. B. (1993). *Persuasion and healing: A comparative study of psychotherapy* (3rd ed.). Baltimore, MD: Johns Hopkins University Press.

Frankl, V. E. (2006). *Man's search for meaning*. Boston: Beacon Press.

Fromm, E., (1956). *The art of loving*. New York: Bantam Books.

Fuertes, J. N., Mislowack, A., Bennett, J., Paul, L., Gilbert, T. C., Fontan, G., et al. (2007). The physician–patient working alliance. *Patient Education and Counseling*, 66(1), 29–36.

Gance-Cleveland, B. (2007). Motivational interviewing: Improving patient education. *Journal of Pediatric Health Care*, 21(2), 81–88.

Gaume, J., Bertholet, N., Faouzi, M., Gmel, G., & Daeppen, J.-B. (2010). Counselor motivational interviewing skills and young adult change talk articulation during brief motivational interventions. *Journal of Substance Abuse Treatment*, 39(3), 272–281.

Gaume, J., Gmel, G., & Daeppen, J.-B. (2008). Brief alcohol interventions: Do counsellors' and patients' communication characteristics predict change? *Alcohol and Alcoholism*, 43, 62–69.

Gaume, J., Gmel, G., Faouzi, M., & Daeppen, J. B. (2009). Counselor skill influences outcomes of brief motivational interventions. *Journal of Substance Abuse Treatment*, 37(2), 151–159.

Gendlin, E. T. (1961). Initiating psychotherapy with "unmotivated" patients. *Psychiatric Quarterly*, 35, 134–139.

Gilmore, S. K. (1973). *The counselor-in-training*. Englewood Cliffs, NJ: Prentice Hall.

Ginott, H. G. (1965). *Between parent and child*. New York: Macmillan.

Gladwell, M. (2007). *Blink: The power of thinking without thinking*. New York: Little, Brown & Company.

Glasser, W. (1975). *Reality therapy: A new approach to psychiatry*. New York: Harper.

Glynn, L. H., Hallgren, K. A., Houck, J. M., McLouth, C. J., Fischer, D. J., & Moyers, T. B. (2011, June). *Introducing the "CACTI" sequential-coding software: A free, open-source program for rating client and provider speech*. Poster presented at the 34th annual meeting of the Research Society on Alcoholism National Conference, Atlanta, GA.

Glynn, L. H., & Moyers, T. B. (2010). Chasing change talk: The clinician's role in evoking client language about change. *Journal of Substance Abuse Treatment*, 39, 65–70.

Goddard, C., & Wierzbicka, A. (1994). *Semantic and lexical universals*. Amsterdam: John Benjamins Publishing.

Golin, C. E., Earp, J. A., Grodensky, C. A., Patel, S. N., Suchindran, C., Kalichman, K. P., et al. (2012). Longitudinal effect of Safe Talk, a motivational interviewing-based program to improve safer sex practices among people living with HIV/AIDS. *AIDS and Behavior*. doi:10.1007/s/10461-011-0029-SC

Gollwitzer, P. M. (1999). Implementation intentions: Simple effects of simple plans. *American Psychologist, 54*, 493–503.

Gollwitzer, P. M., & Schaal, B. (1998). Metacognition in action: The importance of implementation intentions. *Personality and Social Psychology Review, 2*, 124–136.

Gordon, T. (1970). *Parent effectiveness training*. New York: Wyden.

Gordon, T., & Edwards, W. S. (1997). *Making the patient your partner: Communication skills for doctors and other caregivers*. New York: Auburn House Paperback.

Gordon-Reed, A. (2009). Jefferson's vision. *Newsweek, 153*, 61–64.

Graeber, D. A., Moyers, T. B., Griffith, G., Guajardo, E., & Tonigan, S. (2003). A pilot study comparing motivational interviewing and an educational intervention in patients with schizophrenia and alcohol use disorders. *Community Mental Health Journal, 39*(3), 189–202.

Grant, J. E., Donahue, C. B., Odlaug, B. L., Kim, S. W., Miller, M. J., & Petry, N. M. (2009). Imaginal desensitisation plus motivational interviewing for pathological gambling: Randomised controlled trial. *British Journal of Psychiatry, 195*(3), 266–267.

Gray, R., Leese, M., Bindman, J., Becker, T., Burti, L., David, A., et al. (2006). Adherence therapy for people with schizophrenia: European multicentre randomised clinical trial. *British Journal of Psychiatry, 189*, 508–514.

Grodin, J. P. (2006). *Assessing therapeutic change mechanisms in motivational interviewing using the articulated thoughts in simulated situations paradigm*. Unpublished doctoral dissertation, University of Southern California, Los Angeles. Retrieved from *digitallibrary.usc.edu/assetserver/controller/item/etd-Grodin-20060929.pdf*.

Grote, N. K., Swartz, H. A., & Zuckoff, A. (2008). Enhancing interpersonal psychotherapy for mothers and expectant mothers on low incomes: Adaptations and additions. *Journal of Contemporary Psychotherapy, 38*(1), 23–33.

Haddock, G., Beardmore, R., Earnshaw, P., Fitzsimmons, M., Nothard, S., Butler, R., et al. (2012). Assessing fidelity to integrated motivational interviewing and CBT therapy for psychosis and substance use: The MI-CBT fidelity scale (MI-CTS). *Journal of Mental Health, 21*(1), 38–48.

Handmaker, N. S., Miller, W. R., & Manicke, M. (1999). Findings of a pilot study of motivational interviewing with pregnant drinkers. *Journal of Studies on Alcohol, 60*, 285–287.

Handmaker, N. S., & Wilbourne, P. (2001). Motivational interventions in prenatal clinics. *Alcohol Research and Health, 25*(3), 219–229.

Harland, J., White, M., Drinkwater, C., Chinn, D., Farr, L., & Howel, D. (1999). The Newcastle Exercise Project: A randomised controlled trial of methods to promote physical activity in primary care. *British Medical Journal, 319*, 828–832.

Harper, R., & Hardy, S. (2000). An evaluation of motivational interviewing as a method of intervention with clients in a probation setting. *British Journal of Social Work, 30*(3), 393–400.

Harris, K. B., & Miller, W. R. (1990). Behavioral self-control training for problem drinkers: Components of efficacy. *Psychology of Addictive Behaviors, 4,* 82–90.

Harris, K. J., Catley, D., Good, G. E., Cronk, N. J., Harrar, S., & Williams, K. B. (2010). Motivational interviewing for smoking cessation in college students: A group randomized controlled trial. *Preventive Medicine, 51*(5), 387–393.

Hartzler, B., & Espinoza, E. M. (2011). Moving criminal justice organizations toward adoption of evidence-based practice via advanced workshop training in motivational interviewing: A research note. *Criminal Justice Policy Review, 22*(2), 235–253.

Hayes, S. C., Strosahl, K. D., & Wilson, K. G. (1999). *Acceptance and commitment therapy: An experiential approach to behavior change.* New York: Guilford Press.

Heather, N. (2005). Motivational interviewing: Is it all our clients need? *Addiction Research and Theory, 13*(1), 1–18.

Heather, N., Rollnick, S., Bell, A., & Richmond, R. (1996). Effects of brief counselling among male heavy drinkers identified on general hospital wards. *Drug and Alcohol Review, 15*(1), 29–38.

Heather, N., Whitton, B., & Robertson, I. (1986). Evaluation of a self-help manual for media-recruited problem drinkers: Six-month follow-up results. *British Journal of Clinical Psychology, 25,* 19–34.

Heffner, J. L., Tran, G. Q., Johnson, C. S., Barrett, S. W., Blom, T. J., Thompson, R. D., et al. (2010). Combining motivational interviewing with compliance enhancement therapy (MI-CET): Development and preliminary evaluation of a new, manual-guided psychosocial adjunct to alcohol-dependence pharmacotherapy. *Journal of Studies on Alcohol and Drugs, 71*(1), 61–70.

Hendrickson, S. M. L., Martin, T., Manuel, J. K., Christopher, P. J., Thiedeman, T., & Moyers, T. B. (2004). Assessing reliability of the Motivational Interviewing Treatment Integrity behavioral coding system under limited range. *Alcoholism: Clinical and Experimental Research, 28*(5), 74A.

Henry, W. P., Strupp, H. H., Schacht, T. E., & Gaston, L. (1994). Psychodynamic approaches. In A. E. Bergin & S. L. Garfield (Eds.), *Handbook of psychotherapy and behavior change* (4th ed., pp. 467–508). New York: Wiley.

Hester, R. K., Squires, D. D., & Delaney, H. D. (2005). The drinker's check-up: 12-month outcomes of a controlled clinical trial of a stand-alone software program for problem drinkers. *Journal of Substance Abuse Treatment, 28*(2), 159–169.

Hettema, J., Steele, J., & Miller, W. R. (2005). Motivational interviewing. *Annual Review of Clinical Psychology, 1,* 91–111.

Hibbard, J. H., Mahoney, E. R., Stock, R., & Tusler, M. (2007). Do increases in patient activation result in improved self-management behaviors? *Health Services Research, 42*(4), 1443–1463.

Hibbard, J. H., Stockard, J., Mahoney, E. R., & Tusler, M. (2004). Development of the patient activation measure (PAM): Conceptualizing and measuring activation in patients and consumers. *Health Services Research, 39,* 1005–1026.

Hill, C. (2009). *Helping skills: Facilitating exploration, insight and action* (3rd ed.). Washington, DC: American Psychological Association.

Hill, S., & Kavookjian, J. (2012). Motivational interviewing as a behavioral intervention to increase HAART adherence in patients who are HIV-positive: A systematic review of the literature. *AIDS Care: Psychological and Sociomedical Aspects of AIDS/HIV, 24*(5), 583–592.

Hodgins, D. C., Ching, L. E., & McEwen, J. (2009). Strength of commitment language in motivational interviewing and gambling outcomes. *Psychology of Addictive Behaviors, 23*, 122–130.

Hohman, M. M. (2012). *Motivational interviewing in social work practice.* New York: Guilford Press.

Hohman, M. M., & Matulich, W. (2010). Initial validation of the motivational interviewing measure of staff interaction. *Alcoholism Treatment Quarterly, 28*(2), 230–238.

Hohman, M. M. (1998). Motivational interviewing: An intervention tool for child welfare case workers working with substance-abusing parents. *Child Welfare, 77*(3), 275–289.

Hollis, J. F., Polen, M. R., Whitlock, E. P., Lichtenstein, E., Mullooly, J. P., Velicer, W. F., et al. (2005). Teen reach: Outcomes from a randomized, controlled trial of a tobacco reduction program for teens seen in primary medical care. *Pediatrics, 115*(4), 981–989.

Horvath, A. O., & Greenberg, L. S. (1994). *The working alliance: Theory, research, and practice.* New York: Wiley.

Hubble, M. A., Duncan, B. L., & Miller, S. D. (Eds.). (1999). *The heart and soul of change: What works in therapy.* Washington, DC: American Psychological Association.

Hulse, G. K., & Tait, R. J. (2002). Six-month outcomes associated with a brief alcohol intervention for adult inpatients with psychiatric disorders. *Drug and Alcohol Review, 21*(2), 105–112.

Imel, Z. E., Wampold, B. E., & Miller, S. D. (2008). Distinctions without a difference: Direct comparisons of psychotherapies for alcohol use disorders. *Psychology of Addictive Behaviors, 22*(4), 533–543.

Israel, M., & Hay, I. (2006). *Research ethics for social scientists.* Thousand Oaks, CA: Sage.

Ivey, A. E., Ivey, M. B., & Zalaquett, Z. P. (2009). *Intentional interviewing and counseling* (7th ed.). New York: Brooks/Cole.

Janis, I. L., & Mann, L. (1977). *Decision making: A psychological analysis of conflict, choice and commitment.* New York: Free Press.

Jensen, C. D., Cushing, C. C., Aylward, B. S., Craig, J. T., Sorell, D. M., & Steele, R. G. (2011). Effectiveness of motivational interviewing interventions for adolescent substance use behavior change: A meta-analytic review. *Journal of Consulting and Clinical Psychology, 79*(4), 433–440.

Johnson, V. E. (1986). *Intervention: How to help someone who doesn't want help.* Center City, MN: Hazelden.

Juarez, P., Walters, S. T., Daugherty, M., & Radi, C. (2006). A randomized trial of motivational interviewing and feedback with heavy drinking college students. *Journal of Drug Education, 36*(3), 233–246.

Kadden, R., Carroll, K., Donovan, D., Cooney, N., Monti, P., Abrams, D., et al.

(1992). *Cognitive-behavioral coping skills therapy manual* (Vol. 3). Rockville, MD: National Institute on Alcohol Abuse and Alcoholism.

Kanfer, F. H. (1970a). Self-monitoring: Methodological limitations and clinical applications. *Journal of Consulting and Clinical Psychology, 35,* 148–152.

Kanfer, F. H. (1970b). Self-regulation: Research, issues, and speculation. In C. Neuringer & J. L. Michael (Eds.), *Behavior modification in clinical psychology* (pp. 178–220). New York: Appleton-Century-Crofts.

Karno, M. P., & Longabaugh, R. (2004). What do we know? Process analysis and the search for a better understanding of Project MATCH's anger-by-treatment matching effect. *Journal of Studies on Alcohol, 65*(4), 501–512.

Karno, M. P., & Longabaugh, R. (2005a). An examination of how therapist directiveness interacts with patient anger and reactance to predict alcohol use. *Journal of Studies on Alcohol, 66,* 825–832.

Karno, M. P., & Longabaugh, R. (2005b). Less directiveness by therapists improves drinking outcomes of reactant clients in alcoholism treatment. *Journal of Consulting and Clinical Psychology, 73*(2), 262–267.

Karno, M. P., Longabaugh, R., & Herbeck, D. (2009). Patient reactance as a moderator of the effect of therapist structure on posttreatment alcohol use. *Journal of Studies on Alcohol and Drugs, 70*(6), 929–936.

Kass, J. D., & Lennox, S. (2005). Emerging models of spiritual development: A foundation for mature, moral, and health-promoting behavior. In W. R. Miller & H. D. Delaney (Eds.), *Judeo-Christian perspectives on psychology: Human nature motivation and change* (pp. 185–204). Washington, DC: American Psychological Association.

Kay-Lambkin, F. J., Baker, A. L., Lewin, T. J., & Carr, V. J. (2009). Computer-based psychological treatment for comorbid depression and problematic alcohol and/or cannabis use: A randomized controlled trial of clinical efficacy. *Addiction, 104*(3), 378–388.

Kelly, A. B., & Lapworth, K. (2006). The HYP program: Targeted motivational interviewing for adolescent violations of school tobacco policy. *Preventive Medicine, 43*(6), 466–471.

Kertes, A., Westra, H. A., Angus, L., & Marcus, M. (2011). The impact of motivational interviewing on client experiences of cognitive behavioral therapy for generalized anxiety disorder. *Cognitive and Behavioral Practice, 18*(1), 55–69.

Khalsa, S.-R., McCarthy, K. S., Sharpless, B. A., Barrett, M. S., & Barberr, J. P. (2011). Beliefs about the causes of depression and treatment preferences. *Journal of Clinical Psychology, 67*(6), 539–549.

Kiene, S. M., & Barta, W. D. (2006). A brief individualized computer-delivered sexual risk reduction intervention increases HIV/AIDS preventive behavior. *Journal of Adolescent Health, 39*(3), 404–410.

Kiresuk, T. J., Smith, A., & Cardillo, J. E. (Eds.). (1994). *Goal attainment scaling: Applications, theory, and measurement.* Hillsdale, NJ: Erlbaum.

Kistenmacher, B. R., & Weiss, R. L. (2008). Motivational interviewing as a mechanism for change in men who batter: A randomized controlled trial. *Violence and Victims, 23*(5), 558–570.

Klag, S., O'Callaghan, F., Creed, P., & Zimmer-Gembeck, M. (2009). Motivating young people towards success: Evaluation of a motivational interviewing-integrated treatment programme for COD clients in a residential therapeutic community. *Therapeutic Communities, 30*(4), 366–386.

Klein, W. M. P., & Harris, P. R. (2010). Self-affirmation enhances attentional bias toward threatening components of a persuasive message. *Psychological Science, 20*(12), 1463–1467.

Knols, R., Aaronson, N. K., Uebelhart, D., Fransen, J., & Aufdemkampe, G. (2005). Physical exercise in cancer patients during and after medical treatment: A systematic review of randomized and controlled clinical trials [Meta-Analysis Review]. *Journal of Clinical Oncology: Official Journal of the American Society of Clinical Oncology, 23*(16), 3830–3842.

Koerber, A., Crawford, J., & O'Connell, K. (2003). The effects of teaching dental students brief motivational interviewing for smoking-cessation counseling: A pilot study. *Journal of Dental Education, 67*(4), 439–447.

Kristenson, H., Ohlin, H., Hulten-Nosslin, M., Hood, B., & Trell, E. (1983). Identification and intervention of heavy-drinking middle-aged men: Results and follow-up of 24–60 months on long-term studies with randomized centers. *Alcoholism: Clinical and Experimental Research, 7*, 203–209.

Kuchipudi, V., Hobein, K., Flickinger, A., & Iber, F. L. (1990). Failure of a 2-hour motivational intervention to alter recurrent drinking behavior in alcoholics with gastrointestinal disease. *Journal of Studies on Alcohol, 51*(4), 356–360.

Kurtz, E. (1991). *Not-God: A history of Alcoholics Anonymous* (Expanded ed.). Center City, MN: Hazelden.

LaBrie, J. W., Huchting, K., Tawalbeh, S., Pedersen, E. R., Thompson, A. D., Shelesky, K., et al. (2008). A randomized motivational enhancement prevention group reduces drinking and alcohol consequences in first-year college women. *Psychology of Addictive Behaviors, 22*(1), 149–155.

LaBrie, J. W., Lamb, T. F., Pedersen, E. R., & Quinlan, T. (2006). A group motivational interviewing intervention reduces drinking and alcohol-related consequences in adjudicated college students. *Journal of College Student Development, 47*(3), 267–280.

LaChance, H., Feldstein Ewing, S. W., Bryan, A. D., & Hutchison, K. E. (2009). What makes group MET work?: A randomized controlled trial of college student drinkers in mandated alcohol diversion. *Psychology of Addictive Behaviors, 23*(4), 598–612.

Lacrose, S., Chaloux, N., Monaghan, D., & Tarabulsy, G. M. (2010). Working alliance as a moderator of the impact of mentoring relationships among academically at-risk students. *Journal of Applied Social Psychology, 40*(10), 2656–2686.

Laine, C., & Davidoff, F. (1996). Patient-centered medicine: A professional evolution. *Journal of the American Medical Association, 275*(2), 152–156.

Lambert, M. J., Whipple, J., Smart, D., Vermeersch, D., Nielsen, S., & Hawkins, E. (2001). The effects of providing therapists with feedback on patient progress during psychotherapy: Are outcomes enhanced? *Psychotherapy Research, 11*(1), 49–68.

Lander, N. R., & Nelson, D. (2005). *The integrity model of existential psychotherapy in working with the "difficult patient."* New York: Routledge.

Lasser, K. E., Murillo, J., Lisboa, S., Casimir, A. N., Valley-Shah, L., Emmons, K.

M., et al. (2011). Colorectal cancer screening among ethnically diverse, low-income patients: A randomized controlled trial. *Archives of Internal Medicine, 171*(10), 906–912.

Lawson, K., Wolever, R., Donovan, P., & Greene, L. M. (2009). *Health coaching for behavior change: Motivational interviewing methods and practice.* Manasquan, NJ: Healthcare Intelligence Network.

Leak, A., Davis, E. D., Houchin, L. B., & Mabrey, M. (2009). Diabetes management and self-care education for hospitalized patients with cancer. *Clinical Journal of Oncology Nursing, 13*(2), 205–210.

Leake, G. J., & King, A. S. (1977). Effect of counselor expectations on alcoholic recovery. *Alcohol Health and Research World, 11*(3), 16–22.

Lee, C. S., Baird, J., Longabaugh, R., Nirenberg, T. D., Mello, M. J., & Woolard, R. (2010). Change plan as an active ingredient of brief motivational interventions for reducing negative consequences of drinking in hazardous drinking emergency-department patients. *Journal of Studies on Alcohol and Drugs, 71*(5), 726–733.

Lee, K. C. (1991). The problem of appropriateness of the Rokeach Value Survey in Korea. *International Journal of Psychology, 26*(3), 299–310.

Lewis, C. S. (1960). *The four loves.* New York: Harcourt Brace.

Lewis, T. F., & Osborn, C. J. (2004). Solution-focused counseling and motivational interviewing: A consideration of confluence. *Journal of Counseling and Development, 82,* 38–48.

Linehan, M. M. (1993). *Cognitive-behavioral treatment of borderline personality disorder.* New York: Guilford Press.

Linehan, M. M. (1997). Validation and psychotherapy. In A. C. Bohart & L. S. Greenberg (Eds.), *Empathy reconsidered: New directions in psychotherapy* (pp. 353–392). Washington, DC: American Psychological Association.

Linehan, M. M., Dimeff, L. A., Reynolds, S. K., Comtois, K. A., Shaw-Welch, S., Heagerty, P., et al. (2002). Dialectical behavior therapy versus comprehensive validation plus 12-step for the treatment of opioid-dependent women meeting criteria for borderline personality disorder. *Drug and Alcohol Dependence, 67,* 13–26.

Longabaugh, R., & Wirtz, P. W. (Eds.). (2001). *Project MATCH hypotheses: Results and causal chain analyses* (Project MATCH Monograph Series, Vol. 8). Bethesda, MD: National Institute on Alcohol Abuse and Alcoholism.

Longabaugh, R., Wirtz, P. W., Zweben, A., & Stout, R. L. (1998). Network support for drinking, Alcoholics Anonymous, and long-term matching effects. *Addiction, 93,* 1313–1333.

Longabaugh, R., Woolard, R. F., Nirenberg, T. D., Minugh, A. P., Becker, B., Clifford, P. R., et al. (2001). Evaluating the effects of a brief motivational intervention for injured drinkers in the emergency department. *Journal of Studies on Alcohol, 62*(6), 806–816.

Longabaugh, R., Zweben, A., LoCastro, J. S., & Miller, W. R. (2005). Origins, issues and options in the development of the combined behavioral intervention. *Journal of Studies on Alcohol Supplement*(15), 179–187.

Loudenburg, R. (2008). *South Dakota Public Safety DUI program: Four-year evaluation report.* Pierre, SD: Office of Highway Safety, South Dakota Department of Public Safety.

Maclean, L. G., White, J. R., Jr., Broughton, S., Robinson, J., Shultz, J. A., Weeks, D. L., et al. (2012). Telephone coaching to improve diabetes self-management for rural residents. *Clinical Diabetes, 30*(1), 13–16.

Madsen, W. C. (2009). Collaborative helping: A practice framework for family-centered services. *Family Process, 48*(1), 103–116.

Madson, M. B., & Campbell, T. C. (2006). Measures of fidelity in motivational enhancement: A systematic review. *Journal of Substance Abuse Treatment, 31*, 67–73.

Madson, M. B., Loignon, A. C., & Lane, C. (2009). Training in motivational interviewing: A systematic review. *Journal of Substance Abuse Treatment, 36*, 101–109.

Magill, M., Apodaca, T. R., Barnett, N. P., & Monti, P. M. (2010). The route to change: Within-session predictors of change plan completion in a motivational interview. *Journal of Substance Abuse Treatment, 38*, 299–305.

Mallams, J. H., Godley, M. D., Hall, G. M., & Meyers, R. J. (1982). A social-systems approach to resocializing alcoholics in the community. *Journal of Studies on Alcohol, 43*, 1115–1123.

Mann, R. E., & Rollnick, S. (1996). Motivational interviewing with a sex offender who believed he was innocent. *Behavioural and Cognitive Psychotherapy, 24*(2), 127–134.

Mantler, T., Irwin, J. D., & Morrow, D. (2010). Assessing motivational interviewing through co-active life coaching tools as a smoking cessation intervention: A demonstration study. *International Journal of Evidence Based Coaching and Mentoring, 8*(2), 49–63.

Marijuana Treatment Project Research Group. (2004). Brief treatments for cannabis dependence: Findings from a randomized multisite trial. *Journal of Consulting and Clinical Psychology, 72*(3), 455–466.

Markland, D., Ryan, R. M., Tobin, V., & Rollnick, S. (2005). Motivational interviewing and self-determination theory. *Journal of Social and Clinical Psychology, 24*, 785–805.

Marlatt, G. A., & Donovan, D. M. (Eds.). (2005). *Relapse prevention: Maintenance strategies in the treatment of addictive behaviors* (2nd ed.). New York: Guilford Press.

Marsden, J., Stillwell, G., Barlow, H., Boys, A., Taylor, C., Hunt, N., et al. (2006). An evaluation of a brief motivational intervention among young ecstasy and cocaine users: No effect on substance and alcohol use outcomes. *Addiction, 101*(7), 1014–1026.

Martin, J. E., & Sihn, E. P. (2009). Motivational interviewing: Applications to Christian therapy and church ministry. *Journal of Psychology and Christianity, 28*(1), 71–77.

Martino, S., Canning-Ball, M., Carroll, K. M., & Rounsaville, B. J. (2011). A criterion-based stepwise approach for training counselors in motivational interviewing. *Journal of Substance Abuse Treatment, 40*, 357–365.

Maslow, A. H. (1943). A theory of human motivation. *Psychological Review, 50*, 370–396.

Maslow, A. H. (1970). *Motivation and personality* (2nd ed.). New York: Harper & Row.

Mason, M., Pate, P., Drapkin, M., & Sozinho, K. (2011). Motivational interviewing integrated with social network counseling for female adolescents: A random-ized pilot study in urban primary care. *Journal of Substance Abuse Treat-ment, 41*(2), 148–155.

McConnaughy, E. N., Prochaska, J. O., & Velicer, W. F. (1983). Stages of change in psychotherapy: Measurement and sample profiles. *Psychotherapy: Theory, Research and Practice, 20,* 368–375.

McDonald, H. P., Garg, A. X., & Haynes, R. B. (2002). Interventions to enhance patient adherence to medication prescriptions. *Journal of the American Medi-cal Association, 288*(22), 2868–2879.

McGregor, D. (2006). *The human side of enterprise* (Annotated ed.). New York: McGraw-Hill.

McMurran, M. (2002). *Motivating offenders to change: A guide to enhancing engagement in therapy.* Chichester, UK: Wiley.

McMurran, M. (2009). Motivational interviewing with offenders: A systematic review. *Legal and Criminological Psychology, 14*(1), 83–100.

McMurran, M., & Ward, T. (2004). Motivating offenders to change in therapy: An organizing framework. *Legal and Criminological Psychology, 9*(2), 295–311.

McNamara, R., Robling, M., Hood, K., Bennet, K., Channon, S., Cohen, D., et al. (2010). Development and evaluation of a psychosocial intervention for chil-dren and teenagers experiencing diabetes (DEPICTED): A protocol for a clus-ter randomised controlled trial of the effectiveness of a communication skills training programme for healthcare professionals working with young people with type 1 diabetes. *BMC Health Services Research, 10*(36).

Mendel, E., & Hipkins, J. (2002). Motivating learning disabled offenders with alcohol-related problems: A pilot study. *British Journal of Learning Disabili-ties, 30*(4), 153–158.

Merlo, L. J., Storch, E. A., Lehmkuhl, H. D., Jacob, M. L., Murphy, T. K., Good-man, W. K., et al. (2010). Cognitive behavioral therapy plus motivational interviewing improves outcome for pediatric obsessive–compulsive disorder: A preliminary study. *Cognitive Behaviour Therapy, 39*(1), 24–27.

Merton, T. (1960). *Spiritual direction and meditation.* Collegeville, MN: Liturgi-cal Press.

Meyers, R. J., Miller, W. R., Smith, J. E., & Tonigan, J. S. (2002). A randomized trial of two methods for engaging treatment-refusing drug users through con-cerned significant others. *Journal of Consulting and Clinical Psychology, 70,* 1182–1185.

Meyers, R. J., & Smith, J. E. (1995). *Clinical guide to alcohol treatment: The com-munity reinforcement approach.* New York: Guilford Press.

Meyers, R. J., & Wolfe, B. L. (2004). *Get your loved one sober: Alternatives to nagging, pleading and threatening.* Center City, MN: Hazelden Publishing and Educational Services.

Miller, N. H. (2010). Motivational interviewing as a prelude to coaching in health-care settings. *Journal of Cardiovascular Nursing, 25*(3), 247–251.

Miller, S. D., Duncan, B. L., Brown, J., Sorrell, R., & Chalk, M. B. (2006). Using formal client feedback to improve retention and outcome: Making ongoing real-time assessment feasible. *Journal of Brief Therapy, 5*(1), 5–22.

Miller, S. D., Duncan, B. L., Sorrell, R., & Brown, G. S. (2005). The Partners for

Change outcome management system. *Journal of Clinical Psychology, 61*(2), 199–208.

Miller, W. R. (1978). Behavioral treatment of problem drinkers: A comparative outcome study of three controlled drinking therapies. *Journal of Consulting and Clinical Psychology, 46,* 74–86.

Miller, W. R. (1983). Motivational interviewing with problem drinkers. *Behavioural Psychotherapy, 11,* 147–172.

Miller, W. R. (1985a). *Living as if: How positive faith can change your life.* Philadelphia: Westminster Press.

Miller, W. R. (1985b). Motivation for treatment: A review with special emphasis on alcoholism. *Psychological Bulletin, 98,* 84–107.

Miller, W. R. (1994). Motivational interviewing: III. On the ethics of motivational intervention. *Behavioural and Cognitive Psychotherapy, 22,* 111–123.

Miller, W. R. (1996). What is a relapse? Fifty ways to leave the wagon. *Addiction, 91*(Suppl.), S15–S27.

Miller, W. R. (2000). Rediscovering fire: Small interventions, large effects. *Psychology of Addictive Behaviors, 14,* 6–18.

Miller, W. R. (2008). *Living as if: Your road, your life.* Carson City, NV: The Change Companies.

Miller, W. R. (Ed.). (2004). *Combined Behavioral Intervention manual: A clinical research guide for therapists treating people with alcohol abuse and dependence* (Vol. 1). Bethesda, MD: National Institute on Alcohol Abuse and Alcoholism.

Miller, W. R., & Atencio, D. J. (2008). Free will as a proportion of variance. In J. Baer, J. C. Kaufman, & R. F. Baumeister (Eds.), *Are we free?: Psychology and free will* (pp. 275–295). New York: Oxford University Press.

Miller, W. R., & Baca, L. M. (1983). Two-year follow-up of bibliotherapy and therapist-directed controlled drinking training for problem drinkers. *Behavior Therapy, 14,* 441–448.

Miller, W. R., Benefield, R. G., & Tonigan, J. S. (1993). Enhancing motivation for change in problem drinking: A controlled comparison of two therapist styles. *Journal of Consulting and Clinical Psychology, 61,* 455–461.

Miller, W. R., & Brown, J. M. (1991). Self-regulation as a conceptual basis for the prevention and treatment of addictive behaviours. In N. Heather, W. R. Miller, & J. Greeley (Eds.), *Self-control and the addictive behaviours* (pp. 3–79). Sydney: Maxwell Macmillan Publishing Australia.

Miller, W. R., & C'de Baca, J. (2001). *Quantum change: When epiphanies and sudden insights transform ordinary lives.* New York: Guilford Press.

Miller, W. R., & Danaher, B. G. (1976). Maintenance in parent training. In J. D. Krumboltz & C. E. Thoresen (Eds.), *Counseling methods* (pp. 434–444). New York: Holt, Rinehart & Winston.

Miller, W. R., Forcehimes, A. A., & Zweben, A. (2011). *Treating addiction: Guidelines for professionals.* New York: Guilford Press.

Miller, W. R., Gribskov, C. J., & Mortell, R. L. (1981). Effectiveness of a self-control manual for problem drinkers with and without therapist contact. *International Journal of the Addictions, 16,* 1247–1254.

Miller, W. R., & Heather, N. (Eds.). (1986). *Treating addictive behaviors: Processes of change.* New York: Plenum Press.

Miller, W. R., & Heather, N. (Eds.). (1998). *Treating addictive behaviors* (2nd ed.). New York: Plenum Press.

Miller, W. R., & Jackson, K. A. (1995). *Practical psychology for pastors: Toward more effective counseling* (2nd ed.). Englewood Cliffs, NJ: Prentice Hall.

Miller, W. R., & Johnson, W. R. (2008). A natural language screening measure for motivation to change. *Addictive Behaviors, 33*, 1177–1182.

Miller, W. R., Leckman, A. L., Delaney, H. D., & Tinkcom, M. (1992). Long-term follow-up of behavioral self-control training. *Journal of Studies on Alcohol, 53*, 249–261.

Miller, W. R., LoCastro, J. S., Longabaugh, R., O'Malley, S., & Zweben, A. (2005). When worlds collide: Blending the divergent traditions of pharmacotherapy and psychotherapy outcome research. *Journal of Studies on Alcohol, Supplement No. 15*, 17–23.

Miller, W. R., & Manuel, J. K. (2008). How large must a treatment effect be before it matters to practitioners? An estimation method and demonstration. *Drug and Alcohol Review, 27*, 524–528.

Miller, W. R., & Martin, J. E. (Eds.). (1988). *Behavior therapy and religion: Integrating spiritual and behavioral approaches to change.* Newbury Park, CA: Sage.

Miller, W. R., & Mee-Lee, D. (2010). *Self-management: A guide to your feelings, motivation, and positive mental health.* Carson City, NV: The Change Companies.

Miller, W. R., & Meyers, R. J. (1995, Spring). Beyond generic criteria: Reflections on life after clinical science wins. *Clinical Science*, 4–6.

Miller, W. R., Meyers, R. J., & Tonigan, J. S. (1999). Engaging the unmotivated in treatment for alcohol problems: A comparison of three strategies for intervention through family members. *Journal of Consulting and Clinical Psychology, 67*, 688–697.

Miller, W. R., & Mount, K. A. (2001). A small study of training in motivational interviewing: Does one workshop change clinician and client behavior? *Behavioural and Cognitive Psychotherapy, 29*, 457–471.

Miller, W. R., & Moyers, T. B. (2006). Eight stages in learning motivational interviewing. *Journal of Teaching in the Addictions, 5*(1), 3–17.

Miller, W. R., Moyers, T. B., Arciniega, L., Ernst, D., & Forcehimes, A. A. (2005). Training, supervision and quality monitoring of the COMBINE study behavioral interventions. *Journal of Studies on Alcohol, 66*(Suppl. 15), S188–S195.

Miller, W. R., & Muñoz, R. F. (1976). *How to control your drinking.* Englewood Cliffs, NJ: Prentice Hall.

Miller, W. R., & Muñoz, R. F. (2005). *Controlling your drinking: Tools to make moderation work for you.* New York: Guilford Press.

Miller, W. R., & Rollnick, S. (1991). *Motivational interviewing: Preparing people to change addictive behavior.* New York: Guilford Press.

Miller, W. R., & Rollnick, S. (2002). *Motivational interviewing: Preparing people for change* (2nd ed.). New York: Guilford Press.

Miller, W. R., & Rollnick, S. (2009). Ten things that motivational interviewing is not. *Behavioural and Cognitive Psychotherapy, 37*, 129–140.

Miller, W. R., & Rose, G. S. (2009). Toward theory of motivational interviewing. *American Psychologist, 64*, 527–537.

Miller, W. R., & Sanchez, V. C. (1994). Motivating young adults for treatment and lifestyle change. In G. Howard (Ed.), *Issues in alcohol use and misuse by young adults* (pp. 55–82). Notre Dame, IN: University of Notre Dame Press.

Miller, W. R., Sorensen, J. L., Selzer, J., & Brigham, G. (2006). Disseminating evidence-based practices in substance abuse treatment: A review with suggestions. *Journal of Substance Abuse Treatment, 31,* 25–39.

Miller, W. R., & Sovereign, R. G. (1989). The check-up: A model for early intervention in addictive behaviors. In T. Løberg, W. R. Miller, P. E. Nathan, & G. A. Marlatt (Eds.), *Addictive behaviors: Prevention and early intervention* (pp. 219–231). Amsterdam: Swets & Zeitlinger.

Miller, W. R., Sovereign, R. G., & Krege, B. (1988). Motivational interviewing with problem drinkers: II. The Drinker's Check-up as a preventive intervention. *Behavioural Psychotherapy, 16,* 251–268.

Miller, W. R., & Taylor, C. A. (1980). Relative effectiveness of bibliotherapy, individual and group self-control training in the treatment of problem drinkers. *Addictive Behaviors, 5,* 13–24.

Miller, W. R., Taylor, C. A., & West, J. C. (1980). Focused versus broad spectrum behavior therapy for problem drinkers. *Journal of Consulting and Clinical Psychology, 48,* 590–601.

Miller, W. R., Toscova, R. T., Miller, J. H., & Sanchez, V. (2000). A theory-based motivational approach for reducing alcohol/drug problems in college. *Health Education and Behavior, 27,* 744–759.

Miller, W. R., Wilbourne, P. L., & Hettema, J. (2003). What works?: A summary of alcohol treatment outcome research. In R. K. Hester & W. R. Miller (Eds.), *Handbook of alcoholism treatment approaches: Effective alternatives* (3rd ed., pp. 13–63). Boston: Allyn & Bacon.

Miller, W. R., Yahne, C. E., Moyers, T. B., Martinez, J., & Pirritano, M. (2004). A randomized trial of methods to help clinicians learn motivational interviewing. *Journal of Consulting and Clinical Psychology, 72,* 1050–1062.

Miller, W. R., Yahne, C. E., & Tonigan, J. S. (2003). Motivational interviewing in drug abuse services: A randomized trial. *Journal of Consulting and Clinical Psychology, 71,* 754–763.

Miller, W. R., Zweben, A., DiClemente, C. C., & Rychtarik, R. C. (1992). *Motivational enhancement therapy manual: A clinical research guide for therapists treating individuals with alcohol abuse and dependence* (Vol. 2, Project MATCH Monograph Series). Rockville, MD: National Institute on Alcohol Abuse and Alcoholism.

Moe, E. L., Elliot, D. L., Goldberg, L., Kuehl, K. S., Stevens, V. J., Breger, R. K., et al. (2002). Promoting healthy lifestyles: Alternative models' effects (PHLAME). *Health Education Research, 17*(5), 586–596.

Monti, P. M., Barnett, N. P., Colby, S. M., Gwaltney, C. J., Spirito, A., Rohsenow, D. J., et al. (2007). Motivational interviewing versus feedback only in emergency care for young adult problem drinking. *Addiction, 102*(8), 1234–1243.

Monti, P. M., Colby, S. M., Barnett, N. P., Spirito, A., Rohsenow, D. J., Myers, M., et al. (1999). Brief intervention for harm reduction with alcohol-positive older adolescents in a hospital emergency department. *Journal of Consulting and Clinical Psychology, 67*(6), 989–994.

Monti, P. M., Kadden, R. M., Rohsenow, D. J., Cooney, N. L., & Abrams, D. B. (2002). *Treating alcohol dependence: A coping skills training guide* (2nd ed.). New York: Guilford Press.

Morrill, M. I., Eubanks-Fleming, C. J., Harp, A. G., Sollenberger, J. W., Darling, E. V., & Cordova, J. V. (2011). The marriage check-up: Increasing access to marital health care. *Family Process, 50*, 471–485.

Mowrer, O. H. (1966). Integrity therapy: A self-help approach. *Psychotherapy: Theory, Research and Practice, 3*, 114–119.

Mowrer, O. H., Vattano, A. J., & Others. (1974). *Integrity groups: The loss and recovery of community.* Urbana, IL: Integrity Groups.

Mowrer, O. H., & Vattano, A. J. (1976). Integrity groups: A context for growth in honesty, responsibility, and involvement. *Journal of Applied Behavioral Sciences, 12*, 419–431.

Moyers, T. (2004). History and happenstance: How motivational interviewing got its start. *Behavioural and Cognitive Psychotherapy, 18*, 291–298.

Moyers, T. B., Manuel, J. K., Wilson, P. G., Hendrickson, S. M. L., Talcott, W., & Durand, P. (2008). A randomized trial investigating training in motivational interviewing for behavioral health providers. *Behavioural and Cognitive Psychotherapy, 36*(2), 149–162.

Moyers, T. B., & Martin, T. (2006). Therapist influence on client language during motivational interviewing sessions. *Journal of Substance Abuse Treatment, 30*, 245–252.

Moyers, T. B., Martin, T., Catley, D., Harris, K. J., & Ahluwalia, J. S. (2003). Assessing the integrity of motivational interventions: Reliability of the Motivational Interviewing Skills Code. *Behavioural and Cognitive Psychotherapy, 31*, 177–184.

Moyers, T. B., Martin, T., Christopher, P. J., Houck, J. M., Tonigan, J. S., & Amrhein, P. C. (2007). Client language as a mediator of motivational interviewing efficacy: Where is the evidence? *Alcoholism: Clinical and Experimental Research, 31* (Suppl.), 40S–47S.

Moyers, T. B., Martin, T., Houck, J. M., Christopher, P. J., & Tonigan, J. S. (2009). From in-session behaviors to drinking outcomes: A causal chain for motivational interviewing. *Journal of Consulting and Clinical Psychology, 77*(6), 1113–1124.

Moyers, T. B., Martin, T., Manuel, J. K., Hendrickson, S. M., & Miller, W. R. (2005). Assessing competence in the use of motivational interviewing. *Journal of Substance Abuse Treatment, 28*(1), 19–26.

Moyers, T. B., Miller, W. R., & Hendrickson, S. M. L. (2005). How does motivational interviewing work? Therapist interpersonal skill predicts client involvement within motivational interviewing sessions. *Journal of Consulting and Clinical Psychology, 73*, 590–598.

Murphy, C. M., & Maiuro, R. D. (2009). *Motivational interviewing and stages of change in intimate partner violence.* New York Springer.

Murray, E. J., & Segal, D. L. (1994). Emotional processing in vocal and written expression of feelings about traumatic experiences. *Journal of Traumatic Stress, 7*, 391–405.

Naar-King, S., Outlaw, A., Green-Jones, M., Wright, K., & Parsons, J. T. (2009).

Motivational interviewing by peer outreach workers: A pilot randomized clinical trial to retain adolescents and young adults in HIV care. *AIDS Care*, *21*(7), 868–873.

Naar-King, S., & Suarez, M. (Eds.). (2011). *Motivational interviewing with adolescents and young adults*. New York: Guilford Press.

National Research Council. (2009). *On being a scientist* (3rd ed.). Washington, DC: National Academies Press.

Neighbors, C. J., Barnett, N. P., Rohsenow, D. J., Colby, S. M., & Monti, P. M. (2010). Cost-effectiveness of a motivational intervention for alcohol-involved youth in a hospital emergency department. *Journal of Studies on Alcohol and Drugs*, *71*(3), 384–394.

New Revised Standard Version. (1989). New York: Oxford University Press.

Newnham-Kanas, C., Morrow, D., & Irwin, J. D. (2010). Motivational coaching: A functional juxtaposition of three methods for health behaviour change: Motivational interviewing, coaching, and skilled helping. *International Journal of Evidence Based Coaching and Mentoring*, *8*(2), 27–48.

Nock, M. K., & Kazdin, A. E. (2005). Randomized controlled trial of a brief intervention for increasing participation in parent management training. *Journal of Consulting and Clinical Psychology*, *73*(5), 872–879.

Norcross, J. C. (Ed.). (2002). *Psychotherapy relationships that work: Therapist contributions and responsiveness to patients*. New York: Oxford University Press.

Norcross, J. C., & Wampold, B. E. (2011). Evidence-based therapy relationships: Research conclusions and clinical practices. *Psychotherapy*, *48*(1), 98–102.

Nouwen, H. J. M. (2005). *In memoriam*. Notre Dame, IN: Ave Maria Press.

Nowinski, J., Baker, S., & Carroll, K. M. (1992). *Twelve step facilitation therapy manual: A clinical research guide for therapists treating individuals with alcohol abuse and dependence*. Rockville, MD: National Institute on Alcohol Abuse and Alcoholism.

Nuro, K. F., Maccarelli, L., Baker, S. M., Martino, S., Rounsaville, B. J., & Carroll, K. M. (2005). *Yale Adherence and Competence Scale (YACS II) guidelines* (2nd ed.). West Haven, CT: Yale University Press.

O'Leary, C. C. (2001, January). The early childhood family check-up: A brief intervention for at-risk families with preschool-aged children. *Dissertation Abstracts International: Section B: The Sciences and Engineering*, *62*(6-B), 2992.

Olsen, S., Smith, S. S., Oei, T. P., & Douglas, J. (2012). Motivational interviewing (MINT) improves continuous positive airway pressure (CPAP) acceptance and adherence: A randomized clinical trial. *Journal of Consulting and Clinical Psychology*, *80*(1), 151–163.

Ondersma, S. J., Chase, S. K., Svikis, D. S., & Schuster, C. R. (2005). Computer-based brief motivational intervention for perinatal drug use. *Journal of Substance Abuse Treatment*, *28*(4), 305–312.

Ondersma, S. J., Svikis, D. S., & Schuster, C. R. (2007). Computer-based brief intervention a randomized trial with postpartum women. *American Journal of Preventive Medicine*, *32*(3), 231–238.

Ondersma, S. J., Winhusen, T., Erickson, S. J., Stine, S. M., & Wang, Y. (2009).

Motivation enhancement therapy with pregnant substance-abusing women: Does baseline motivation moderate efficacy? *Drug and Alcohol Dependence, 101*(1–2), 74–79.

Pantalon, M. V. (2011). *Instant influence: How to get anyone to do anything—FAST.* New York: Little, Brown.

Parks, G. A., & Woodford, M. S. (2005). CHOICES about alcohol: A brief alcohol abuse prevention and harm reduction program for college students. In G. R. Walz & R. K. Rep (Eds.), *Vistas: Compelling perspectives on counseling 2005* (Article 36). Alexandria, VA: American Counseling Association.

Parr, G., Haberstroh, S., & Kottler, J. (2000). Interactive journal writing as an adjunct in group work. *Journal for Specialists in Group Work, 25*(3), 229–242.

Parsons, J. T., Golub, S. A., Rosof, E., & Holder, C. (2007). Motivational interviewing and cognitive-behavioral intervention to improve HIV medication adherence among hazardous drinkers: A randomized controlled trial. *Journal of Acquired Immune Deficiency Syndromes, 46*(4), 443–450.

Passmore, J. (2007). Addressing deficit performance through coaching: Using motivational interviewing for performance improvement at work. *International Coaching Psychology Review, 2*(3), 265–275.

Passmore, J., & Whybrow, A. (2008). Motivational interviewing: A specific approach for coaching psychologists. In S. Palmer & A. Whybrow (Eds.), *Handbook of coaching psychology: A guide for practitioners* (pp. 160–173). New York: Routledge.

Patel, S. H., Lambie, G. W., & Glover, M. M. (2008). Motivational counseling: Implications for counseling male juvenile sex offenders. *Journal of Addictions and Offender Counseling, 28*(2), 86–100.

Patterson, G. R. (1974). *Living with children: New methods for parents and teachers.* New York: Research Press.

Patterson, G. R. (1975). *Families: Applications of social learning to family life* (rev. ed.). New York: Research Press.

Patterson, G. R., & Chamberlain, P. (1994). A functional analysis of resistance during patient training therapy. *Clinical Psychology: Science and Practice, 1*(1), 53–70.

Patterson, G. R., & Forgatch, M. S. (1985). Therapist behavior as a determinant for client noncompliance: A paradox for the behavior modifier. *Journal of Consulting and Clinical Psychology, 53,* 846–851.

Pennebaker, J. W. (1997). Writing about emotional experiences as a therapeutic process. *Psychological Science, 8*(3), 162–165.

Persson, L.-G., & Hjalmarson, A. (2006). Smoking cessation in patients with diabetes mellitus: Results from a controlled study of an intervention programme in primary healthcare in Sweden. *Scandinavian Journal of Primary Health Care, 24*(2), 75–80.

Pettinati, H. M., Weiss, R. D., Dundon, W., Miller, W. R., Donovan, D. M., Ernst, D. B., et al. (2005). A structured approach to medical management: A psychosocial intervention to support pharmacotherapy in the treatment of alcohol dependence. *Journal of Studies on Alcohol and Drugs, Supplement 15,* 170–178.

Pierson, H. M., Hayes, S. C., Gifford, E. V., Roget, N., Padilla, M., Bissett, R., et al. (2007). An examination of the Motivational Interviewing Treatment Integrity code. *Journal of Substance Abuse Treatment, 32,* 11–17.

Polcin, D. L., Galloway, G. P., Palmer, J., & Mains, W. (2004). The case for high-dose motivational enhancement therapy. *Substance Use and Misuse, 39*(2), 331–343.

Pollak, K. I., Alexander, S. C., Coffman, C. J., Tulsky, J. A., Lyna, P., Dolor, R. J., et al. (2010). Physician communication techniques and weight loss in adults: Project CHAT. *American Journal of Preventive Medicine, 39*(4), 321–328.

Pollak, K. I., Alexander, S. C., Østbye, T., Lyna, P., Tulsky, J. A., Dolor, R. J., et al. (2009). Primary care physicians' discussions of weight-related topics with overweight and obese adolescents: Results from the Teen CHAT Pilot Study. *Journal of Adolescent Health, 45*(2), 205–207.

Premack, D. (1972). Mechanisms of self-control. In W. A. Hunt (Ed.), *Learning mechanisms in smoking* (pp. 107–123). Chicago: Aldine.

Prochaska, J. O., & DiClemente, C. C. (1984). *The transtheoretical approach: Crossing traditional boundaries of therapy.* Homewood, IL: Dow/Jones Irwin.

Proctor, S. L., Cowin, C. J., Hoffmann, N. G., & Allison, S. (2009). A tool to engage jail inmates: A trademarked journaling process shows promise in giving offenders insight on their substance use. *Addiction Professional, 7*(1), 22–26.

Proctor, S. L., Hoffman, N. G., & Allison, S. (2012). The effectiveness of interactive journaling in reducing recidivism among substance dependent jail inmates. *International Journal of Offender Therapy and Comparative Criminology, 56*(2), 317–332.

Progoff, I. (1975). *At a journal workshop.* New York: Dialogue House Library.

Project MATCH Research Group. (1993). Project MATCH: Rationale and methods for a multisite clinical trial matching patients to alcoholism treatment. *Alcoholism: Clinical and Experimental Research, 17,* 1130–1145.

Project MATCH Research Group. (1997a). Matching alcoholism treatments to client heterogeneity: Project MATCH posttreatment drinking outcomes. *Journal of Studies on Alcohol, 58*(1), 7–29.

Project MATCH Research Group. (1997b). Project MATCH secondary *a priori* hypotheses. *Addiction, 92,* 1671–1698.

Project MATCH Research Group. (1998a). Matching alcoholism treatments to client heterogeneity: Project MATCH three-year drinking outcomes. *Alcoholism: Clinical and Experimental Research, 22,* 1300–1311.

Project MATCH Research Group. (1998b). Matching alcoholism treatments to client heterogeneity: Treatment main effects and matching effects on drinking during treatment. *Journal of Studies on Alcohol, 59*(6), 631–639.

Project MATCH Research Group. (1998c). Therapist effects in three treatments for alcohol problems. *Psychotherapy Research, 8,* 455–474.

Quenk, N. L. (2009). *Essentials of the Myers-Briggs Type Indicator assessment* (2nd ed.). New York: Wiley.

Rachman, A. W. (1990). Judicious self-disclosure in group analysis. *Group, 14*(3), 132–144.

Rao, S. A. (1999). *The short-term impact of the family check-up: A brief motivational intervention for at-risk families.* Ph.D. Dissertation, University of Oregon, Eugene.

Reid, A. E., Cialdini, R. B., & Aiken, L. S. (2010). Social norms and health behavior. In A. Steptoe (Ed.), *Handbook of behavioral medicine: Methods and approaches* (pp. 263–274). New York: Springer.

Reinke, K., Herman, K. C., & Sprick, R. (2001). *Motivational interviewing for effective classroom management: The classroom check-up.* New York: Guilford Press.

Resnicow, K., Jackson, A., Blissett, D., Wang, T., McCarty, F., Rahotep, S., et al. (2005). Results of the healthy body healthy spirit trial. *Health Psychology, 24*(4), 339–348.

Resnicow, K., Jackson, A., Braithwaite, R., Diiorio, C., Blisset, D., Rahotep, S., et al. (2002). Healthy Body/Healthy Spirit: A Church-Based Nutrition and Physical Activity Intervention. *Health Education Research, 17*(5), 562–573.

Resnicow, K., Jackson, A., Wang, T., De, A. K., McCarty, F., Dudley, W. N., et al. (2001). A motivational interviewing intervention to increase fruit and vegetable intake through Black churches: Results of the Eat for Life trial. *American Journal of Public Health, 91*(10), 1686–1693.

Resnicow, K., Kramish Campbell, M., Carr, C., McCarty, F., Wang, T., Periasamy, S., et al. (2004). Body and soul: A dietary intervention conducted through African-American churches. *American Journal of Preventive Medicine, 27*(2), 97–105.

Richardson, L. (2012). Motivational interviewing: Helping patients move toward change. *Journal of Christian Nursing, 29*(1), 18–24.

Rise, J., Thompson, M., & Verplanken, B. (2003). Measuring implementation intentions in the context of the theory of planned action. *Scandinavian Journal of Psychology, 44,* 87–95.

Roberts, M. (2001). *Horse sense for people.* Toronto, ON: Knopf.

Robles, R. R., Reyes, J. C., Colon, H. M., Sahai, H., Marrero, C. A., Matos, T. D., et al. (2004). Effects of combined counseling and case management to reduce HIV risk behaviors among Hispanic drug injectors in Puerto Rico: A randomized controlled study. *Journal of Substance Abuse Treatment, 27*(2), 145–152.

Roffman, R. A., Edleson, J. L., Neighbors, C., Mbilinyi, L., & Walker, D. (2008). The men's domestic abuse check-up: A protocol for reaching the nonadjudicated and untreated man who batters and who abuses substances. *Violence Against Women, 14*(5), 589–605.

Rogers, C. R. (1942). *Counseling and psychotherapy.* Boston: Houghton Mifflin.

Rogers, C. R. (1954). *Psychotherapy and personality change.* Chicago: University of Chicago Press.

Rogers, C. R. (1959). A theory of therapy, personality, and interpersonal relationships as developed in the client-centered framework. In S. Koch (Ed.), *Psychology: The study of a science (Vol. 3). Formulations of the person and the social contexts* (pp. 184–256). New York: McGraw-Hill.

Rogers, C. R. (1962). The nature of man. In S. Doniger (Ed.), *The nature of man in theological and psychological perspective* (pp. 91–96). New York: Harper & Brothers.

Rogers, C. R. (1965). *Client-centered therapy.* New York: Houghton Mifflin.

Rogers, C. R. (1967). The interpersonal relationship: The core of guidance. In C. R. Rogers & B. Stevens (Eds.), *Person to person: The problem of being human* (pp. 89–103). Moab, UT: Real People Press.

Rogers, C. R. (1980a). Beyond the watershed: And where now? In C. R. Rogers (Ed.), *A way of being* (pp. 292–315). New York: Houghton Mifflin.

Rogers, C. R. (Ed.). (1980b). *A way of being.* Boston: Houghton Mifflin.

Rogers, C. R. (1989). The interpersonal relationship: The core of guidance. In C. R. Rogers & B. Stevens (Eds.), *Person to person: The problem of being human* (pp. 89–103). Moab, UT: Real People Press.

Rogers, C. R., & Sanford, R. (1989). Client-centered psychotherapy. In H. I. Kaplan & B. J. Sadock (Eds.), *Comprehensive textbook of psychiatry* (5th ed.). Baltimore, MD: Williams & Wilkins.

Rogers, R. W. (1975). A protection motivation theory of fear appeals and attitude change. *Journal of Psychology, 91,* 93–114.

Rohsenow, D. J., Monti, P. M., Martin, R. A., Colby, S. M., Myers, M. G., Gulliver, S. B., et al. (2004). Motivational enhancement and coping skills training for cocaine abusers: Effects on substance use outcomes. *Addiction, 99*(7), 862–874.

Rokeach, M. (1973). *The nature of human values.* New York: Free Press.

Rollnick, S., Mason, P., & Butler, C. (1999). *Health behavior change: A guide for practitioners.* New York: Churchill Livingstone.

Rollnick, S., & Miller, W. R. (1995). What is motivational interviewing? *Behavioural and Cognitive Psychotherapy, 23,* 325–334.

Rollnick, S., Miller, W. R., & Butler, C. C. (2008). *Motivational interviewing in health care: Helping patients change behavior.* New York: Guilford Press.

Rollnick, S., Miller, W. R., & Heather, N. (1998). Readiness, importance, and confidence: Critical conditions of change in treatment *Treating addictive behaviors* (2nd ed., pp. 49–60). New York: Plenum Press.

Rosen, P. J., Hiller, M. L., Webster, J. M., Staton, M., & Leukefeld, C. (2004). Treatment motivation and therapeutic engagement in prison-based substance use treatment. *Journal of Psychoactive Drugs, 36*(3), 387–396.

Rosenblum, A., Foote, J., Cleland, C., Magura, S., Mahmood, D., & Kosanke, N. (2005). Moderators of effects of motivational enhancements to cognitive behavioral therapy. *American Journal of Drug and Alcohol Abuse, 31*(1), 35–58.

Rosengren, D. B. (2009). *Building motivational interviewing skills: A practitioner workbook.* New York: Guilford Press.

Rubak, S., Sandbaek, A., Lauritzen, T., & Christensen, B. (2005). Motivational interviewing: A systematic review and meta-analysis. *British Journal of General Practice, 55*(513), 305–312.

Rubino, G., Barker, C., Roth, T., & Fearon, P. (2000). Therapist empathy and depth of interpretation in response to potential alliance ruptures: The role of therapist and patient attachment styles. *Psychotherapy Research, 10,* 408–420.

Runyon, M. K., Deblinger, E., & Schroeder, C. M. (2009). Pilot evaluation of outcomes of combined parent–child cognitive-behavioral group therapy for families at risk for child physical abuse. *Cognitive and Behavioral Practice, 16*(1), 101–118.

Rush, B. R., Dennis, M. L., Scott, C. K., Castel, S., & Funk, R. R. (2008). The interaction of co-occurring mental disorders and recovery management checkups on substance abuse treatment participation and recovery. *Evaluation Review, 32*(1), 7–38.

Safran, J. D., Crocker, P., McMain, S., & Murray, P. (1990). Therapeutic alliance rupture as a therapy event for empirical investigation. *Psychotherapy: Theory, Research, Practice, Training, 27*(2), 154–165.

Safren, S. A., Otto, M. W., Worth, J. L., Salomon, E., Johnson, W., Mayer, K., et al. (2001). Two strategies to increase adherence to HIV antiretroviral medication: Life-steps and medication monitoring. *Behaviour Research and Therapy, 39*(10), 1151–1162.

Sanders, L. (2011). *Values-based motivational interviewing: Effectiveness for smoking cessation among New Mexico veterans.* Doctoral Dissertation, University of New Mexico, Albuquerque.

Santa Ana, E. J., Wulfert, E., & Nietert, P. J. (2007). Efficacy of group motivational interviewing (GMI) for psychiatric inpatients with chemical dependence. *Journal of Consulting and Clinical Psychology, 75*(5), 816–822.

Schaus, J. F., Sole, M. L., McCoy, T. P., Mullett, N., & O'Brien, M. C. (2009). Alcohol screening and brief intervention in a college student health center: A randomized controlled trial. *Journal of Studies on Alcohol and Drugs Supplement*(16), 131–141.

Schermer, C. R. (2005). Feasibility of alcohol screening and brief intervention. *Journal of Trauma: Injury, Infection, and Critical Care, 59*(Suppl. 3), S119–S123.

Schermer, C. R., Moyers, T. B., Miller, W. R., & Bloomfield, L. A. (2006). Trauma center brief interventions for alcohol disorders decrease subsequent driving under the influence arrests. *Journal of Trauma, 60*(1), 29–34.

Schermer, C. R., Qualls, C. R., Brown, C. L., & Apodaca, T. R. (2001). Intoxicated motor vehicle passengers: An overlooked at-risk population. *Archives of Surgery, 136*, 1244–1248.

Schmidt, U., & Treasure, J. (1997). *Clinician's guide to getting better bit(e) by bit(e): A survival kit for sufferers of bulimia nervosa and binge eating disorders.* Hove, UK: Psychology Press/Erlbaum.

Schmiege, S. J., Broaddus, M. R., Levin, M., & Bryan, A. D. (2009). Randomized trial of group interventions to reduce HIV/STD risk and change theoretical mediators among detained adolescents. *Journal of Consulting and Clinical Psychology, 77*(1), 38–50.

Scholl, M. B., & Schmitt, D. M. (2009). Using motivational interviewing to address college client alcohol abuse. *Journal of College Counseling, 12*(1), 57–70.

Scott, C. K., & Dennis, M. L. (2009). Results from two randomized clinical trials evaluating the impact of quarterly recovery management checkups with adult chronic substance users. *Addiction, 104*(6), 959–971.

Secades-Villa, R., Fernánde-Hermida, J. R., & Arnáez-Montaraz, C. (2004). Motivational interviewing and treatment retention among drug user patients: A pilot study. *Substance Use and Misuse, 39*(9), 1369–1378.

Sellman, J. D., MacEwan, I. K., Deering, D. D., & Adamson, S. J. (2007). A comparison of motivational interviewing with non-directive counseling. In G. Tober & D. Raistrick (Eds.), *Motivational dialogue: Preparing addiction professionals for motivational interviewing practice* (pp. 137–150). New York: Routledge.

Sellman, J. D., Sullivan, P. F., Dore, G. M., Adamson, S. J., & MacEwan, I. (2001). A randomized controlled trial of motivational enhancement therapy (MET) for mild to moderate alcohol dependence. *Journal of Studies on Alcohol, 62*(3), 389–396.

Senft, R. A., Polen, M. R., Freeborn, D. K., & Hollis, J. F. (1997). Brief intervention in a primary care setting for hazardous drinkers. *American Journal of Preventive Medicine, 13*(6), 464–470.

Severson, H. H., Peterson, A. L., Andrews, J. A., Gordon, J. S., Cigrang, J. A., Danaher, B. G., et al. (2009). Smokeless tobacco cessation in military personnel: A randomized controlled trial. *Nicotine and Tobacco Research, 11*(6), 730–738.

Sherman, D. A. K., Nelson, L. D., & Steele, C. M. (2000). Do messages about health risks threaten self?: Increasing the acceptance of threatening health messages via self-affirmation. *Personality and Social Psychology Bulletin, 26*(9), 1046–1058.

Sherman, M. D., Fischer, E., Bowling, U. B., Dixon, L., Ridener, L., & Harrison, D. (2009). A new engagement strategy in a VA-based family psychoeducation program. *Psychiatric Services, 60*(2), 254–257.

Simmons, R. G., Marine, S. K., & Simmons, R. L. (1987). *Gift of life: The effect of organ transplantation on individual, family, and societal dynamics* (2nd ed.). New Brunswick, NJ: Transaction.

Simon, S. B. (1978). *Negative criticism: Its swath of destruction and what you can do about it.* Niles, IL: Argus Communications.

Sinclair, K. S., Campbell, T. S., Carey, P. M., Langevin, E., Bowser, B., & France, C. R. (2010). An adapted postdonation motivational interview enhances blood donor retention. *Transfusion, 50*(8), 1778–1786.

Slagle, D. M., & Gray, M. J. (2007). The utility of motivational interviewing as an adjunct to exposure therapy in the treatment of anxiety disorders. *Professional Psychology: Research and Practice, 38*(4), 329–337.

Slavet, J. D., Stein, L. A., Klein, J. L., Colby, S. M., Barnett, N. P., & Monti, P. M. (2005). Piloting the family check-up with incarcerated adolescents and their parents. *Psychological Services, 2*(2), 123–132.

Smart, R. G. (1974). Employed alcoholics treated voluntarily and under constructive coercion: A follow-up study. *Quarterly Journal of Studies on Alcohol, 35*, 196–209.

Smith, D. C., Hall, J. A., Jang, M., & Arndt, S. (2009). Therapist adherence to a motivational-interviewing intervention improves treatment entry for substance-misusing adolescents with low problem perception. *Journal of Studies on Alcohol and Drugs, 70*(1), 101–105.

Smith, D. E., Heckemeyer, C. M., Kratt, P. P., & Mason, D. A. (1997). Motivational interviewing to improve adherence to a behavioral weight-control program for older obese women with NIDDM: A pilot study. *Diabetes Care, 20*(1), 52–54.

Smith, J. E., & Meyers, R. J. (2004). *Motivating substance abusers to enter treatment: Working with family members.* New York: Guilford Press.

Snyder, C. R. (1994). *The psychology of hope.* New York: Free Press.

Sobell, L. C., Sobell, M. B., & Agrawal, S. (2009). Randomized controlled trial of a cognitive-behavioral motivational intervention in a group versus individual format for substance use disorders. *Psychology of Addictive Behaviors, 23*(4), 672–683.

Soria, R., Legido, A., Escolano, C., Lopez Yeste, A., & Montoya, J. (2006). A randomised controlled trial of motivational interviewing for smoking cessation. *British Journal of General Practice, 56*(531), 768–774.

Spirito, A., Monti, P. M., Barnett, N. P., Colby, S. M., Sindelar, H., Rohsenow, D. J., et al. (2004). A randomized clinical trial of a brief motivational intervention for alcohol-positive adolescents treated in an emergency department. *Journal of Pediatrics, 145*(3), 396–402.

Squires, D. D., & Hester, R. K. (2004). Using technical innovations in clinical practice: The Drinker's Check-up software program. *Journal of Clinical Psychology, 60*(2), 159–169.

Steele, C. M. (1988). The psychology of self-affirmation: Sustaining the integrity of the self. *Advances in Experimental Social Psychology, 21*, 261–302.

Stein, L. A. R., Colby, S. M., Barnett, N. P., Monti, P. M., Golembeske, C., & Lebeau-Craven, R. (2006). Effects of motivational interviewing for incarcerated adolescents on driving under the influence after release. *American Journal on Addictions, 15*(Suppl. 1), S50–S57.

Stein, M. D., Charuvastra, A., Maksad, J., & Anderson, B. J. (2002). A randomized trial of a brief alcohol intervention for needle exchangers (BRAINE). *Addiction, 97*(6), 691–700.

Stephenson, W. (1953). *The study of behavior: Q-technique and its methodology.* Chicago: University of Chicago Press.

Stitzer, M., & Petry, N. (2006). Contingency management for treatment of substance abuse. *Annual Review of Clinical Psychology, 2*, 411–434.

Stitzer, M. L., Petry, N. M., & Peirce, J. (2010). Motivational incentives research in the National Drug Abuse Treatment Clinical Trials Network. *Journal of Substance Abuse Treatment, 38*(Suppl. 1), S61–S69.

Stott, N., Rollnick, S., Rees, M., & Pill, R. (1995). Innovation in clinical method: Diabetes care and negotiating skills. *Family Practice, 12*(4), 413–418.

Stotts, A. L., Schmitz, J. M., Rhoades, H. M., & Grabowski, J. (2001). Motivational interviewing with cocaine-dependent patients: A pilot study. *Journal of Consulting and Clinical Psychology, 69*(5), 858–862.

Strang, J., & McCambridge, J. (2004). Can the practitioner correctly predict outcome in motivational interviewing? *Journal of Substance Abuse Treatment, 27*(1), 83–88.

Suarez, M. (2011). Application of motivational interviewing to neuropsychology practice: A new frontier for evaluations and rehabilitation. In M. R. Schoenberg & J. G. Scott (Eds.), *The little black book of neuropsychology: A syndrome-based approach* (pp. 863–872). New York: Springer.

Sullivan, H. S. (1970). *The psychiatric interview.* New York: Norton.

Swan, M., Schwartz, S., Berg, B., Walker, D., Stephens, R., & Roffman, R. (2008). The teen marijuana check-up: An in-school protocol for eliciting voluntary self-assessment of marijuana use. *Journal of Social Work Practice in the Addictions, 8*(3), 284–302.

Switzer, G. E., Simmons, R. G., & Dew, M. A. (1996). Helping unrelated strangers:

Physical and psychological reactions to the bone marrow donation process among anonymous donors. *Journal of Applied Social Psychology, 26,* 469–490.

Taveras, E. M., Gortmaker, S. L., Hohman, K. H., Horan, C. M., Kleinman, K. P., Mitchell, K., et al. (2011). Randomized controlled trial to improve primary care to prevent and manage childhood obesity: The High Five for Kids study. *Archives of Pediatric Adolescent Medicine, 165*(8), 714–722.

Tevyaw, T. O., Borsari, B., Colby, S. M., & Monti, P. M. (2007). Peer enhancement of a brief motivational intervention with mandated college students. *Psychology of Addictive Behaviors, 21*(1), 114–119.

Tevyaw, T. O., & Monti, P. M. (2004). Motivational enhancement and other brief interventions for adolescent substance abuse: Foundations, applications, and evaluations. *Addiction, 99*(Suppl. 2), S63–S75.

The Dalai Lama, & Ekman, P. (2008). *Emotional awareness.* New York: Times Books.

Thevos, A. K., Kaona, F. A., Siajunza, M. T., & Quick, R. E. (2000). Adoption of safe water behaviors in Zambia: Comparing educational and motivational approaches. *Education for Health, 13*(3), 366–376.

Thevos, A. K., Olsen, S. J., Rangel, J. M., Kaona, F. A. D., Tembo, M., & Quick, R. E. (2002). Social marketing and motivational interviewing as community interventions for safe water behaviors: Follow-up surveys in Zambia. *International Quarterly of Community Health Education, 21*(1), 51–65.

Thevos, A. K., Quick, R. E., & Yanduli, V. (2000). Motivational interviewing enhances the adoption of water disinfection practices in Zambia. *Health Promotion International, 15*(3), 207–214.

Thomas, M. L., Elliott, J. E., Rao, S. M., Fahey, K. F., Paul, S. M., & Miaskowski, C. (2012). A randomized, clinical trial of education or motivational-interviewing-based coaching compared to usual care to improve cancer pain management. *Oncology Nursing, 39*(1), 39–49.

Thrasher, A. D., Golin, C. E., Earp, J. A., Tien, H., Porter, C., & Howie, L. (2006). Motivational interviewing to support antiretroviral therapy adherence: The role of quality counseling. *Patient Education and Counseling, 62*(1), 64–71.

Trice, H. M., & Beyer, J. M. (1984). Work-related outcomes of the constructive-confrontation strategy in a job-based alcoholism program. *Journal of Studies on Alcohol, 45,* 393–404.

Truax, C. B. (1966). Reinforcement and non-reinforcement in Rogerian psychotherapy. *Journal of Abnormal Psychology, 71,* 1–9.

Truax, C. B., & Carkhuff, R. R. (1967). *Toward effective counseling and psychotherapy.* Chicago: Aldine.

Uebelacker, L. A., Hecht, J., & Miller, I. W. (2006). The family check-up: A pilot study of a brief intervention to improve family functioning in adults. *Family Process, 45*(2), 223–236.

UKATT Research Team. (2001). United Kingdom alcohol treatment trial (UKATT): Hypotheses, design and methods. *Alcohol and Alcoholism, 36*(1), 11–21.

UKATT Research Team. (2005). Effectiveness of treatment for alcohol problems: Findings of the randomized UK alcohol treatment trial (UKATT). *British Medical Journal, 331,* 541–544.

Vader, A. M., Walters, S. T., Prabhu, G. C., Houck, J. M., & Field, C. A. (2010).

The language of motivational interviewing and feedback: Counselor language, client language, and client drinking outcomes. *Psychology of Addictive Behaviors, 24*(2), 190–197.

Valanis, B., Lichtenstein, E., Mullooly, J. P., Labuhn, K., Brody, K., Severson, H. H., et al. (2001). Maternal smoking cessation and relapse prevention during health care visits. *American Journal of Preventive Medicine, 20*(1), 1–8.

Valanis, B., Whitlock, E. E., Mullooly, J., Vogt, T., Smith, S., Chen, C., et al. (2003). Screening rarely screened women: Time-to-service and 24-month outcomes of tailored interventions. *Preventive Medicine, 37*(5), 442–450.

Valle, S. K. (1981). Interpersonal functioning of alcoholism counselors and treatment outcome. *Journal of Studies on Alcohol, 42*, 783–790.

van Keulen, H. M., Mesters, I., Ausems, M., van Breukelen, G., Campbell, M., Resnicow, K., et al. (2011). Tailored print communication and telephone motivational interviewing are equally successful in improving multiple lifestyle behaviors in a randomized controlled trial. *Annals of Behavioral Medicine, 41*, 104–118.

Van Ryzin, M. J., Stormshak, E. A., & Dishion, T. J. (2012). Engaging parents in the family check-up in middle school: Longitudinal effects on family conflict and problem behavior through the high school transition. *Journal of Adolescent Health.*

VanWormer, J. J., & Boucher, J. L. (2004). Motivational interviewing and diet modification: A review of the evidence. *The Diabetes Educator, 30*(3), 404–406, 408–410, 414–406, passim.

Velasquez, M. M., von Sternberg, K., Dodrill, C., Kan, L., & Parsons, J. (2005). The transtheoretical model as a framework for developing substance abuse interventions. *Journal of Addictions Nursing, 16*(1), 31–40.

Velasquez, M. M., Maurer, G. G., Crouch, C., & DiClemente, C. C. (2001). *Group treatment for substance abuse: A stages of change therapy manual.* New York: Guilford Press.

Villanueva, M., Tonigan, J. S., & Miller, W. R. (2007). Response of Native American clients to three treatment methods for alcohol dependence. *Journal of Ethnicity in Substance Abuse, 6*(2), 41–48.

Viscott, D. S. (1972). *The making of a psychiatrist.* Westminster, MD: Arbor House.

Vong, S. K., Cheing, G. L., Chan, F., So, E. M., & Chan, C. C. (2011). Motivational enhancement therapy in addition to physical therapy improves motivational factors and treatment outcomes in people with low back pain: A randomized controlled trial. *Archives of Physical Medicine and Rehabilitation, 92*(2), 176–183.

Vuchinich, R. E., & Heather, N. (Eds.). (2003). *Choice, behavioral economics, and addiction.* New York: Pergamon.

Wagener, T. L., Leffingwell, T. R., Mignogna, J., Mignogna, M. R., Weaver, C. C., Cooney, N. J., et al. (2012). Randomized trial comparing computer-delivered and face-to-face personalized feedback interventions for high-risk drinking among college students. *Journal of Substance Abuse Treatment.*

Wagner, C. C., & Ingersoll, K. S. (2009). Beyond behavior: Eliciting broader change with motivational interviewing. *Journal of Clinical Psychology, 65*(11), 1180–1194.

Wagner, C. C., & Ingersoll, K. S. (in press). *Motivational interviewing in groups.* New York: Guilford Press.

Wahab, S., Menon, U., & Szalacha, L. (2008). Motivational interviewing and colorectal cancer screening: A peek from the inside out. *Patient Education and Counseling, 72,* 210–217.

Waldron, H. B., Miller, W. R., & Tonigan, J. S. (2001). Client anger as a predictor of differential response to treatment. In R. Longabaugh & P. W. Wirtz (Eds.), *Project MATCH hypotheses: Results and causal chain analyses* (Vol. 8, pp. 134–148). Bethesda, MD: National Institute on Alcohol Abuse and Alcoholism.

Walker, D. D., Roffman, R. A., Picciano, J. F., & Stephens, R. S. (2007). The check-up: In-person, computerized, and telephone adaptations of motivational enhancement treatment to elicit voluntary participation by the contemplator. *Substance Abuse Treatment, Prevention, and Policy, 2,* 2.

Walker, D. D., Roffman, R. A., Stephens, R. S., Wakana, K., Berghuis, J., & Kim, W. (2006). Motivational enhancement therapy for adolescent marijuana users: A preliminary randomized controlled trial. *Journal of Consulting and Clinical Psychology, 74*(3), 628–632.

Walters, S. T., Clark, M. D., Gingerich, R., & Meltzer, M. L. (2007). *Motivating offenders to change: A guide for probation and parole.* Washington, DC: National Institute of Corrections, U.S. Department of Justice.

Walters, S. T., Hester, R. K., Chiauzzi, E., & Miller, E. (2005). Demon rum: High-tech solutions to an age-old problem. *Alcoholism: Clinical and Experimental Research, 29*(2), 270–277.

Walters, S. T., Ogle, R., & Martin, J. E. (2002). Perils and possibilities of group-based motivational interviewing. In W. R. Miller & S. Rollnick (Eds.), *Motivational interviewing: Preparing people to change* (2nd ed., pp. 377–390). New York: Guilford Press.

Walters, S. T., Vader, A. M., Nguyen, N., Harris, T. R., & Eells, J. (2010). Motivational interviewing as a supervision strategy in probation: A randomized effectiveness trial. *Journal of Offender Rehabilitation, 49*(5), 309–323.

Walton, M. (1986). *The Deming management method.* New York: Perigee.

Wampold, B. E. (2007). Psychotherapy: The humanistic (and effective) treatment. *American Psychologist, 62*(8), 855–873.

Watkins, C. L., Auton, M. F., Deans, C. F., Dickinson, H. A., Jack, C. I., Lightbody, C. E., et al. (2007). Motivational interviewing early after acute stroke: A randomized, controlled trial. *Stroke, 38*(3), 1004–1009.

Watkins, C. L., Wathan, J. V., Leathley, M. J., Auton, M. F., Dickinson, H. A., Sutton, C. J., et al. (2011). The 12-month effects of early motivational interviewing after acute stroke: A randomized controlled trial. *Stroke, 42*(7), 1956–1961.

Webber, K. H., Tate, D. F., & Quintiliani, L. M. (2008). Motivational interviewing in internet groups: A pilot study for weight loss. *Journal of the American Dietetic Association, 108*(6), 1029–1032.

Weinstein, P., Harrison, R., & Benton, T. (2004). Motivating parents to prevent caries in their young children: One-year findings. *Journal of the American Dental Association, 135*(6), 731–738.

Weinstein, P., Harrison, R., & Benton, T. (2006). Motivating mothers to prevent caries: Confirming the beneficial effect of counseling. *Journal of the American Dental Association, 137*(6), 789–793.

Welch, G., Rose, G., Hanson, D., Lekarcyk, J., Smith-Ossman, S., Gordon, T., et al. (2003). Changes in Motivational Interviewing Skills Code (MISC) scores following motivational interviewing training for diabetes educators. *Diabetes, 52*(Suppl. 1), A421.

Welch, G., Zagarins, S. E., Feinberg, R. G., & Garb, J. L. (2011). Motivational interviewing delivered by diabetes educators: Does it improve blood glucose control among poorly controlled type 2 diabetes patients? *Diabetes Research and Clinical Practice, 91*(1), 54–60.

Westerberg, V. S., Miller, W. R., & Tonigan, J. S. (2000). Comparison of outcomes for clients in randomized versus open trials of treatment for alcohol use disorders. *Journal of Studies on Alcohol, 61,* 720–727.

Westra, H. A. (2012). *Motivational interviewing in the treatment of anxiety.* New York: Guilford Press.

White, W. L., & Miller, W. R. (2007). The use of confrontation in addiction treatment: History, science, and time for a change. *The Counselor, 8*(4), 12–30.

Woodall, W. G., Delaney, H., Rogers, E., & Wheeler, D. (2000). A randomized trial of victim impact panels' DWI deterrence effectiveness. *Alcoholism: Clinical and Experimental Research, 24*(Suppl.), 113A (abstract).

Woodall, W. G., Delaney, H. D., Kunitz, S. J., Westerberg, V. S., & Zhao, H. (2007). A randomized trial of a DWI intervention program for first offenders: Intervention outcomes and interactions with antisocial personality disorder among a primarily American-Indian sample. *Alcoholism: Clinical and Experimental Research, 31*(6), 974–987.

Worthington, E. L., Jr. (2003). *Forgiving and reconciling: Bridges to wholeness and hope.* Downers Grove, IL: InterVarsity Press.

Worthington, E. L., Jr. (Ed.). (2005). *Handbook of forgiveness.* New York: Routledge.

Wulfert, E., Blanchard, E. B., Freidenberg, B. M., & Martell, R. S. (2006). Retaining pathological gamblers in cognitive behavior therapy through motivational enhancement: A pilot study. *Behavior Modification, 30*(3), 315–340.

Yahne, C. E., & Miller, W. R. (1999). Evoking hope. In W. R. Miller (Ed.), *Integrating spirituality into treatment: Resources for practitioners* (pp. 217–233). Washington, DC: American Psychological Association.

Yevlahova, D., & Satur, J. (2009). Models for individual oral health promotion and their effectiveness: A systematic review. *Australian Dental Journal, 54*(3), 190–197.

Zweben, A. (1991). Motivational counseling with alcoholic couples. In W. R. Miller & S. Rollnick (Eds.), *Motivational interviewing: Preparing people to change addictive behavior* (pp. 225–235). New York: Guilford Press.

Index

471